Hemodynamic Rounds, Second Edition

Hemodynamic Rounds, Second Edition

Edited by
Morton J. Kern, M.D.

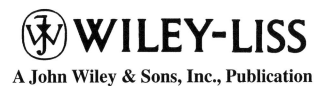

WILEY-LISS

A John Wiley & Sons, Inc., Publication

New York • Chichester • Weinheim • Brisbane • Singapore • Toronto

For ordering and customer service, call 1-800-CALL-WILEY.

Library of Congress Cataloging-in-Publication Data:

Hemodynamic rounds / edited by Morton J. Kern. — 2nd ed.
        p.   cm.
     Includes bibliographical references and index.
     ISBN 0-471-34759-0 (pbk. : alk. paper)
     1. Hemodynamic monitoring.   2. Cardiovascular system—Diseases—
Diagnosis.   I. Kern, Morton J.   II. Kern, Morton J.   Hemodynamic
rounds.
     [DNLM: 1. Coronary Circulation—physiology Collected Works.
2. Coronary Disease—physiopathology Collected Works.
3. Hemodynamics—physiology Collected Works.   WG 106 H498 1999]
RC670.5.H45H45   1999
617.4'12059—dc21
DNLM/DLC
for Library of Congress   99-25101
                                                              CIP

Printed in the United States of America.

10 9 8 7 6 5 4 3

To Margaret and Anna Rose, the systole of my life

The following chapters originally appeared in the Journal of Catheterization and Cardiovascular Diagnosis. The Journal is the only appropriate literature citation for the articles printed on these pages.

Chapter 1	27:147-154 (1992)
Chapter 2	43:90-94 (1998)
Chapter 3	21:112-120 (1990)
Chapter 4	43:201-205 (1998)
Chapter 5	26:232-240 (1992)
Chapter 6	44:336-340 (1998)
Chapter 7	28:244-248 (1993)
Chapter 8	28:167-172 (1993)
Chapter 9	26:308-315 (1992)
Chapter 10	27:52-56 (1992)
Chapter 11	43:313-317 (1998)
Chapter 12	45:70-75 (1998)
Chapter 13	43:466-471 (1998)
Chapter 14	23:211-218 (1991)
Chapter 15	21:278-286 (1990)
Chapter 16	24:209-213 (1991)
Chapter 17	24:111-120 (1991)
Chapter 18	44:227-234 (1998)
Chapter 19	25:336-342 (1992)
Chapter 20	26:34-40 (1992)
Chapter 21	26:152-158 (1992)
Chapter 22	(in press)
Chapter 23	(in press)
Chapter 24	45:287-291 (1998)
Chapter 25	27:223-227 (1992)
Chapter 26	24:22-27 (1991)
Chapter 27	22:145-152 (1992)
Chapter 28	44:438-442 (1998)
Chapter 29	(in press)
Chapter 30	25:57-60 (1992)
Chapter 31	25:154-160 (1992)
Chapter 32	26:204-211 (1992)
Chapter 33	45:174-182 (1998)
Chapter 34	44:70-74 (1998)
Chapter 35	28:51-55 (1993)
Chapter 36	27:147-154 (1992)
Chapter 37	25:241-248 (1992)
Chapter 38	24:315-319 (1991)
Chapter 39	22:197-204 (1991)
Chapter 40	22:302-306 (1991)
Chapter 41	23: 50-53 (1991)
Chapter 42	27:291-297 (1992)

Contents

Contributors

Frank V. Aguirre, MD, Professor of Medicine, Southern Illinois University, Prairie Cardiovascular Consultants, Springfield, MO 62701

Elie Azrak, MD, Fellow in Cardiology, Saint Louis University Hospital, St. Louis, MO 63110

Richard G. Bach, MD, Associate Professor of Medicine, Saint Louis University Hospital, St. Louis, MO 63110

Thomas Christopher, MD, Fellow in Cardiology, Emory University, 2314 Harper Landing, Rozwell, GA 30076 (770) 649-1233

W. Randall Craig, MD, Heart Care Associates, Joplin, MO 64804

Sharon G. Cresci, MD, Cardiology, Washington University School of Medicine, St. Louis, MO 63110

Ubeydullah Deligonul, MD, Professor of Medicine, University of Texas Health Center at Tyler, Tyler, TX 75708

Thomas J. Donohue, MD, Associate Professor of Medicine, Saint Louis University, St. Louis, MO 63110

Krystof J. Godlewski, MD, Assistant Professor of Medicine, University of Louisville, Louisville, KY 40202

James A. Goldstein, MD, Associate Professor of Medicine, William Beaumont Hospital, Royal Oak, MI 48073

Marco Guerrero, MD, Fellow in Cardiology, St. Louis University, St. Louis, MO 63110

Stuart T. Higano, MD, Cardiovascular Diseases and Internal Medicine, Mayo Clinic, Rochester, MN 55905

Frank J. Hildner, MD, Professor of Medicine, University of Miami School of Medicine, Miami, FL; Editor-in-Chief, Catheterization and Cardiovascular Interventions, Ocala Heart Institute, Ocala, FL 34470

Thomas C. Hilton, MD, Jacksonville Heart Center, Jacksonville, FL 32204

Morton J. Kern, MD, Professor of Medicine, Director J.G. Mudd Cardiac Catheterization Laboratory, Saint Louis University Hospital, St. Louis, MO 63110

Leslie W. Miller, MD, Professor of Medicine, University of Minnesota, Minneapolis, MN 55455

Glenn T. Morris, MD, Fellow in Cardiology, University of Louisville School of Medicine, Louisville, KY 40202

Sanjeev Puri, MD, Cardiology, University of Arkansas, Little Rock, AR 72205

Hassan Rajjoub, MD, Fellow in Cardiology, Saint Louis University Hospital, St. Louis, MO 63110

W. Jeffrey Schoen, MD, Fellow in Cardiology, University of Louisville School of Medicine, Louisville, KY 40202

Naeem K. Tahirheli, MD, Fellow, Division of Cardiovascular Diseases and Internal Medicine, Mayo Clinic, Rochester, MN 55905

J. David Talley, MD, Associate Professor of Medicine, Associate Director, Division of Cardiology, University of Arkansas for Medical Sciences, Little Rock, AR 72205

Preface

Hemodynamics continue to be an integral part of the invasive cardiology experience. However, increased attention to angiographic detail of the coronary arteries for various and novel catheter-based interventions has left the role of hemodynamics in the catheterization laboratory in a secondary, or occasionally forgotten position. In some institutions echocardiography has replaced invasive hemodynamics for the study of valvular disorders. While it is true that the clinical basis for echocardiographic decisions is derived from direct correlation to pressure measurements, the application of direct hemodynamics has failed to back translate to the catheterization laboratory in some, especially busy graduate training programs.

The first edition of the Hemodynamic Rounds emphasized the interpretation of hemodynamics for clinical decisions in a case management format and has been used as a text of hemodynamic study for many cardiovascular trainees and cardiologists in practice. In this second edition of the Hemodynamic Rounds, we extend an already large base of interesting hemodynamic case examples and re-organize the format to include the new sections in a more logical approach to the study of pressure waves associated with various pathophysiologic situations.

To set the background for all waveform interpretation, Section I on valvular hemodynamics initiates the reader with descriptions of pressure wave artifacts and pitfalls of right heart hemodynamics (Chapters 1 and 2). The interpretation of low gradient aortic valve stenosis (Chapter 4) and abnormal hemodynamics related to aortic root reconstruction (Chapter 6) are new in examining common yet perplexing clinical problems. Additional case discussions involving mitral valve gradients, bioprosthetic valves, and double-valve prosthesis hemodynamic studies have now been included.

In Section II, the descriptions of valvuloplasty hemodynamics have been expanded and include a detailed examination of pressure waveforms during pulmonic balloon valvuloplasty. Section III, constrictive physiology, places new emphasis on the hemodynamic criteria involving dynamic respiratory variations of ventricular pressure interaction. This criteria should be incorporated into the standard hemodynamic data acquired in such cases. The recording of simultaneous left and right ventricular pressures during respiration will become another valuable criteria for the hemodynamic diagnosis of constrictive physiology.

An additional section on hypertrophic cardiomyopathy (Section V) has been established. The use of dual-chamber pacing, surgical myectomy, and the most recent technique of alcohol septal infarction for control of symptomatic hypertrophic obstructive cardiomyopathy is discussed.

Section VI on coronary hemodynamics has also been expanded. The new concepts involving absolute and relative coronary velocity reserve and pressure-derived fractional flow reserve are compared to help the practitioner understand the practical in-laboratory coronary hemodynamic measurements for decision making.

In the last section, Section VII – unusual hemodynamics, we have added a focused discussion on the left ventricular diastolic pressure which, at first glance, is a simple measurement. As will be discovered, the accurate interpretation of the left ventricular pressure goes beyond the left ventricular end-diastolic pressure now and requires more detailed study to appreciate its true significance in several specialized circumstances.

I would like to thank my colleagues in the J.G. Mudd Cardiac Catheterization Laboratory, Dr. Frank Aguirre, Dr. Richard Bach, Dr. Eugene Caracciolo, and Dr. Thomas Donohue, and the cardiology fellows who participated in collecting these hemodynamics during our clinical practice. I would also like to thank the continued efforts of Donna Sander in the preparation of all my materials. I could not complete this work without her effort. I continue to thank Dr. Frank Hildner, editor of *Catheterization and Cardiovascular Interventions* (formerly *Catheterization and Cardiovascular Diagnosis*), for his continued support, encouragement, and friendship involving this work. Finally, I again dedicate this book to my wife Margaret, and my daughter, Anna Rose, who remain the systole of my life. I hope this Hemodynamic Rounds, Second Edition, will be as enjoyable and educational as the first.

Morton J. Kern, MD

Introduction

Morton J. Kern, MD, and Frank J. Hildner, MD

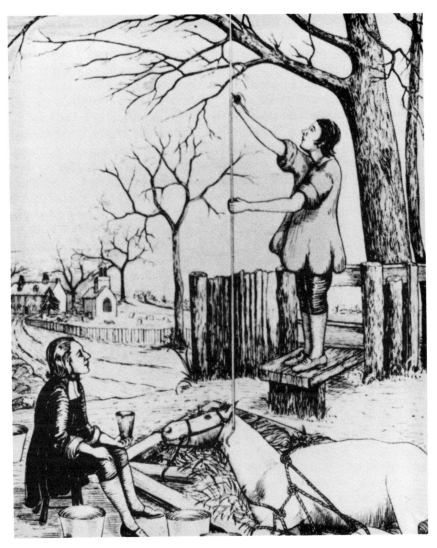

Drawing depicting Dr. Stephen Hales (seated) directing and observing the measurement of arterial pressure in a sedated horse circa 1730. (Reproduced with permission from: "Medicine: An Illustrated History," Lyons AS, Petrucelli RJ II (eds), New York, Harry N. Abrams, Inc., 1987.)

HISTORICAL REVIEW

On February 28, 1733, the president of the Council of the Royal Society, Sir Hans Sloane, requested that Stephen Hales, one of the counselors, present his information on the mechanics of blood circulation from a previous presentation of a series of hemodynamic experiments reported in his book *Haemastaticks* [1]. Mr.

Hales took his place in medical history next to William Harvey with regard to studies of the human and animal circulation. *De Motu Cordis* [2] and *Haemastaticks* stimulated scientists interested in the newly developed principles and mathematical computations of fluid mechanics as applied to circulatory physiologic events. The simple measurement of blood pressure now became a subject of great scientific interest.

From such basic interests, experimental physiologists at Oxford University in the 1800s, investigating the physiology of the circulation, began estimating the output of ventricular contraction and velocity of blood flow in the aorta based on relatively primitive measurements of cardiovascular structures. These data remain valid and correspond to currently accepted data obtained by computerized quantitative techniques. Cardiologists interested in hemodynamics should continue to emulate Stephen Hales who relied on direct measurements and observations repeatedly checked and applied on simple and repeatedly confirmed computations. The numerous original achievements in hemodynamics provided to us by Hales are remarkable even by today's standards and included the first direct and accurate measurement of blood pressure in different animals (Fig. 1) under different physiologic conditions such as hemorrhage and respiration; cardiac output estimated by left ventricular systolic stroke volume measured from the diastolic volume after death of the animal; calculations of pressure measured on the internal surface of the left ventricular at the beginning of systole; determination of blood flow velocity in the aorta approximating 0.5m/sec. Stephen Hales introduced the concept of the wind castle or capacitance effect in the transformation of pulsatile flow in large vessels to continuous flow in smaller vessels. Hales also made the first direct measurement of venous blood pressure and correct interpretation of venous return on cardiac output in relation to contraction and respirations. Since recording equipment documenting the observations of Hales was lacking, understanding the unique collection of data depends on interpreting descriptive material.

Our current appreciation of hemodynamics as provided in this book stems directly from a small group of modern physiologists active in the 1920s, among whom Dr. Carl Wiggers, from Western Reserve University in Ohio, emerges. Major advances in hemodynamic research arose from the development of recording instruments with improved fidelity able to capture and reproduce the waveforms of rapidly changing pressures during the various phases of cardiac contractions in the various heart chambers. Dr. Wiggers and colleagues also employed the newly developed electrocardiogram to obtain simultaneous pressure waveforms and electrical activity and thus, establish the fundamental electrical-mechan-

ical intervals and relationships which are the benchmark against which the observations of the pressure tracings of classical diseased conditions, some of which are described herein, can be compared [3].

An interval of sixty years separates the originators of clinical cardiovascular anatomy and physiology from present day practitioners. What happened during that time should not be forgotten because it still affects us today. However, some of the lessons that have been learned, while still valid, tend to be ignored. From the time Claude Bernard coined the phrase "cardiac catheterization" (1840) [4], laboratories of that type and name have been hemodynamic and physiology laboratories. After Forssman performed the first documented human cardiac catheterization—on himself [5], the nature of the work did not change, only the subjects. In the late 1930s, Cournand and Ranges [6] used the new right heart catheterization technique to investigate pulmonary physiology. With World War II, the scope and direction of their work changed to include hemorrhagic shock and drug effects on the circulation. But in those days, the most serious problems presented by patients related to congenital and rheumatic heart disease. Accordingly, laboratories around the world began publishing data on the hemodynamics and physiology of atrial septal defects [7], ventricular septal defects [8], stenotic and insufficient mitral and aortic valves and ventricular function. The beginning of invasive cardiology had come to an end.

Without doubt, the most important and crucial development needed for the advancement of the field of cardiovascular diseases was the cathode ray tube, a direct result of the war. Before the image intensifier [9,10], cardiac fluoroscopy utilized high dose radiation and required the physician to accommodate his eyes to a green fluorescent screen by wearing red goggles for 15-20 minutes before starting. Indeed, the faintly glowing image in a completely dark room frequently failed to reveal even the position of the catheter [11]. Without the additional light provided by the image intensifier, "angiocardiography" was nothing more than a simple flat plate radiograph, or perhaps a sequence of cut films obtained on the newly developed serial film changer [12]. Cineangiography was developed in the late fifties through the persistent efforts of Janker (1954) [13] and Sones (1958) [14]. The addition of advanced imaging spurred the progress of catheter invasive techniques, which then permitted investigation of heretofore unapproachable anatomical sites, clinical conditions, and disease entities which in turn resulted in effective cardiac surgery. Once again hemodynamic analysis was needed to explain what was being newly observed and to assist the development of medical and surgical interventions. After the basic mechanics of congenital anomalies and rheumatic abnormalities were confirmed, conditions related to occlusive coronary artery disease such as myocardial infarction, left ventricular aneurysms, mitral chordal, and septal rupture were investigated. Soon thereafter, newer concepts of systolic and diastolic myocardial mechanical function, hypertrophic obstructive and non-obstructive cardiomyopathy, electrophysiologic relations, and other previously unappreciated conditions came under scrutiny. The final result was a body of knowledge that permitted development and use of the newly conceived non-invasive techniques including advanced physical examination (phonocardiographs, ballistocardiographs, etc.), exercise stress testing, radionuclide imaging, and echocardiography. In this age of imaging, even as it was during the previous fifty or sixty years, hemodynamic analysis remains absolutely necessary for a proper understanding and appreciation of all cardiovascular conditions and situations.

APPROACH TO HEMODYNAMIC WAVEFORM INTERPRETATION

With this background, we turn our attention from pressure waveforms to the interpretation of cardiac pathophysiology. Each chapter has been published or will soon appear in *Catheterization and Cardiovascular Diagnosis* and will serve to provide both novice and advanced cardiologists with classical and, at times, unique pressure tracings to emphasize the value of careful observation as the waveforms relate to different cardiac pathophysiology states.

It is clear that good quality hemodynamic data is required for the quantitative determinations of pathophysiologic conditions for most cardiovascular maladies. As in the days of Dr. Hales, some hemodynamic data is extraordinarily simple, such as using a sphygmomanometer for indirect assessment of systemic arterial pressure. Some hemodynamic data may also be complex, requiring catheterization with placement of multiple catheters within several chambers of the heart. Such data can then be used in the precise computations of pressure and flow to determine valvular gradients, myocardial contraction, relaxation, compliance, impedance and work [15–17]. Additional techniques, unknown to physiologists and cardiologists in decades earlier, have recently provided insight into the physiology of the coronary circulation. Intracoronary Doppler and vascular ultrasound imaging catheters can now provide information complementary to but previously unavailable through traditional angiographic methodologies.

As with all laboratory data, the significance of various hemodynamic findings should be placed in context of the ancillary historical, clinical, echocardiographic, roentgenographic, and electrocardiographic data. Acting on isolated laboratory values is dangerous and has been the nemesis of all technical innovations in medicine.

METHODOLOGIES INVOLVED IN HEMODYNAMIC DATA COLLECTION

Each laboratory, and preferably all physicians, should establish protocols for right and left heart catheterization. A uniform and consistent approach to data collection insures complete, accurate and reliable data for the majority of clinical problems. The standardized routine also obviates missing easily overlooked data collection steps. Time is also saved during procedure setup and data recording. The technical staff does not have to rethink what will happen for a unique and personal hemodynamic protocol of each different operator. Right heart catheterization, sometimes performed sequentially with left heart catheterization, may often be combined simultaneously with left heart catheterization to provide the most complete data. In most academic laboratories, a combined methodology is preferred.

The methodology for performing right heart catheterization has been reviewed previously [18], but the indications have become a subject for controversy [18,19]. While some quarters feel routine right heart catheterization is unjustified, others are equally adamant that patient care demands our maximum effort to provide optimum results. Unexpected congenital and hemodynamic abnormalities are found at right heart catheterization even with previous echocardiography. This has been pointed out by Shanes et al.[20] and Barron et al. [21] even though they come to opposite opinions. However, there is no debate if right heart catheterization is performed to evaluate patients with previous congenital heart disease, valvular heart disease, left or right heart failure, previous myocardial infarction, cardiomyopathy or any unexplained significant clinical historical or physical findings.

Left heart hemodynamic protocols most often use a single pressure transducer, but simultaneous measurements of left ventricular and arterial pressure can easily be obtained through the side arm of an arterial sheath and the smaller catheter residing within using two transducers. Pressure obtained from an arterial sheath is satisfactory when at least a one French size larger sheath than the arterial catheter is used. After collecting the hemodynamic data, computations are made to clarify and enhance quantitative cardiac function. Measurements of cardiac work, calculation of flow resistance, valve areas, and shunt calculations are based on accurate hemodynamic data, arterial and venous blood oxygen saturations, and cardiac output determinations.

If the information is considered important enough to perform hemodynamic measurements, the operators should take the time to obtain pressure waveforms that are reliable and unequivocal, separating artifact from pathology. To achieve this goal, operators must be familiar with the equipment producing the waveforms and the sources of error found in recording techniques, tubing, transducers and catheters. The following section will highlight the important considerations for equipment used in daily hemodynamic measurements.

EQUIPMENT FOR HEMODYNAMIC STUDIES

A set of transducers, tubing and manifolds are employed for hemodynamic measurements which should be cost efficient, familiar, accurate, and simple to use for the laboratory. Although a variety of manifolds exist which are both disposable and reusable, the variety of transducers, tubing, and injection syringes should be cost efficient and easy to operate. Optimal hemodynamic pressure waves should be properly damped to reduce sinusoid "ringing" or overshoot artifact. Short, stiff tubing with a minimal distance from the end of the catheter to the transducer is desirable. Long tubing contributes to poor quality tracings, introducing "fling" artifact due to the momentum of fluid through the tube. The zero position for hemodynamic measurements is also important. In some laboratories, the zero level is set at mid chest, measured in the AP diameter of the patient (divided by 2) with the transducer connected by a fluid-filled tube to the zero level fixed at the table. When the transducer is raised above the zero level, pressure is lower. When the transducer is lower than the zero level, the pressure is higher. Setting an accurate zero before and at the conclusion of each measurement is minimally time consuming and assures accuracy by eliminating recordings with erroneous zero baselines or transducer systems that have zero drift errors over time. The zero position at the mid chest level can also be obtained by using two fluid-filled tubes connected to transducers. One tube is placed on top of the chest and the other at the back. The zero line manifold is then set at bedside height so that the two pressures are equidistant from this height. Artifacts related to under- and over-damping and suggestions to reduce these artifacts are described in Chapter 2.

Pressure Transducers

For most laboratories, table-mounted fluid-filled transducers produce acceptable clinical studies. Other devices are available which are suitable for special situations or requirements. Among these are miniaturized transducers mounted on the pressure manifold or placed in the pressure line. Some are disposable which obviates the need for sterilization but also adds to the cost. Other transducers are mounted on the end of the catheter and are inserted into the vessel or chamber being studied. These can be zeroed but require another pressure sensing device for calibration. The specialized reusable micromanometer transducer-tipped catheters producing high fidelity pressure recordings are required in the computation of the rate of rise of pressure with time (dP/dt) or relaxation (-dP/dt). Catheter reuse requires careful and meticulous cleaning which is difficult and tedious at best. The cost of these devices usually prevents use in other than investigational pursuits.

Pressure Manifolds

Three and four port manifolds are available in disposable or reusable plastic configurations. In general, most laboratories set the first 3 ports for pressure, flush solution and radiographic contrast media. A four port manifold is also available and offers the advantage of an attached fourth port closed system for disposal of flush solutions. The waste fluid port (fourth port) minimizes contamination of personnel and laboratory equipment. The clear plastic manifolds are safe, practical and disposable.

Physiologic Recorders

Every laboratory is equipped with a physiologic recorder with a multichannel photographic oscilloscope, electrocardiographic and pressure amplifiers and hard copy printer capability. Some use analog to digital signal converters to store and reproduce waveforms. A variety of specialized amplifiers (e.g., green dye curve calculators or signal differentiators) permit additional data collection. Multichannel (2–20 channels) units can process, display and record electrocardiographic, pressure signals and direct inputs from a variety of external sources, such as thermodilution green dye, coronary sinus thermodilution or coronary Doppler velocity catheters. Although the number of recorded channels may be less than the number that can be displayed, for routine cardiac catheterization at least one electrocardiogram and one to three pressure signals are required. In complex cases such as electrophysiologic studies, congenital, valvular heart disease or hemodynamic research studies it is common to use between 6 and 18 channels. The physiologic recorder should be set up with amplifiers calibrated to reference pressure or voltage standards before each case. After the recorder is ready, pressure transducers are calibrated to a common pressure source. Differences in amplifiers or transducers can then be easily identified.

Recording artifacts may be responsible for confusing data. Examples of recording artifacts producing abnormal hemodynamic tracings are included in several chapters. The recording technician should demonstrate pressure scale changes and insure correct time line positioning to assist the physician in observing and collecting accurate and complete information.

CARDIAC OUTPUT METHODOLOGY

Critical to the calculations of nearly all hemodynamic data (systemic and pulmonary vascular resistances, as well as valve areas) is the accurate determination of cardiac output. The two methods most widely accepted for determining cardiac output have been reviewed [15,16]. The Fick method assesses oxygen consumption with a polarographic cell or Douglas bag and blood oxygen saturations. The second method is indicator dilution technique, most commonly employing room temperature or iced saline using cold as the indicator. Green dye cardiac output curves are equally accurate but less commonly used in most laboratories. Methods and limitations of these techniques have been described in detail [22.] The operators in the cardiac catheterization laboratory should familiarize themselves with the limitations and potential sources of error with both techniques.

REVIEWING WAVEFORMS

Pressure waveforms may be confusing for the cardiovascular fellow-in-training. After an intense training period in which the components of all pressure waves found in cardiovascular structures are incorporated, the young physician must be encouraged to continue practicing pattern recognition and deductive analysis. He should continue to strengthen his skills by performing systematic analysis of complete pressure data obtained on all indicated cases. This systematic examination includes a comparison of the pressure values across valves, an analysis of the pressure in all adjacent chambers and the determination of whether the abnormalities are internally consistent with the clinical questions to be addressed. Finally, pressure calculation of resistance values and valve areas need to be confirmed (manual calculations to verify computer-managed data will, at times, be required). When reviewing physiologic tracings, every operator, whether expert or novice, should consider the following key points.

First, identify the cardiac rhythm. Most cardiac events can be identified by their timing from within the R-R cycle. Hemodynamic data obtained during arrhythmias may be confusing since the various irregular contraction sequences distort pressure waves. Next, determine the pressure scale on which the waveform is recorded and verify the pressure per division to be certain there is no recording artifact. Also, note the recording speed to assess the appropriate cardiac rhythm and timing of events occurring within one cardiac cycle. The comparison of waveforms for the chamber of interest should be made against known waveforms of normal physiology. The right atrial A and V waves are commonly deformed by various arrhythmias, valvular disease or pericardial and respiratory pathophysiologic states. Right and left ventricular waveforms are generally unaffected by most diseases, but the rate and position of the upslope and downslope of the pressure waves (relative to each other) should be brisk and characteristic. Electrocardiographic conduction abnormalities may alter the activation sequence of ventricular pressure. The presence of an exaggerated A wave in the ventricular tracings may identify chamber stiffness increased above normal limits. The early appearance of the A wave may also indicate first degree AV conduction block, a commonly observed phenomenon. Pressure artifacts should then be differentiated from true pathophysiologic waveforms. The type of artifacts due to catheter fling, over or underdamping will be discussed in Chapter 2.

Finally, the interpretation of the waveforms should be made in conjunction with the clinical presentation and suspected diseased conditions of the patient. A large V wave does not always represent valvular regurgitation. The equilibration of right and left ventricular diastolic pressures may be hypovolemia rather than pericardial constriction. Consider alternative clinical and physiologic explanations.

The examination and consideration of possible mechanisms of the various waveform phenomena forms the basis for the chapters in this book. The information will hopefully enhance the reader's appreciation of seemingly trivial, but often important confirmatory data for patients in discovery and confirmation of their cardiac pathophysiology.

REFERENCES

1. Hales S (ed): "Statical Essays: Containing Haemastaticks," New York, Hafner Publishing Company, Inc., 1964.
2. Harvey W (ed): "Movement of the Heart and Blood in Animals," Springfield, IL, Charles C. Thomas, 1962.
3. Wiggers CJ (ed): "The Pressure Pulses in the Cardiovascular System," New York, Longmans, Green and Co., 1928.
4. Grmek MD: Catalogue des manuscrits de Claude Bernard. Paris: Masson et Cie, 1967.
5. Forssman W: Die sondierung des rechten herzens. Klin Wochenschr 8:2085-2087, 1929.
6. Cournand A, Ranges HA: Catheterization of the right auricle in man. Proc Soc Exp Biol Med 46:462, 1941.
7. Brannon ES, Weens HS, Warren JV: Atrial septal defect. Study of hemodynamics by the technique of right heart catheterization. Am J Med Sci 210:480, 1945.
8. Baldwin E deF, Moore LV, Noble RP: The demonstration of ventricular septal defect by means of right heart catheterization. Am Heart J 32:152, 1944.
9. Sturm RE, Morgan RH: Screen intensification systems and their limitations. Am J Roentgenol 62:617, 1949.
10. Moon RJ: Amplifying and intensifying fluoroscopic images by means of scanning X-ray tube. Science 112:339, 1950.
11. Zimmerman HA: Presentation at the Twenty-second Annual Scientific Session of the American Heart Association, Atlantic City, NJ, June 4, 1949.

12. Sanchez-Perez JM, Carter RA: Time factors in cerebral angiography and an automatic seriograph. Am J Roentgenol 62:509–518, 1949.

13. Janker R: "Roentgenotogische Funktionsdiagnostic Wupper." Elberfeld: Garandit, 1954.

14. Sones FM Jr: Cinecardioangiography. Pediatr Clin North Am 5:945, 1958.

15. Grossman E, Baim DS (eds): "Cardiac Catheterization, Angiography and Intervention," 4th Edition, Philadelphia, Lea & Febiger, 1991.

16. Pepine CJ, Hill JA, Lambert CR (eds): "Diagnostic and Therapeutic Cardiac Catheterization," Baltimore, Williams & Wilkins, 1989.

17. Miller G (ed): "Invasive Investigation of the Heart," London, Blackwell Scientific Publications, 1989.

18. Green DG and Society for Cardiac Angiography officers and Trustees: Right heart catheterization and temporary pacemaker insertion during coronary arteriography for suspected coronary artery disease. Cathet Cardiovasc Diagn 10:429–430, 1984.

19. Samet P: The complete cardiac catheterization. Cathet Cardiovasc Diagn 10:431–432, 1984.

20. Shanes JG, Stein MA, Dierenfeldt BJ, Kondos GT: The value of routine right heart catheterization in patients undergoing coronary arteriography. Am Heart J 113:1261–1263, 1987.

21. Barron JT, Ruggie N, Uretz E, Messer JV: Findings on routine right heart catheterization in patients with suspected coronary artery disease. Am Heart J 115:1193, 1988.

22. Kern MJ, Deligonul U, Gudipati C: Hemodynamic and ECG data. In Kern MJ (ed): "The Cardiac Catheterization Handbook," St. Louis, Mosby Year Book, 1991, pp 119–177.

PART I: VALVULAR HEMODYNAMICS

The question of abnormal valvular hemodynamics is probably the most common indication for right and left heart catheterization. This section details not only the hemodynamics of the valvular lesions associated with aortic, mitral, pulmonic, and tricuspid valves, but importantly describes artifacts of all pressure measurements and pitfalls of right heart pressure waveforms. Understanding these basic hemodynamic principles will enhance the reader's appreciation of subtle but important unusual or questionable waveforms. I direct the reader to the new material in this section including the examination of low gradient aortic valve stenosis, the hemodynamics associated with prosthetic aortic root reconstruction and aortic insufficiency, mitral stenosis with pulsus alternans, and evaluation of bioprosthetic single and double valves.

Morton J. Kern, MD

Chapter 1

Pressure Wave Artifacts

Morton J. Kern, MD, Frank V. Aguirre, MD, and Thomas Donohue, MD

INTRODUCTION

If the measurement of blood pressure were automatically available without having to attend to transducer flushing, pressure line and manifold connections, and missettings on the recorders or kinks in catheters, the study of hemodynamics would be as routine and reliable as that of electrocardiography. However, as with any recording system which requires specially trained personnel and multiple combinations of different types of connectors, the mechanical and electrical artifacts of both fluid-filled tubes and high fidelity recording instruments produce pressure wave artifacts which must be recognized as the major flaw in accurate hemodynamic data interpretation.

In an earlier hemodynamic rounds, we addressed the most common of the pressure wave artifacts of fluid-filled systems, exaggerated "ringing" or underdamping, and overly damped "rounded" waveforms. We will now examine several of the more obscure artifacts produced by catheters, recorders, and amplifiers alone or in combination which may contribute to the misinterpretation of hemodynamic data.

PRESSURE SYSTEM RESONANCE: THE UNDER AND OVERDAMPED WAVEFORM

An "underdamped" pressure tracing is one in which the pressure wave is rapidly reflected within the system and produces an oscillating sinusoidal distortion of the pressure waveform [1]. This underdamped tracing is also called "ringing" as in continued bounding of sound waves in a bell with a characteristic demonstration of the physics of reflected waves [2]. Commonly, an air bubble

in the pressure line will be small enough to be rapidly accelerated and decelerated, moving the fluid column back and forth, resulting in ringing of the pressure tracing. The effect of a bubble in the pressure line connected to a 7F pigtail catheter and fluid-filled transducer used to measure left ventricular pressure is illustrated in Figure 1 (left panel). The bubble causes a high spike on the left ventricular upstroke and a large negative overshoot wave on the left ventricular pressure downstroke. When the pressure line and transducer are properly flushed, the left ventricular pressure (Fig. 1, right panel) shows an excellent and normal waveform which should be expected with modern fluid-filled systems.

An overdamped waveform reduces the impact of the pressure wave, rounding the contours and delaying the upstroke and downstroke of the pressure wave. An example of pressure overdamping will be described below.

HIDDEN ARTIFACTS

Observe the underdamped pressure waveform on Figure 2. The pulmonary capillary wedge (PCW) and pulmonary artery pressures were recorded during the balloon catheter deflation. The fluid-filled transducer was properly flushed. Note the oscillations making precise waveform analysis difficult. The ringing was due to vigorous catheter movement in the right heart. This amount of underdamping is common with the right heart balloon-tipped catheters and can be reduced with instillation of a 50% saline/contrast flush. However, there are two additional artifacts which will contribute to misinterpretation. While looking for the hidden artifacts, consider what is the maximal pressure of the V wave, the pulmonary ar-

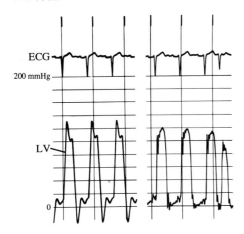

Fig. 1. Left ventricular (LV) pressure with 7F pigtail catheter using fluid-filled transducers. Left panel demonstrates "ringing" artifact. See text for details.

tery diastolic pressure, and the heart rate? Check the pressure scale again. How many lines from 0–50 mm Hg? The recording technician inadvertently omitted line 10. Nine lines are placed on the screen with the standard notations of 0, 25, and 50 mm Hg. The V wave is 24 mm Hg if the "25 mm Hg" marker is low and line 10 is omitted from the top. Otherwise, the V wave = 27 mm Hg (50/9 mm Hg = 5.6 × 4.8) if nine divisions are equal to 50 mm Hg. In most settings, this degree of error is clinically unimportant, but in cases where valve areas are considered worthwhile hemodynamically, this error is unacceptable. The pulmonary artery pressure is computed as for the V wave.

What is the heart rate? Traditional teaching methods count the RR intervals in 10 seconds and multiply by 6. Unfortunately, this recording is also missing the time lines. The heart rate might be estimated by assuming the usual recording speed of 25 mm/sec and measuring the distance on the paper. However, this patient may have had tachycardia and the recording speed could be 50 mm/sec. Again, although minimally important for clinical decisions, the operator's confidence in his data is not optimal. These deficiencies should be minimized for accurate and trustworthy data collection.

Consider the hemodynamics obtained in a 60-yr-old man who has mild dyspnea, chest pain, and a systolic murmur (Fig. 3). Central aortic and femoral arterial pressures were matched using fluid-filled catheters (6F arterial sheath and 5F pigtail catheter) before assessing the aortic valve gradient. Report your readings of left ventricular and aortic pressures, heart rate, estimated valve gradient, and quick area calculations given a thermodilution cardiac output of 3.0 liters/min. A problem again arises because of the two recording artifacts discussed on Figure 2. Left ventricular systolic pressure is either 140

mm Hg or 155 mm Hg (200/9 × 7 = 22.2 × 7). The aortic pressure is 130 mm Hg or 144 mm Hg (22.2 × 6.5). The peak to peak gradient is 10 or 11 mm Hg with valve area of $3.0/\sqrt{10} = 0.95$ or $3.0/\sqrt{11} = 0.90$ cm^2, respectively. The heart rate on Figure 3 must be estimated as discussed for Figure 2 since the time lines were again omitted.

Pressure lines can also be malpositioned if the switch which controls the pressure line scale is accidentally moved during recording (Fig. 4). On some recorders this switch is next to the dial controlling the number of pressure lines displayed and the event marker button. A slip of the technician's finger will change pressure data. Note that the aortic pressure is artificially higher when the pressure scale is shifted downward. We know aortic pressure is not truly different because of the unchanged zero base starting and ending points (arrows).

One additional note on time lines: physiologic recorders provide options whether the vertical lines should be only at the edges, top, bottom, or fully across the page (Fig. 5A). Use of the full page lines is preferable as timing markers for hemodynamic events in our laboratory. Partial page time lines make confirmation of waveform events more difficult and possibly erroneous to the imprecise observer. The selection of interval markers (e.g., one line every sec) for clinical purposes is usually standard. Use of more frequent markers (e.g., one line every 0.04 sec) is helpful for research studies or high speed recordings to measure hemodynamic events (Fig. 5B).

A TRANSIENTLY WIDE PULSE PRESSURE: EPISODIC AORTIC INSUFFICIENCY?

A continuous hemodynamic tracing was recorded during 7F left ventricular catheter pullback after ventriculography (Fig. 6A). The pullback was easily and smoothly, but slowly, performed. The operator noted a wide pulse pressure which appeared to diminish over the next several beats. Should the operator reload for aortography to demonstrate transient aortic insufficiency? To a new student of hemodynamics, this mystifying physiology of waxing aortic insufficiency might require more study. However, a slow pigtail catheter pullback from the left ventricle might be incomplete leaving a portion of the uncoiled pigtail in the left ventricle with several side holes still transmitting the lower left ventricular diastolic pressure falsely reducing aortic diastolic pressure. This phenomenon is demonstrated again with simultaneous femoral arterial and pigtail catheter pressures (Figs. 6B,C). The changing diastolic pressure is due to catheter movement with a different number of pigtail catheter side holes moving across the aortic valve.

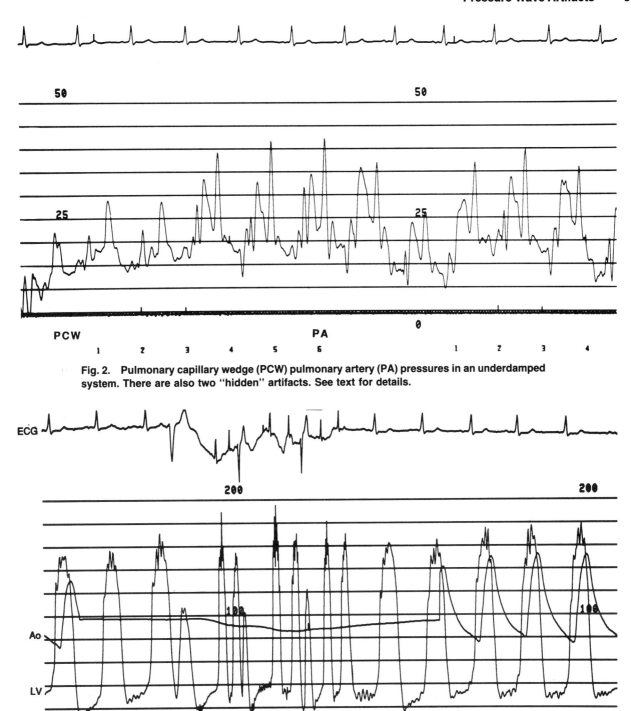

Fig. 2. Pulmonary capillary wedge (PCW) pulmonary artery (PA) pressures in an underdamped system. There are also two "hidden" artifacts. See text for details.

Fig. 3. Left ventricular (LV) and aortic (Ao) pressures in a patient with mild aortic stenosis. What is the left ventricular pressure and heart rate? See text for details.

With complete catheter removal, two systemic pressures match without the diastolic pressure artifact (Fig. 6C, right side). This artifact can be easily recognized by the unusual diastolic waveform with a late diastolic shoulder and rapid dip differentiating it from a wide pulse pressure of valvular insufficiency.

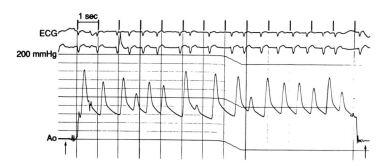

Fig. 4. Aortic (Ao) pressure recording. Pressure at left side is 140/60 mm Hg; at right 160/85 mm Hg. Why? See text for details.

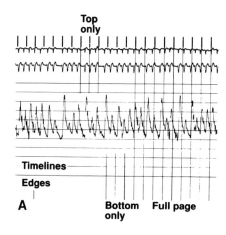

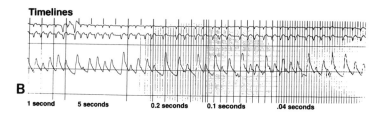

Fig. 5. A: Demonstration of time line presentations on recording paper. (Left to right): time lines are at edges only, top only, bottom only, and full page. Hemodynamic events are most easily timed with full page lines. B: Demonstration of time line interval spacing. Five full page lines occur between dark divisions of 0.2, 0.1, and 0.04 sec intervals.

CAUSES OF DELAYED OR LATE RISING CENTRAL AORTIC PRESSURE

The most proximally measured aortic pressure wave rise before pressure waves measured more distally. This constant physiologic requirement may be disturbed only by pressure waveform artifacts. Consider the hemodynamic data obtained in a 72-yr-old man with aortic stenosis (Fig. 7). Because of mild peripheral vascular disease, simultaneous pressures were initially obtained with a 6F femoral arterial sheath and a 5F pigtail catheter with fluid-filled transducers. The pressures measured before crossing the aortic valve demonstrated a good correspondence with two notable features: a slightly reduced femoral pressure overshoot consistent with mild peripheral vascular disease and a slow central aortic pressure upstroke consistent with aortic stenosis. These pressure waveforms are acceptable for routine clinical use. Crossing the heavily calcified valve in the enlarged aortic root was accomplished with the pigtail catheter and a 0.038″ straight guidewire as previously described [3]. Mild difficulty in advancing the pigtail catheter over the valve and into the left ventricle was encountered.

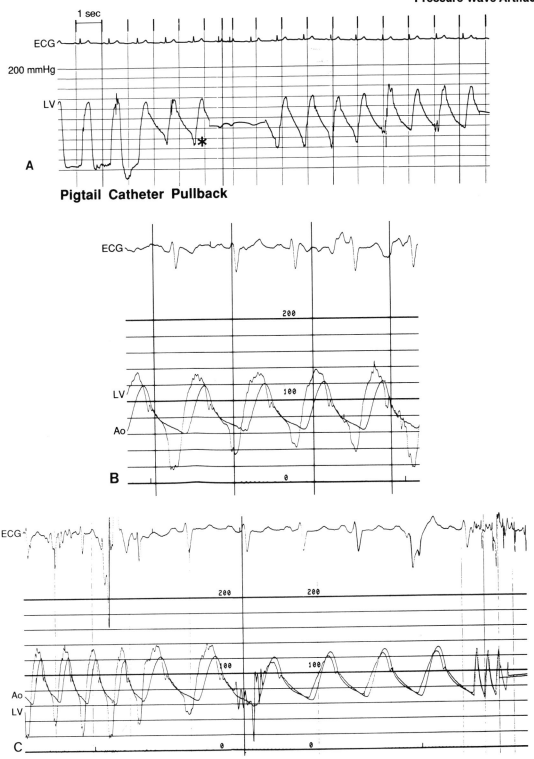

Pigtail Catheter Pullback

Fig. 6.   A: Left ventricular (LV) catheter pullback with transient aortic insufficiency. Note unusual diastolic waveform. See text for details. **B,C:** Left ventricular (LV) and simultaneous aortic (Ao) pressures. See text for details.

Examine the simultaneous left ventricular and aortic pressures (Fig. 5, lower panel). Why does left ventricular pressure rise after aortic pressure? Why is aortic pressure different from the above noted femoral pressure? The left ventricular pressure is overly damped with a rounded contour. A delay in pressure transmission is

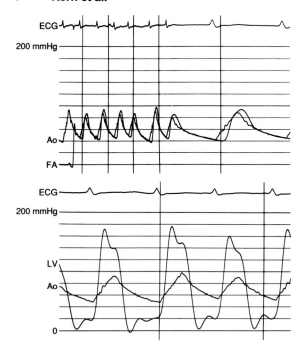

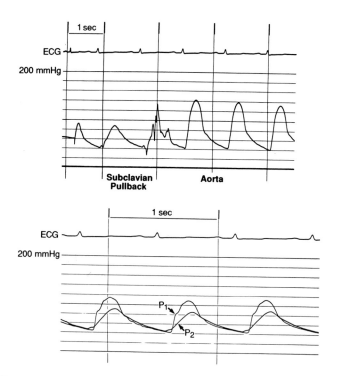

Fig. 7.   Top: Central and femoral (FA) pressures. Bottom: Left ventricular (LV) and aortic (Ao) pressures in a patient with aortic stenosis. Note delay and unusual waveform in left ventricular pressure. Explain? See text for details.

Fig. 8.   Upper panel: Catheter pullback from subclavian artery to aorta. Note gradient and waveform change. Lower panel: Two central aortic pressures. P_1 is in the aorta at the level of the left subclavian origin. Where is P_2? See text for details.

caused by a catheter kink in crossing the valve which could not be eliminated by vigorous flushing. Pressure overdamping can be caused by inadequate flushing, leaving an air bubble or blood in the line reducing the fidelity of pressure transmission. This problem may be exaggerated in small diameter tubes and catheters. Increasing the fluid viscosity with contrast media would also produce the damped and delayed tracing. This artifact was eliminated by changing catheters, in this case, to a 7F or 8F sheath with a 6F or 7F pigtail. A second arterial puncture or the transseptal approach as discussed in an earlier rounds [4] are also alternative solutions. Because of the peripheral vascular disease, a second small pigtail catheter was placed in the central aortic position to use for gradient measurement, explaining the differences between the aortic pressures.

Another example of a late rising proximal aortic pressure is shown on Figure 8 (lower panel). P_1 and P_2 are pressure tracings from two fluid-filled catheters located in the thoracic aorta. P_1 has a brisk upstroke with an anacrotic shoulder and dicrotic notch. P_2 is an earlier rising tracing with a considerably slower upslope and attenuated resonant waveform characteristics. What conditions produced this pattern and from which locations are these pressures obtained? P_1 is in the descending aorta below the left subclavian artery origin. P_2 is just beyond the ostial portion of the left subclavian artery

which had a significant narrowing producing a 30–40 mm Hg systolic gradient, slow upstroke, and loss of the anacrotic shoulder and dicrotic notch. On pullback from the subclavian artery to the aorta, the systolic gradient and changing waveform are evident (Fig. 8, upper panel). Subclavian stenosis and coarctation are the two conditions which can cause this pressure with catheters in the central aorta.

In the consideration of aortic coarctation (Fig. 9), one pressure waveform should be delayed with a slightly slower upstroke, but this pressure waveform will occur with the most distal pressure (e.g., not with P_2 but with P_1) since the delay in pulse transmission usually occurs in the aorta below the subclavian take-off narrowing, not as above in the subclavian artery as shown on Figure 8.

DISEQUILIBRATION

Differences in transducer signal response to the same pressure can cause false readings, artifactual gradients, and erroneous clinical decisions. Precision in measurement requires equisensitive amplifier settings and matched transducer gain settings. Matching of peripheral with central aortic pressure to assess the aortic valve gradient requires properly flushed transducers with equisensitive pressure responses. Although most transducers

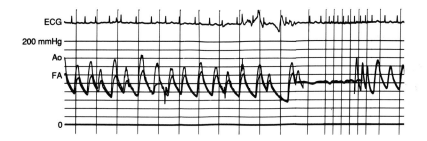

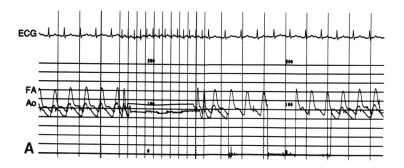

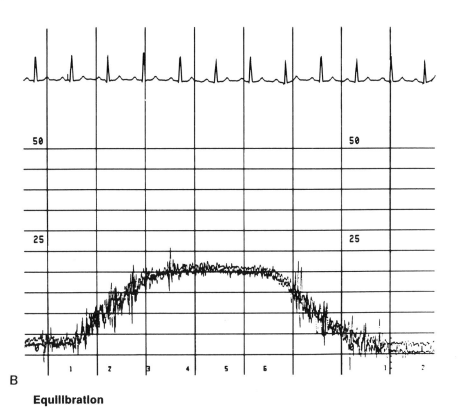

Equilibration

Fig. 9.   A: Unmatched central (Ao) and femoral (FA) arterial pressures despite matched zero points. Why? See text for details. B: Demonstration of equisensitivity and calibration of three fluid-filled transducers.

are highly reliable, an occasionally defective product or loose connection may produce a disparity in pressures expected to be equivalent. Examine the femoral artery sheath and central aortic pressures on Figure 10A. The pressure differences were not attributable to a loose pressure connection, overdamped or unflushed tubing, or unmatched amplifier settings. The aortic pressure transducer was faulty and subsequently replaced, permitting matching of the pressures similar to that shown in Figure 7. One way to quickly check equisensitivity of pressure transducers is shown on Figure 10B. Hold all manifolds (in this example three manifolds are connected to three transducers) at the same level then raise and lower the manifolds together observing the equivalency of pressure responses. A separation of one of the transducer tracings indicates a faulty calibration or defective transducer.

CONCLUSIONS

Pressure waveform artifacts are produced by mechanical (tubing, connections, stopcocks, catheters), electrical (amplifier settings, loose cable fittings) or technician-induced (recording without proper pressure or time lines or paper speed, or scale) artifacts. Recognition of these artifacts will save time and prevent hemodynamic data misinterpretation.

ACKNOWLEDGMENTS

The authors wish to thank the J.G. Mudd Cardiac Catheterization Team, Robert Roth, RN, and Donna Sander for manuscript preparation.

REFERENCES

1. Lambert CR, Pepine CJ, Nichols WW: Pressure measurements. In Pepine CJ (ed): "Diagnostic and Therapeutic Cardiac Catheterization." Baltimore: Williams & Wilkins, 1989, pp 283–293.
2. Nichols WW, O'Rourke MF (eds): Measuring principles of arterial waves. In "McDonald's Blood Flow In Arteries: Theoretical, Experimental and Clinical Practices, 3rd edition." Philadelphia: Lea & Febiger, 1990, pp 143–161.
3. Kern MJ: Catheter selection for the stenotic aortic valve. Cathet Cardiovasc Diagn 17:190–191, 1989.
4. Kern MJ, Deligonul U: Hemodynamic rounds: Interpretation of cardiac pathophysiology from pressure waveform analysis. I. The stenotic aortic valve. Cathet Cardiovasc Diagn 21:112–120, 1990.

Chapter 2

Pitfalls of Right-Heart Hemodynamics

Morton J. Kern, MD

INTRODUCTION

One of the most common pitfalls in the interpretation of hemodynamic data is the failure to appreciate abnormalities in cardiac rhythms often accounting for the alteration and, at times, misinterpretation of pressure waveforms [1,2]. Examine the right-heart hemodynamics in a patient undergoing evaluation for shortness of breath. The right atrial pressure (Fig. 1, left and middle) demonstrates an alteration in the phasic waveform. At left, the "V" wave or "S" wave suggests tricuspid regurgitation. However, this waveform is significantly different during the measurements made only a few minutes later (Fig. 1, middle). How has the physiology been affected?

Examining the electrocardiogram, a paced rhythm is responsible for the initially regurgitant wave in the right atrial pressure. The peak of the pressure wave corresponds to the QRS (the trace lines the time from the electrocardiogram to the pressure wave). As the rhythm changes to a sinus mechanism (Fig. 1, center of middle panel), the normal right atrial waveform is restored and the regurgitant waveform is eliminated. The changing rhythm also affects the determination of maximal pulmonary artery pressures (Fig. 1, right). During pacing, the pulmonary artery pressure has a larger respiratory variation and is higher than pressures obtained during normal sinus rhythm.

Examine the right heart hemodynamics obtained in a patient undergoing evaluation for ischemia-induced ventricular dysrhythmia and congestive heart failure (Fig. 2). The mean right atrial pressure (Fig. 2, top left) is 9 mm Hg with large "V" waves. Why is the right atrial waveform different between the left and right panels of Figure 2? Note the electrocardiogram. When sinus rhythm is restored (note "P" waves), the "V" wave is attenuated and a normal right atrial pressure waveform can be seen with a reduction in right atrial pressure to a mean value of 7 mm Hg (Fig. 2, top right). A similar response can be appreciated in the pulmonary capillary wedge pressure (Fig. 2, lower left). During sinus rhythm, pulmonary capillary wedge averages 18 mm Hg, with a "V" wave up to 24 mm Hg. However, during ventricular tachycardia, the mean pulmonary capillary wedge pressure markedly increases to 24 mm Hg with "V" waves up to 40 mm Hg (Fig. 2, lower right). Interpretation of the hemodynamic waveform is thus critically dependent on the particular cardiac rhythm which reflects the physiologic responses generating the cardiac pressure [3,4].

A 39-year-old man with congestive heart failure and cardiomyopathy undergoes hemodynamic evaluation. The influence of cardiac rhythm on right-heart hemodynamics can be appreciated in Figure 3. Examine the right atrial waveform at top right (Fig. 3). Note the alteration of the "V" wave configuration. How does one explain the large pointed waveforms at left side in contrast to the smaller, broader waveforms demonstrated at the right? While considering the possibilities, examine the differences in right ventricular pressures obtained during this study (Fig. 3, upper right and lower left panels). Compare the effects of the cardiac rhythm to the generation of right ventricular pressure.

The right atrial pressure "V" waves (Fig. 3, top left) occur during junctional rhythm with atrial superimposition on the QRS and third-degree heart block. As the atrial time delay permits normal sinus mechanisms to intervene, the waveform changes into a sinus-type rhythm with a larger "A" wave and small "V" wave. Note the

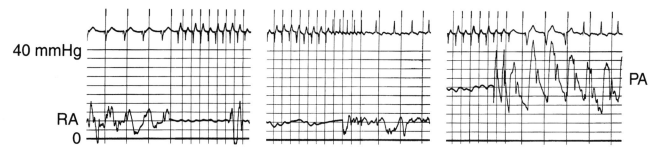

Fig. 1.   (Left) Right atrial (RA) pressure (0–40 mm Hg scale) during alterations in cardiac rhythm (middle). (Far right), change in pulmonary artery (PA) pressure.

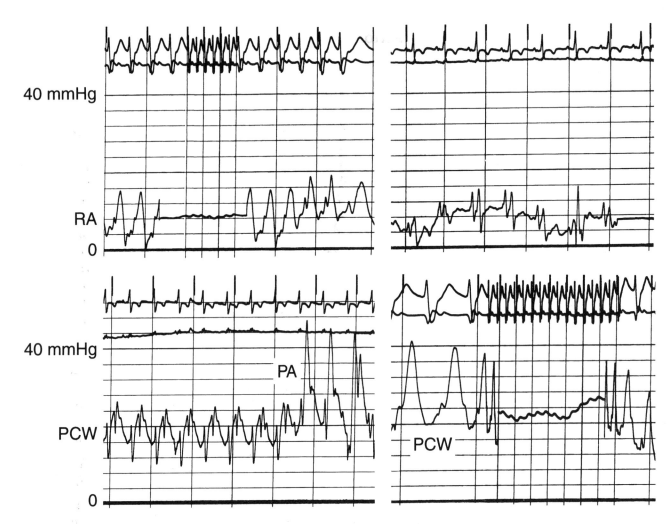

Fig. 2.   Right-heart hemodynamics during changes in cardiac rhythm. (Top left and right) RA, right atrial; PCWP, pulmonary capillary wedge pressure; PA, pulmonary artery (Bottom left and right).

decrease in mean right atrial pressure from 10–12 mm Hg to <8 mm Hg when sinus rhythm is in play.

The evaluation of right ventricular pressure is also interesting in that the accelerated junctional rhythm during complete heart block has a lower peak systolic pressure of approximately 38 mm Hg (Fig. 3, top right,

right side). When the rhythm changes, the peak systolic right ventricular pressure increases to approximately 50 mm Hg and the initiation of the atrial wave can be seen as a deflection on the QRS (Fig. 3, midportion at upper right). As the sinus mechanism contributes to the filling of the ventricle and precedes QRS activation of ventricular

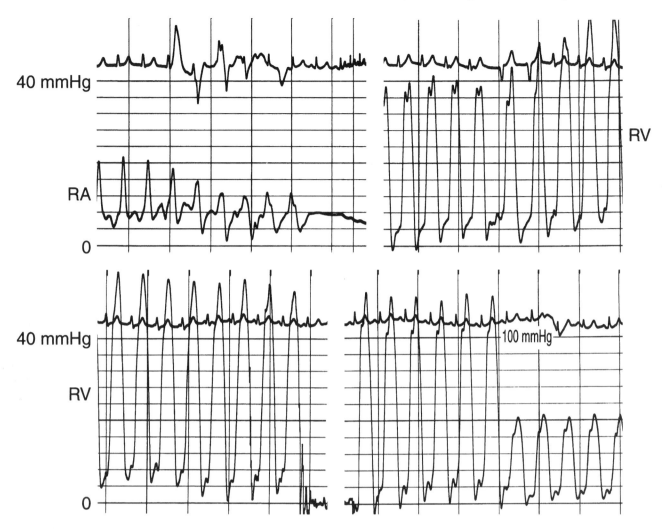

Fig. 3. (Top right) Right atrial (RA) and (Top left and lower right) right ventricular (RV) pressures (0–40 mm Hg scale) during alterations in cardiac rhythm. Lower right: RV pressure scale change from 0–40 mm Hg to 0–100 mm Hg (far right).

contraction, the systolic pressure increases and remains in excess of 50 mm Hg. The rhythm changes explain the wide variations in right atrial and ventricular pressure waveforms and should be important functional clues in the evaluation of hemodynamics for such individuals.

EXAMINATION OF VENA CAVAL PRESSURE WAVEFORMS IN TRICUSPID REGURGITATION

Tricuspid regurgitation often produces distinct waveforms in the right atrial pressure [3–6]. Sometimes, transmission of the regurgitant wave can be detected beyond the vena cava (i.e., transmitted to the jugular veins) [7]. However, it is uncommon to observe changing waveforms in the inferior vena cava compared to those in the right atrium. For purposes of demonstration, we recorded the inferior vena caval pressure and compared the waveforms to those of the right atrial and ventricular

pressures in a patient with modest tricuspid regurgitation (Fig. 4).

A 61-year-old woman had tricuspid regurgitation of unknown etiology which was associated with mild pulmonary hypertension and dyspnea. Coronary arteriography was normal. Left ventriculography demonstrated mild global hypokinesis with an ejection fraction of 55%. Aortic pressure was 125/70 mm Hg, left ventricular pressure was 125/12 mm Hg, and pulmonary capillary wedge pressure was 20 mm Hg with normal "A" and "V" wave configurations. The effects of tricuspid regurgitation on the right atrium and inferior vena cava were assessed by measuring two pressures simultaneously, one from each of the two lumens of a balloon-tipped pulmonary artery catheter. The systolic wave of regurgitation could be appreciated in both the right atrium and inferior vena cava. The right atrial pressure was measured with the tip of the balloon-tipped catheter looped within the

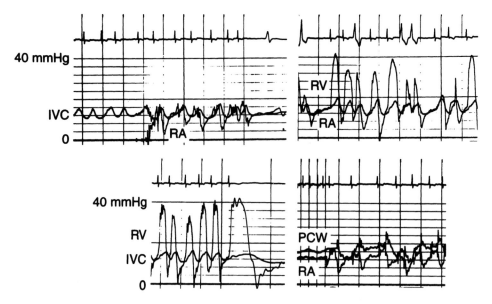

Fig. 4.   (Top left) Right atrial (RA) and inferior vena cava (IVC) pressures in a patient with tricuspid regurgitation. (Top right) RA and RV pressures. (Lower left) RV and IVC pressures. (Lower Right) Pulmoncapillary wedge (PCW) and RA pressures.

right atrium (Fig. 4, upper left). The inferior vena cava pressure was measured approximately 10 cm below the inferior border of the right atrium. The pressure wave fidelity between the two systems was demonstrated to be equivalent by comparing the right ventricular and right atrial pressures measured with the same transducers on advancement of the catheter into the right ventricular apex (Fig. 4, top right).

The waveform of the inferior vena cava is slower in upstroke and downstroke, with reduced velocity. The blunted waveform is due, in part, to the considerably higher capacity and compliance of the vena cava compared to those of the right atrium. It is also important to note that the right atrial pressure mean, as expected, is lower than the vena cava, with a 2–4 mm Hg pressure gradient required for maintenance of normal blood flow. The pressure gradient between the inferior vena cava and right atrium occurs predominantly during the end of atrial diastole (Fig. 4, top left).

The severity of tricuspid regurgitation can be appreciated when comparing the right ventricular and right atrial pressures (Fig. 4, top right), showing the regurgitant "S" wave and large "V" wave of tricuspid regurgitation. Tricuspid regurgitation is, by waveform characteristics, most severe during the ventricular couplet appearing in the midportion of this tracing, in which the pressure during systole is achieved for both beats. When comparing the vena cava and right ventricular pressures (Fig. 4, lower left), the delay in waveform and transmission of the vena cava can be appreciated. Of interest, the differences between the mean pulmonary capillary wedge (16 mm Hg) and mean right atrial (12 mm Hg) (Fig. 4, lower right) demonstrate the larger "Y"

descent in right atrial pressure which drives the inferior vena cava flow. Inferior vena cava flow in most cases parallels that of superior vena cava flow, and thus large "V" waves in the jugular vein on clinical examination can reflect either significant tricuspid regurgitation or functional regurgitation during cardiac arrhythmias [7].

The jugular pulse closely reflects events in right atrial pressure and also parallels changes observed in the vena cava [8,9]. However, one must remember that the change in pressure within the right atrium is reflected principally by a change in volume for the venous system. It is thought that the pulse wave transmission from the right atrium to the jugular veins has the least disparity for pressure waves which are positive and are thought to be conducted more rapidly as compared to negative pressure waves [10]. The venous pulse "A" and "C" waves have an average delay from right atrial pressures of approximately 60 msec, the "V" wave 80 msec, the "Y" trough 90 msec, and the "X" trough 110 msec [10]. It requires 60 msec for the right atrial "A" wave to reach the right ventricle and cause a positive defection in this chamber. These delays should be considered when examining the jugular venous pulse, as well as inferior vena caval pressure waves as a reflection of right atrial pressure [4].

Jugular vein pulsations may have induced artifact by carotid arterial pressure waves. This artifact can be recognized by an irregular pulsation often obscuring the "X" descent. The irregular wave shows a carotid-like contour, with the dicrotic notch recognized in the middle of the "X" descent [4]. As in the case example, Tavel [7] also notes that tricuspid insufficiency often produces a prominent "V" wave beginning early and tending to obliterate the "X" descent. In severe tricuspid regurgitation, the "V" wave corresponds and begins with the "C" wave and shows a broad plateau terminating in a steep "Y" descent. This wave has been termed the regurgitant or "S" wave. In the setting of atrial fibrillation, nearly complete obliteration of the "X" descent is required before making the diagnosis of tricuspid insufficiency from a venous pulse wave. In patients with normal sinus rhythm, changes in the venous pulse suggesting tricuspid regurgitation may demonstrate only slight decrease in the "X" descent equal to or above the level of the "Y" trough. In some patients, a separate systolic wave may appear on the "V" wave ascent and may be an obscured clue to the presence of tricuspid regurgitation [6]. In addition, in tricuspid regurgitation there may be a relatively normal venous pulse wave; hence, the diagnostic accuracy of the waveform is helpful in that a normal curve cannot be used to exclude tricuspid disease. The characteristic pulse waves may be absent at rest but brought on by inspiratory maneuvers or increasing heart rate [6].

CONCLUSIONS

Careful examination of hemodynamics requires examination not only of individual pressure waves and their timing to the QRS, but also of the electrocardiogram and its various components. It would not be unusual to have different and obscured electrocardiographic waveforms present without an appreciation on the hemodynamic tracing, since often only one lead is recorded. When the electrocardiographic waveform is in question, various leads should be recorded with the hemodynamic tracing. Changing leads of the 12-lead electrocardiogram can be helpful in determining whether a certain rhythm is accurately identified. This approach has important implications for the genesis of right-heart pressure waveforms, as well as accurate reporting of absolute systolic and diastolic pressures. Careful examination of right-heart hemodynamics may reveal unanticipated pathophysiologic mechanisms.

ACKNOWLEDGMENTS

The author thanks the J.G. Mudd Cardiac Catheterization Laboratory for technical support, and Donna Sander for manuscript preparation.

REFERENCES

1. Kern MJ (ed): "Hemodynamic Rounds: Interpretation of Pathophysiology From Pressure Waveform Analysis." New York: Wiley-Liss, 1993. pp 1–6
2. Kern MJ, Deligonul U, Donohue T, Caracciolo E, Feldman T: Hemodynamic data. In Kern MJ (ed): "The Cardiac Catheterization Handbook," 2nd ed. St. Louis: Mosby-YearBook, 1995, pp 108–207.
3. Grossman W: Profiles in valvular heart disease. Grossman W. In: "Cardiac Catheterization and Angiography." Philadelphia: Lea & Febiger, 1986, p 378.
4. Tavel ME: Normal sounds and pulses: Relationships and intervals between the various events. Tavel M In: "Clinical Phonocardiography and External Pulse Recording," 2nd ed. Chicago: Year Book Medical Publishers, 1972, pp 35–58.
5. Lingamneni R, Cha SD, Maranhao V, Gooch AS, Goldberg H. Tricuspid regurgitation: Clinical and angiographic assessment. Cathet Cardiovasc Diagn 5:7–17, 1979.
6. Mueller O, Shillingford J: Tricuspid incompetence. Br Heart J 16:195–204, 1954.
7. Tavel ME (ed): The jugular pulse tracing: Its clinical application. In: "Clinical Phonocardiography and External Pulse Recording," 2nd ed. Chicago: Year Book Medical Publishers, 1972, pp 207–226.
8. Morgan BC, Abel FL, Mullins GL, Guntheroth WG: Flow patterns in cavae, pulmonary artery, pulmonary vein and aorta in intact dogs. Am J Physiol 210:903–909, 1966.
9. Brecher GA, Hubay CA: Pulmonary blood flow and venous return during spontaneous respiration. Circ Res 3:210–214, 1955.
10. Willems J, Roelandt J, Kesteloot H: The jugular venous pulse tracing. Proceedings of the Fifth European Congress of Cardiology, Sept 1968; p 433.

Chapter 3

The Stenotic Aortic Valve

Morton J. Kern, MD, and Ubeydullah Deligonul, MD

THE STENOTIC AORTIC VALVE

The most commonly encountered hemodynamic valvular problems are those related to aortic stenosis. This first hemodynamic rounds will focus on techniques and tracings utilized in this large patient subgroup.

Case Presentation

Hemodynamic tracings were obtained in a 75 year old man with a history of mild shortness of breath and exertional chest pain (Figure 1). The patient has had a known heart murmur since the age of 50. The patient has mild hypertension, smokes 1 pack of cigarettes per day and is taking no medications. Electrocardiogram showed predominant normal sinus rhythm, left ventricular hypertrophy. Chest x-ray showed borderline moderate sized cardiac silhouette. Echocardiography was consistent with aortic stenosis and the patient was referred for cardiac catheterization. Prior to contrast ventriculography, pressures in the left ventricle and aorta were measured with fluid-filled catheters. Before discussing these findings, examine the tracings and consider the following questions: From which locations are these pressures obtained? What is responsible for the increase in pressure gradient and peak left ventricular pressure on beat #3? If this patient went into atrial fibrillation, would hemodynamic compromise occur? Does this patient have aortic insufficiency combined with aortic stenosis from pressure tracings?

Measuring Pressure Gradients in Aortic Stenosis

There are four invasive methods to measure aortic-left ventricular pressure gradients:

1) A single arterial puncture using a peripheral (femoral or brachial) artery pressure matched to central aortic pressure through a side arm of a larger sheath through which passes a one French size smaller left ventricular catheter (commonly a pigtail).

2) Two arterial punctures with one catheter in the left ventricle and one positioned just above the aortic valve.

3) Femoral venous approach for transseptal entry to the left ventricle with central aortic pressure obtained from an arterial catheter above the aortic valve.

4) A single arterial puncture (or cutdown) with a single catheter, 2 transducers; one left ventricular, one aortic pressure (most commonly 2 high fidelity micromanometer transducers or a double lumen pigtail, fluid-filled catheter). All pressures are matched before positioning across the valve.

From the methods noted above, how can one determine the location of pressure measurements for this patient (Figure 1)? By observing the timing of upstroke of the aortic (Ao) pressure, one sees the aortic pressure rises immediately (i.e., without time delay) with left ventricular pressure and must therefore be measured from the most proximal (central aorta) chamber to the left ventricle. The left ventricular pressure was obtained via the transseptal approach. All pressures using a centrally positioned arterial catheter will have this immediate upstroke. Compare this pressure tracing to that in Figure 2 (panel A) in which the femoral artery pressure (FA) (through a side-arm of an 8 French sheath with a 7 French pigtail catheter in the left ventricle) is used. After matching the femoral artery pressure with the catheter in the central aortic position, femoral artery pressure is used for comparison against left ventricular pressure. The time delay (usually 40–50 msec after upstroke of left ventricular pressure) of the femoral artery pressure indicates the distance away from the heart.

When assessing hemodynamics using the peripheral arterial pressure for central aortic pressure, Folland et al [1] examined femoral artery-left ventricular systolic gradients with and without pressure realignment (shifting the upstroke to match). Without realignment, left ventricular-femoral artery gradient over estimated the left ventricular-aortic mean gradient by approximately 9mmHg. When the left ventricular-femoral artery gradients were aligned, under estimation of the left ventricular-aortic mean gradient by approximately 10mmHg was noted, representing the fact that peak systolic (femoral) arterial pressure is higher and the upstroke faster for the peripheral arterial than central aortic pressure tracings with a planimetered gradient smaller when using aligned

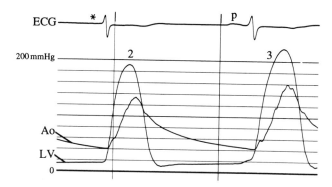

Fig. 1. Simultaneous aortic (Ao) and left ventricular (LV) pressure tracings obtained (0–200mmHg scale) in a patient with dyspnea and chest pain. See text for details.

left ventricular-femoral artery pressures. One solution proposed was to average the aligned and non-aligned gradients to most closely approximate true left ventricular aortic valve gradients. Whenever there is a significant discrepancy using a peripheral pressure, we recommend a second (usually small) arterial catheter be positioned above the aortic valve.

Because of spontaneous changes in cardiac cycle length, especially evident in atrial fibrillation, determination of left ventricular-aortic valve gradients with a single catheter pullback technique is not recommended. When a single catheter is used as the only pressure measurement available, then closely matched R–R cycle lengths should be planimetered for valve area calculations.

Does the presence of a catheter across the valve significantly influence the gradient? Carabello et al [2] observed an increase of >10mmHg in peripheral arterial pressure when a catheter is withdrawn from the left ventricle across severely (<0.6cm²) stenotic aortic valves. This observation is thought to be due to catheter cross-sectional area contribution to reduced aortic valve area. In view of recent experience with aortic valvuloplasty, transient reduction in aortic valve area (and in some cases, near occlusion of aortic outflow) is generally tolerated. Calculations of aortic valve area consider reduction by catheter cross-sectional area insignificant.

In general, selection of catheters for crossing stenotic aortic valves is based on operator training and experience. Standard configurations and guidewires may not always cross stenotic aortic valves. Use of a pigtail catheter (one size smaller than the femoral arterial sheath) is our first choice [3].

Disappearing Gradients During Data Collection

A 49 year old man with mild early fatigue, vague atypical chest pain syndrome and systolic murmur underwent hemodynamic study (Figure 2). The femoral (sheath) and left ventricular pressures (pigtail catheter) were matched at the central aortic position prior to crossing into the left ventricle. In panel A, significant aortic stenosis is demonstrated. Within a few minutes after inserting the pigtail catheter into the left ventricle, the hemodynamic pressures on panel B were obtained. On fluoroscopy, the pigtail catheter appeared to be in nearly the identical position within the ventricle on both tracings. How can one explain the loss of gradient? If panel B was your initial tracing, is there significant aortic stenosis?

Observe the left ventricular-end diastolic pressure on panel B. The left ventricular pressure continues to decline throughout diastole and increases just at the A wave. Compare this pressure tracing to panel A. The left ventricular diastolic waveform is flat or slightly increasing before the prominent "A" wave. The aortic (FA) pressure is unchanged in both panels so this cannot account for the change in the stenotic gradient. The explanation for the loss of gradient is that one of the side holes of the pigtail catheter is now residing in the aorta, evidenced by the continual decline of diastolic left ventricular pressure. This highly abnormal diastolic pressure configuration may be rarely seen in patients who have hypertrophic cardiomyopathy [4]. Had panel B been the first tracing recorded, one might have concluded that aortic stenosis was not significant. For this reason, repositioning the pigtail catheter within the ventricle in all cases, especially those with questionable pressure tracings relative to clinical findings, is mandatory. This catheter artifact is easily recognized if more side holes have their opening in the aorta with the left ventricular diastolic pressure even more elevated, approaching that of aortic diastolic pressure.

Cardiac Rhythms and Aortic Pressure Gradients

Returning to Figure 1, what role does the cardiac rhythm play with respect to aortic-left ventricular gradients? Atrial contraction increases left ventricular-end diastolic volume and results in increased peak left ventricular pressure, as well as the aortic pressure. Beat #2 is a junctional beat (no "P" wave) without atrial contraction. Beat #3 is a normal sinus beat ("P" wave on the electrocardiographic tracing) and an "A" wave visible on the left ventricular pressure. The atrial contribution to left ventricular filling increases the aortic pressure by approximately 25% (for aortic from 134mmHg to 160mmHg and for left ventricular pressures from 190mmHg to 220mmHg). In the full cycle beat (#3), the valve area calculation, however, does not change appreciably since both the left ventricular pressure and the aortic pressure increase together. A post extrasystolic beat with an augmented filling period also has a marked increase in the left ventricular systolic pressure with no

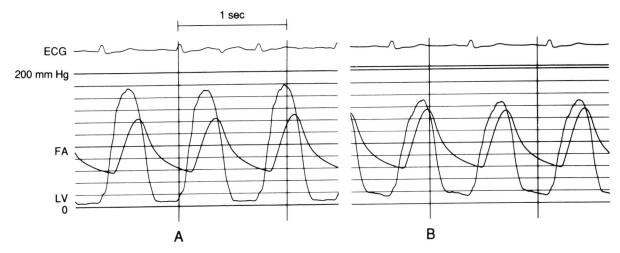

Fig. 2. Simultaneous femoral artery (FA) and left ventricular (LV) pressure tracings (0–200mmHg scale) in a patient with systolic murmur. See text for details.

change or a slight increase in the aortic pressure. In view of the junctional beat and its hemodynamics, it would be unlikely if this patient decompensated in atrial fibrillation if the ventricular response could be controlled.

Types of Aortic-Left Ventricular Gradients

For aortic stenosis, aortic-left ventricular gradients are described in three ways: 1) peak left ventricular pressure minus maximum aortic pressure, "peak to peak" gradient; 2) peak "instantaneous" left ventricular-aortic (usually reported from Doppler flow velocity); 3) mean left ventricular-aortic gradient [planimetered area under aortic-left ventricular curves (shifted to match aortic upstroke, if needed)].

The "peak to peak" gradient is a convenient catheterization laboratory number used to convey quickly the magnitude of the gradient. It has no meaning in physiologic terms since these peaks do not occur at the same time. In severe aortic stenosis, "peak to peak" gradients approximate planimetered mean gradients.

One of the most precise hemodynamic methods of measuring aortic valvular gradients was used in a 55 year old woman with a systolic murmur and long standing hypertension (Figure 3). An 8 French dual micromanometer-tipped catheter with two miniaturized pressure transducers separated by approximately 5–7cm was inserted across the aortic valve. The precisely defined upstroke of both the aortic and left ventricular pressure accurately demonstrate an early pressure gradient of minimal aortic stenosis. The upstroke of aortic pressure with a high frequency vibration coincides precisely with left ventricular pressure upstroke during ejection of blood from the left ventricle. Simultaneous high fidelity pressures may detect the early systolic gradients of an "im-

pulse type" [5] (Figure 4A) which may be normal in many younger patients with vigorous hearts, especially during high flow states such as exercise [6,7] (Figure 4B). The peak to peak gradient on Figure 3 is obviously much smaller than the mean or peak instantaneous gradient.

The peak instantaneous gradient is more difficult to obtain from the hemodynamic data alone, but occurs early in ejection (Figure 3, just after the J point of the electrocardiogram well before the peak pressure) and is the maximal distance (pressure) between left ventricular and aortic pressures [8]. This value is most easily obtained by Doppler techniques and correlates with aortic valve planimetered areas [9]. Peak instantaneous gradients can be estimated as planimetered mean gradient/

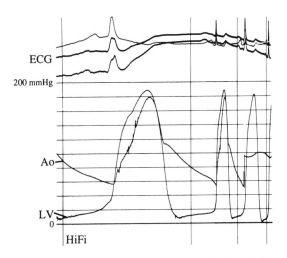

Fig. 3. Simultaneous measurements of aortic (Ao) and left ventricular (LV) pressures (0–200mmHg scale) in a patient with hypertension. See text for details.

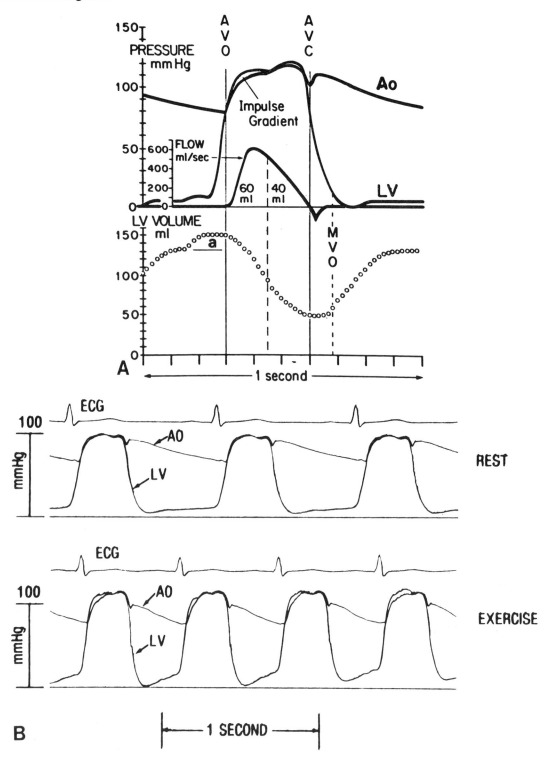

Fig. 4.   A: Impulse-type gradient in a normal left ventricle. Left ventricular (LV) and aortic (Ao) pressures, aortic outflow and ventricular volumes are displayed. Solid vertical lines indicate aortic valve opening (AVO) and aortic valve closure (AVC). Dashed lines indicate mid point of systole and mitral valve opening (MVO). A=atrial contribution to ventricular filling. See text for details. Reproduced from Criley et al (5) with permission. B: Representative aortic (Ao) and left ventricular (LV) micromanometer pressures at rest and during exercise in normal human left ventricle. An impulse gradient can be seen during exercise. ECG=electrocardiogram. Reproduced from Pasipoularides (7) with permission.

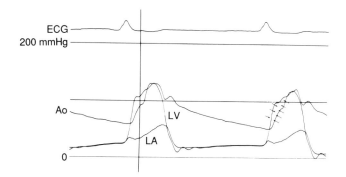

Fig. 5. Aortic (Ao) and left ventricular (LV) pressure tracings in a patient with an intrinsic "impulse-type" aortic valve gradient (arrow). Left atrial (LA) pressure was obtained through a sheath. See text for details.

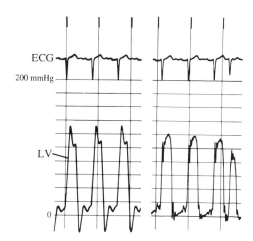

Fig. 6. Left ventricular pressure tracings before (left) and after (right) pressure system manipulation. See text for details.

0.70 (9). Similarly, the mean planimetered gradient can be estimated as 0.71 × "peak to peak" gradient + 17mmHg [9].

The Dilemma of Small Aortic-Left Ventricular Gradients and Low Aortic Flow

A complete discussion of issues regarding aortic valve area calculations is the subject of a future hemodynamic rounds. It is worth noting, however, that a continuing dilemma exists in patients with low cardiac output and small aortic-left ventricular gradients (e.g., the patient with dyspnea, poor left ventricular function and a 20mmHg aortic-left ventricular gradient with cardiac output of 3L/min; aortic valve area = 0.7cm^2) [10,11]. Should this valve be replaced with a prosthetic valve which has an intrinsic gradient of 10–20mmHg? As Carabello [2] discusses, the Gorlin formula for aortic valve area calculations uses an empiric constant (K) which now must be considered a variable under low flow conditions. Although some laboratories attempt to increase cardiac output and reassess gradients (and valve areas) under low and high flow states, there is no data indicating augmented cardiac output calculations are better than those at rest.

A 62 year old man undergoes cardiac catheterization 5 years after implantation of a prosthetic mechanical aortic valve. On examination of the hemodynamic tracings (Figure 5), a small (and predominantly early) systolic left ventricular-aortic gradient is apparent. Cardiac output is 4.0L/minute. One can appreciate the intrinsic "impulse type" left ventricular-aortic gradient and clinical limitations of a tilting disc prosthesis in patients with small gradients of the aortic valve. This gradient occurs in a well functioning valve and has no significant pathologic implications. Dyspnea was due to development of new mitral regurgitation ('V' wave on left atrial pressure). As

an aside, from which locations were the pressures obtained? (See discussion for Figure 1.)

Aortic Regurgitation Complicating Aortic Stenosis

Hemodynamic characteristics consistent with chronic aortic regurgitation, always a consideration, only include wide pulse pressure (see Figure 1). A wide pulse pressure can commonly be seen during a long cardiac cycle. The aortic diastolic pressure declines toward left ventricular pressure so that at the end of diastole (40mmHg), the pulse pressure is 70mmHg. This wide pulse pressure is consistent with aortic insufficiency but can also be due to bradycardia alone in patients with non-compliant vascular beds (e.g., systolic hypertension) without aortic regurgitation. The slow heart rate (<60 beats/minute) is indicated by the RR interval longer than the 1 second time line interval. This patient (Figure 1) had no angiographic or Doppler evidence of aortic regurgitation.

Hemodynamic Artifacts of Aortic and Left Ventricular Pressures

Whenever fluid-filled systems are used, artifacts from the transducer chambers, catheters, pressure tubing, or manifolds may confound waveform analysis. Although familiar to many, the tracing on Figure 6 (left panel) demonstrates a prominent high frequency "overshoot" of the left ventricular tracing in early systole and a marked overshoot on the early diastolic portion. The overshoot is characteristically called "ringing," representing the resonating frequency of the pressure system. The tracing on the right is obtained after manipulation of the fluid-filled system. What artifact produced the overshoot? The left hand tracing is characteristic of an un-

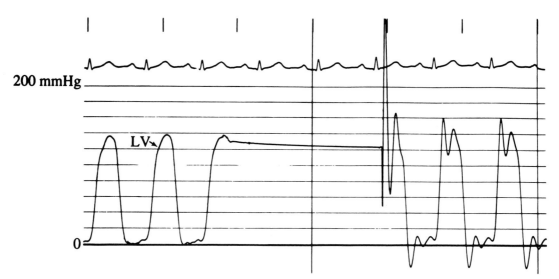

Fig. 7.   Left ventricular (LV) pressure after ventriculography. See text for details.

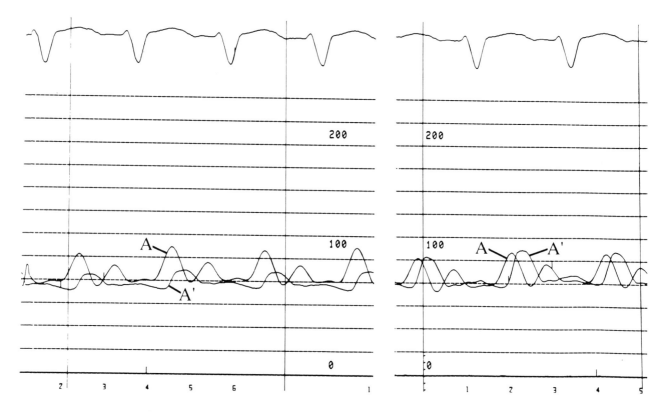

Fig. 8.   Simultaneous central aortic pressure measurement (A) with pigtail catheter and femoral artery sheath (A'). Zero pressures ("checks") are the same. Note differences in delay and overshoot of femoral artery tracing. See text for details.

derdamped (i.e., too much ringing) fluid-filled system with a bubble in the fluid line to the transducer. On flushing the bubble, the system now shows the normal, correctly damped, resonant pattern of left ventricular pressure.

Examine the left ventricular pressure tracing on Figure 7. The pressure waveform on the left was obtained through the pigtail catheter immediately after contrast ventriculography. There is no evidence of ringing as shown earlier. The waveform is slightly rounded. After flushing the catheter, the continuous tracing to the right shows the ringing artifact. What conditions explain this

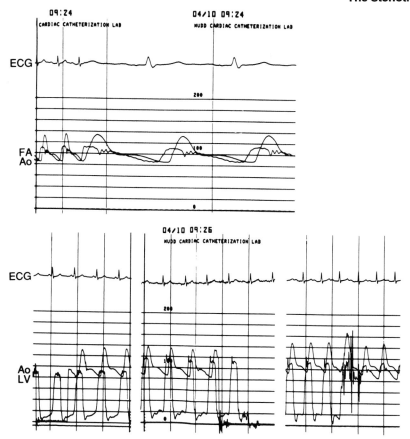

Fig. 9. Simultaneous femoral artery and aortic pressures measured with the 8F femoral artery sheath and 7F pigtail catheter before crossing the aortic valve (top panel). Note the delay in femoral artery pressure and marked overshoot of the peripheral pressure. Both zero and mean pressures were matched. (Lower panel left) aortic pressure markedly higher than left ventricular pressure. Rezero indicated zero drift of the transducer. (Middle panel) matching of left ventricular and aortic pressures, both zeros are now again correct (last beat, right hand side of middle panel). Prior to pullback from left ventricle to aorta, there is again drift of the aortic pressure and on pullback, the disparity between peripheral arterial pressure and aortic pressure can be seen. This is an example of a drifting and faulty transducer. See text for details.

transition in pressure waveform? The contrast media in the catheter remaining after ventriculography has a higher viscosity than saline, thus, damps the system. On flushing the catheter through with saline, the underdamped ringing pattern of the left ventricular pressure appears. When using fluid-filled systems and these pressure tracings, assess the degree of ringing that is acceptable. Flush the catheter to purge bubbles or, if needed, instill contrast media to provide a higher quality pressure signal for more accurate interpretation of the waveforms.

Peripheral Arterial Wave Summation and Zero Drift

Whenever using the femoral artery pressure to assess aortic valve gradients, always match pressures in both transducers prior to obtaining aortic-left ventricular gradients. Zero alignment of both systems and simultaneous pressure recording (both phasic and mean) with a zero position check against transducer drift from baseline af-

ter recording will insure accuracy. A discrepancy should be reconciled or transducers changed.

Femoral and central aortic pressures were measured in a 30 year old woman (Figure 8). A pressure difference was evident with significantly lower femoral artery pressure (left panel). (Remember the later upstroke of the pressure wave marks the more distal location). To reconcile these differences, carefully flush both systems (catheters, manifolds, transducers, zero lines) with special attention to the arterial sheath. After flushing (right panel), the tracings were more closely matched and used for hemodynamics. Note the femoral artery (A') is now higher than central aortic (A) pressure, despite underdamped waveforms.

Although matching of pressures at the beginning of the study is precise, some transducers may drift from zero. Figure 9 (top) shows matched femoral artery-aortic pressures. Femoral artery pressure did not match left ventricular pressure during simultaneous measurements (first

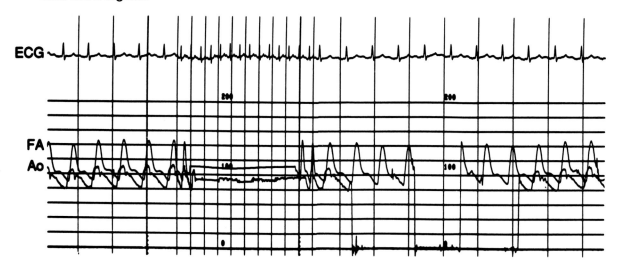

Fig. 10. Simultaneous 8F femoral artery (FA) sheath pressure and central aortic pressure measured through a 7F pigtail catheter. The disparity between pressures is evident on both phasic and mean differences of pressure, despite an accurate "zero" of both transducers. The disparity remained after recalibration. This tracing demonstrates the differences in sensitivity of pressures due to a faulty transducer which was replaced. See text for details.

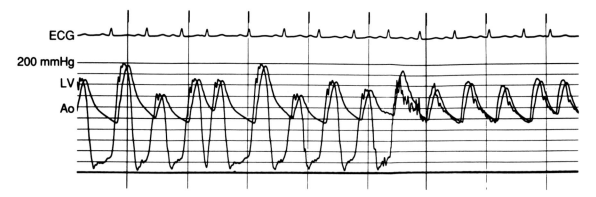

Fig. 11. Simultaneous left ventricular (LV) and aortic (Ao) pressures measured through a 7F pigtail catheter and 8F sheath. The patient has peripheral vascular disease. See text for details.

and second lower panels). Reflushing after initial pressures produced satisfactory measurements with both pressures returning to zero (right edge, bottom middle panel). However, on pullback drift of femoral artery pressure (last panel, bottom) was again evident due to a faulty transducer and zero baseline drift.

Femoral or peripheral arterial pressure does not, and usually should not be equal to central aortic pressure. The overshoot of femoral artery pressure is due to summation of the pressure wave reflections generated by the expansion and recoil characteristics of the central aortic and large artery elasticity. The peripheral or femoral artery pressure is almost always higher than central aortic pressure.

Unequal sensitivity of transducers may cause differences in femoral artery-aortic pressures (Figure 10). Despite precise zeros, the femoral artery-aortic pressures

could not be matched. Recalibrate both transducers with a mercury manometer as a standard to identify a faulty transducer.

When using the peripheral arterial sheath for pressure matching in the determination of aortic valve gradients, artifactual small aortic-left ventricular gradients may be present due to sheath pressure problems. Left ventricular and aortic pressures were measured in a 74 year old man with a heart murmur and severe peripheral vascular disease (Figure 11). Left ventricular pressure was obtained through a 7 French pigtail catheter, passing through the 8 French sheath as customarily performed with our hemodynamic studies. The initial matchup of aortic and central aortic pressures was satisfactory. On recording left ventricular-aortic pressures, a small, early systolic gradient was present. It is evident on pullback of the left ventricular catheter that the gradient is due to a delay and reduced upstroke of the femoral artery pressure (right hand panel, Figure 11). This sheath pressure can be due to 1) pressure artifact with damping within the sheath, 2) significant arterial disease with aortic coarctation or iliac or femoral arterial disease or 3) inadequate pressure transmission outside the sheath. In this patient with peripheral vascular disease and no clinical or echocardiographic signs of aortic stenosis other than an ejection murmur, a second arterial catheter insertion was not performed. Reflushing the sheath rectified the problem.

However, if there is a major discrepancy between the femoral artery and central aortic pressure tracings after all steps to insure good pressures are made, introduction of a second arterial catheter to the central aortic position for precise transvalvular gradient measures should be performed.

ACKNOWLEDGMENT

The authors wish to thank Donna Sander for manuscript preparation.

REFERENCES

1. Folland ED, Parisi AF, Carbone C. Is peripheral arterial pressure a satisfactory substitute for ascending aortic pressure when measuring aortic valve gradients? J Am Coll Cardiol 4:1207–1212, 1984.
2. Carabello BA. Advances in the hemodynamic assessment of stenotic cardiac valves. J Am Coll Cardiol 10:912–919, 1987.
3. Kern MJ. Catheter selection for the stenotic aortic valve. Cathet Cardiovasc Diagn 17:190–191, 1989.
4. Lorell BH, Paulus WJ, Grossman W, Wynne J, Cohn PF, Braunwald E. Improved diastolic function and systolic performance in hypertrophic cardiomyopathy after nifedipine. N Engl J Med 303: 801–803, 1980.
5. Criley JM, Siegel RJ. Has 'obstruction' hindered our understanding of hypertrophic cardiomyopathy? Circulation 72:1148–1154, 1985.
6. Murgo JP, Altobelli SA, Dorethy JF, Logdson JR, McGranahan GM. Normal ventricular ejection dynamics in man during rest and exercise. Am Heart Asso Mongr 46:92, 1975.
7. Pasipoularides A. Clinical assessment of ventricular ejection dynamics with and without outflow obstruction. J Am Coll Cardiol 15:859–882, 1990.
8. Oh JK, Taliercio CP, Holmes DR Jr, Reeder GS, Bailey KR, Seward JB, Tajik AJ. Prediction of the severity of aortic stenosis by Doppler aortic valve area determination: prospective Doppler-catheterization correlation in 100 patients. J Am Coll Cardiol 11:1227–1234, 1988.
9. Gordon JB, Folland ED. Analysis of aortic valve gradients by transseptal technique: implications for noninvasive evaluation. Cathet Cardiovasc Diagn 17:144–151, 1989.
10. Gorlin WB, Gorlin R. A generalized formulation of the Gorlin formula for calculating the area of the stenotic mitral valve and other stenotic cardiac valves. J Am Coll Cardiol 15:246–247, 1990.
11. Wallace AG. Pathophysiology of cardiovascular disease. In Smith LH Jr, Thier SO eds. Pathophysiology. The biological principles of disease. Philadelphia, WB Saunders, 1981, p 1200.

Chapter 4

Low-Gradient Aortic Valve Stenosis

Morton J. Kern, MD, and Sanjeev Puri, MD

INTRODUCTION

The management of most patients with aortic stenosis is generally straightforward. Patients with transvalvular gradients ≥50 mm Hg, or a calculated aortic valve area of ≤0.7 cm², and who complain of angina, syncope, or symptoms of congestive heart failure, require surgery [1]. Asymptomatic patients usually do not require surgery, regardless of their hemodynamics [1–5]. An exceptional group consists of those symptomatic patients who have a small transvalvular gradient and a low cardiac output, with a calculated aortic valve area of ≤0.7 cm² [5]. In these patients, substantial clinical doubt exists regarding whether the aortic valve is sufficiently stenotic to account for the symptoms, or whether the patient has only mild aortic valvular disease and the symptom complex is due to a secondary cardiac problem (e.g., myopathic). The doubt regarding low-gradient aortic stenosis is justified, since the Gorlin formula is flow-dependent at a cardiac output of <4 l/min. The calculated valve area by the Gorlin formula is extremely flow-dependent at flows <3 l/min [6,7]. Because cardiac output at time of cardiac catheterization greatly influences the clinical evaluation and subsequent management decisions, the use of valvular resistance and recalculation of the aortic valve area after a pharmacologic stimulation of cardiac output are often required to facilitate the decision regarding surgery in these patients [8].

AORTIC VALVE RESISTANCE

Aortic valve resistance is related to stenosis as follows: Valve resistance >300 dynes.sec.cm^{-5} indicates severe disease, while resistance <250 dynes.sec.cm^{-5} indicates less critical disease, with resistances of 250–300 dynes.sec.cm^{-5} as intermediate. If a severe valvular stenosis exists, a pharmacologic challenge increasing cardiac output to >4.5 l/min should not alter the valve area from the baseline value [9].

CASE REPORT

Consider the findings in a 57-year-old man with increasing dyspnea and fatigue over the last 6 mo. Three years ago he was noted to have mild aortic stenosis (30 mm Hg gradient, valve area >1.8 cm²) and moderately decreased left ventricular function (global hypokinesis, ejection fraction of 48%). Coronary angiography showed normal coronary arteries. Right-heart hemodynamics demonstrated increased right atrial pressure (12 mm Hg), and mildly elevated right ventricular systolic and pulmonary artery pressures (42/12 mm Hg and 42/28 mm Hg, respectively). Cardiac output by thermodilution was 3.1 l/min. Examine the hemodynamics of the simultaneous femoral artery (previously matched to central aortic pressure before crossing the valve) and left ventricular pressures (Fig. 1, top). The rhythm is atrial fibrillation. Aortic pressure varied between 144/70 mm Hg and 120/80 mm Hg, with corresponding left ventricular pressures between 165/35 mm Hg to 130/22 mm Hg. Peak-to-peak and mean aortic valve gradients fluctuated from 25 mm Hg to 15 mm Hg. Valve resistance calculations ranged from 200–175 units. What recommendation should be made?

Before making a decision, dobutamine (10 μg/kg/min for 3 min) was infused and hemodynamic data were reexamined (Fig. 1, bottom, and Fig. 2). During dobutamine infusion, heart rate increased to 120 beats/min. Aortic pressure averaged 118/65 mm Hg, left ventricular pressure averaged 150/22 mm Hg, and cardiac output

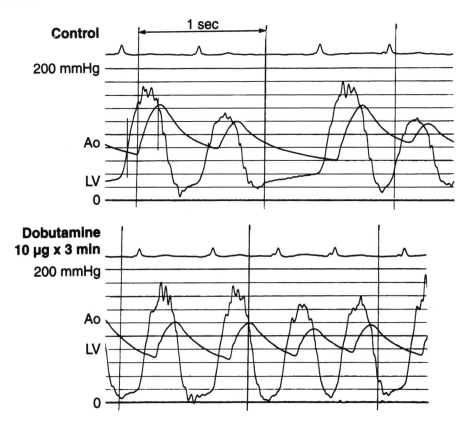

Fig. 1. Aortic (Ao) pressure (femoral artery) and left ventricular (LV) pressure at baseline (control, top) and after dobutamine 10 µg intravenous for 3 min (bottom). Scale, 0–200 mm Hg.

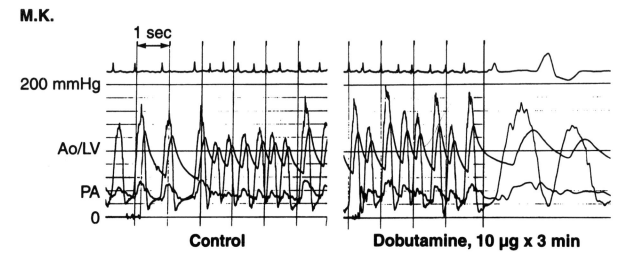

Fig. 2. Aortic (Ao) pressure (femoral artery), left ventricular (LV) pressure, and pulmonary artery (PA) pressure at baseline (control, left) and after dobutamine 10 µg intravenous for 3 min (right). Scale, 0–200 mm Hg.

increased to 4.2 l/min. Valve resistance was calculated at 178 units. Figure 2 shows aortic, left ventricular, and pulmonary artery pressures before (control) and after dobutamine infusion. Note the mild decline in systolic pulmonary artery (Fig. 2) and left ventricular end-diastolic pressures (Fig. 1, bottom). Based on these data (Table I), a recommendation for continued medical therapy without surgery was made.

TABLE I. Hemodynamic Data

	Heart rate (bpm)	Aortic pressure (mm Hg)	Left ventricular pressure (mm Hg)	Mean gradient (mm Hg)	Cardiac output (l/min)	Aortic valve area (cm^2)	Aortic valve resistance*
Baseline	85–100	120/80	135/30	18	3.1	1.0	200
Dobutamine	120	125/78	150/25	28	4.2	1.0	178

*dynes · sec · cm^{-5}

LOW OUTPUT AND VALVE AREAS

Patients with relatively mild aortic-left ventricular pressure gradients appear to have severe stenosis when valve area is calculated in the setting of low cardiac output. However, when cardiac output is increased by vasopressor infusions (e.g., dobutamine) or vasodilator agents (e.g., nitroprusside), a large increase in calculated aortic valve area can be observed [10]. In some cases, increased cardiac output physically produces a greater valve orifice through improvement in leaflet mobility. More commonly, increasing valve area is related to the flow dependence of the Gorlin formula [6].

In severe valvular stenosis, increased cardiac output generally does not increase the calculated valve area, so much that it falls outside the critical range >0.8 cm^2. The constant within the Gorlin formula appears to be variable at different flow rates. Historically, the Gorlin constant was calculated only for the mitral valve where flow dependence is less marked than with aortic stenosis. Flow dependence is not generally a problem in the midrange of cardiac outputs between 4.0–5.0 l/min, or when the aortic stenosis gradient exceeds 50 mm Hg. If improvement in the patient with low-gradient aortic stenosis can be identified from vasodilator therapy during hemodynamic evaluation, chronic vasodilator therapy on an outpatient basis may be highly beneficial.

KEY POINTS

As noted by Carabello [10],

1. Severely stenotic aortic valve areas can be obtained when both cardiac output and pressure gradient are low.
2. Maneuvers which increase cardiac output will almost always increase calculated valve area, except in truly severe aortic stenosis. In mild aortic valve disease, calculated valve area will increase, indicating that the stenosis is only mild and that surgery may not be beneficial.
3. Aortic valve resistance may be a useful adjunct to the Gorlin formula in assessing the severity of aortic stenosis.

ADDRESSING CONFLICTING DATA

In some patients, echocardiographic findings may be in conflict with the hemodynamic data. High systolic flow velocities in the aortic valve region may be due to either valvular or subvalvular obstruction or, at times, may be confused with mitral regurgitation. In most patients with suspected aortic stenosis suggested by transthoracic or transesophageal echo-Doppler, transvalvular pressure gradients using simultaneous peripheral artery and left ventricular pressures are usually confirmatory. However, in patients with aortic stenosis who have small or moderate transvalvular gradients, a more accurate assessment of pressure should be obtained with centrally placed catheters or transseptal technique. In clinical practice, micromanometer-tipped high-fidelity catheters are rarely used, but do provide the most precise pressure-gradient determinations. In patients with peripheral vascular disease, hemodynamic data can be obtained with a single arterial puncture using a long (90-cm) sheath to measure pressures, and a pigtail catheter can be passed into the left ventricle for gradient measurements.

Although the standard has been the transvalvular gradient, Doppler echocardiography remains a highly accurate test for hemodynamic assessment in patients with aortic stenosis. Adele et al. [11] evaluated the significance of transvalvular catheter gradients in patients with aortic stenosis, comparing them to Doppler echocardiographic determinations of the gradient in 18 patients.

The peak instantaneous Doppler pressure gradient was higher with the catheter across the aortic valve compared to that after withdrawal of the aortic catheter, and the mean pressure gradient was also higher before the catheter was withdrawn. The relation of change in Doppler peak instantaneous pressure gradient to the initial peak instantaneous pressure gradient before catheter pullback demonstrated good correspondence and a positive correlation slope, indicating that the catheter *did* contribute to an increased aortic gradient. Although the cross-sectional area of an 8F catheter is 10% that of a valve area measuring 0.5 cm^2, the effective area of a catheter may be greater, depending on its orientation across the narrowed valve orifice. The motion of the catheter may also create turbulence in transvalvular flow, contributing to pressure loss in the poststenotic region. Pliable valves may have an artificial increase in the valve orifice area with such a catheter. Discrepancies between measurements may be due to the catheter placed across the aortic valve, contributing to an already diminished orifice area and leading to overestimation of the transvalvular gradient. Alternatively, the catheter may contribute to prying open one of the cusps, thereby increasing the effective valve area, reducing the transvalvular gradient.

This finding is in agreement with that of Carabello et al. [12], where a >5-mm Hg increase in peripheral arterial pressure could be observed during left ventricular catheter withdrawal in patients with severe aortic stenosis, postulated to be due to catheter cross-sectional area. In most patients, the presence of a catheter across the stenotic aortic valve does result in a significant increase in measured transvalvular pressure gradients, and the catheter effect is proportional to the severity of the underlying aortic stenosis. Systematic over- or underestimation of the actual transvalvular gradient should always be considered.

ASYMPTOMATIC AORTIC STENOSIS

Otto et al. [13] examined the prospective outcomes of patients with valvular aortic stenosis who were asymptomatic. One hundred twenty-three patients with asymptomatic aortic stenosis were followed on an annual basis for 2.5 ± 1.4 yr. Doppler aortic jet velocity increased by 0.32 ± 0.34 m/sec/yr, with a mean gradient increase of 7 ± 7 mm Hg/yr and a valve area decrease of 0.12 ± 0.19 cm^2/yr. At 3-yr follow-up, survival was $62 \pm 8\%$, and $26 \pm 10\%$ at 5-yr follow-up. Predictors of outcome included jet velocity, mean gradient, valve area, and rate of increase in jet velocity, but not age, gender, or etiology of aortic stenosis. The authors concluded that in asymptomatic patients with aortic stenosis, the rate of hemodynamic progression and clinical outcome are predicted by jet velocity, rate of change in jet velocity, and functional status of the patient. Carabello [4,10] suggested that asymptomatic patients can be safely followed until symptoms or changes in hemodynamics occur.

The natural history of aortic stenosis in the modern era has been examined in only a limited number of reports and appears to be related to the rapid development of symptoms which follow with sudden death in short periods of time [3,14]. In the absence of extracardiac comorbidity and coronary artery disease, aortic valve replacement has a 2–3% operative mortality, with an 85% age-corrected 10-yr survival. The timing of aortic valve replacement, therefore, is predicated on symptoms. In patients without cardiac symptoms, survival with medical therapy alone is excellent [1,3,10,14]. Because the risk of

operative death and prosthetic valve-related complications is inherent in the procedure, the risk-benefit ratio is not favorable to the asymptomatic patient.

The study of Otto et al. [13] reinforces the concept that no single discrete valve area defining the critical valve exists, but that this area varies from patient to patient depending on cardiac output and problems of the calculation of valve area. Patients may become symptomatic in the range of 0.6–0.8 cm^2, whereas asymptomatic patients may reside comfortably with valve areas of 0.8–1.0 cm^2. In general, patients with valve areas >1.0 cm^2 are often symptomatic due to other noncardiac sources, especially if the mean transvalvular gradient is <30 mm Hg.

CONCLUSIONS

Before accepting hemodynamic data indicating the critical severity of aortic stenosis in individuals with left ventricular dysfunction and low cardiac output, evaluation of valve function with inotropic agents or vasodilators [6] and their effect on aortic valve area and resistance should be considered.

ACKNOWLEDGMENTS

The author thanks the J.G. Mudd Cardiac Catheterization Laboratory Team for technical support, and Donna Sander for manuscript preparation.

REFERENCES

1. Ross J Jr, Braunwald E: Aortic stenosis. Circulation [supp 1] 38:61–67, 1968.
2. Connolly HM, Oh JK, Orszulak TA, Osborn SL, Roger VL, Hodge DO, Bailey KR, Seward JB, Tajik AJ: Aortic valve replacement for aortic stenosis with severe left ventricular dysfunction: Prognostic indicators. Circulation 95:2395–2400, 1997.
3. Kelly TA, Rothbart RM, Cooper CM, Kaiser DL, Smucker ML, Gibson RS: Comparison of outcome of asymptomatic to symptomatic patients older than 20 years of age with valvular aortic stenosis. Am J Cardiol 61:123–130, 1988.
4. Carabello BA: Timing of valve replacement in aortic stenosis: Moving closer to perfection. Circulation 95:2241–2243, 1997.
5. Carabello BA: Advances in hemodynamic assessment of stenotic cardiac valves. J Am Coll Cardiol 10:912–919, 1987.
6. Cannon JD Jr, Zile MR, Crawford FA Jr, Carabello BA: Aortic valve resistance as an adjunct to the Gorlin formula in assessing the severity of aortic stenosis in symptomatic patients. J Am Coll Cardiol 20:1517–1523, 1992.
7. Cannon SR, Richards KL, Crawford M: Hydraulic estimation of stenotic orifice area: A correction of the Gorlin formula. Circulation 71:1170–1178, 1989.
8. Ford LE, Feldman T, Chiu YC, Carroll JD: Hemodynamic resistance as a measure of functional impairment in aortic valvular stenosis. Circ Res 66:1–7, 1990.

9. Kern MJ, Deligonul U, Donohue T, Caracciolo E, Feldman T: Hemodynamic data. In Kern MJ (ed): "The Cardiac Catheterization Handbook." St. Louis: Mosby-Year Book, 1995, pp 108–207.

10. Carabello BA: Indications for valve surgery in asymptomatic patients with aortic and mitral stenosis. Chest 108:1678–1682, 1995.

11. Adele C, Vaitkus PT, Tischler MD: Evaluation of the significance of a transvalvular catheter on aortic valve gradient in aortic stenosis: A direct hemodynamic and Doppler echocardiographic study. Am J Cardiol 79:513–516, 1997.

12. Carabello BA, Barry WH, Grossman W: Changes in arterial pressure during left heart pullback in patients with aortic stenosis: A sign of severe aortic stenosis. Am J Cardiol 44:424–427, 1979.

13. Otto CM, Burwash IG, Legget ME, Munt BI, Fujioka M, Healy NL, Kraft CD, Miyake-Hull CY, Schwaeggier RG: Prospective study of asymptomatic valvular aortic stenosis: Clinical, echocardiographic, and exercise predictors of outcome. Circulation 95:2262–2270, 1997.

14. Pellika PA, Nishimura RA, Bailey KR, Tajik AJ: The natural history of adults with asymptomatic, hemodynamically significant aortic stenosis. J Am Coll Cardiol 15:1012–1017, 1990.

Chapter 5

Aortic Regurgitation

Morton J. Kern, MD, and Frank V. Aguirre, MD

INTRODUCTION

Aortic regurgitation is one of the most common valvular lesions studied in the cardiac catheterization laboratory. Patients with aortic regurgitation may present under dramatically different circumstances with, at times, confusing clinical findings and symptoms [1–3]. Depending on the primary cause and extent of disease of the aortic valve leaflets and/or aortic root, some patients may require only valve replacement or undergo a combined procedure replacing both the aortic root and valve. An overview of the major mechanisms and etiologies of aortic regurgitation is provided on Table I.

Aortic root disease has been steadily increasing over decades past with the use of combined echocardiographic and hemodynamic assessment of nearly all patients becoming the current standard of diagnosis [4]. The echocardiographic determination of the severity of aortic regurgitation is equal to and, at times, even more sensitive than angiographic and hemodynamic characteristics used for daily clinical decisions [5]. The influence of aortic regurgitation on the calculation of aortic valve area in patients with combined aortic stenosis is controversial. This rounds will illustrate several hemodynamic fingerprints as clues in the various clinical presentations and determinations of the severity of the regurgitant aortic valve.

Three Patients With a Diastolic Murmur

Patient A is a 63-yr-old man with symptoms of left ventricular failure and a loud decrescendo aortic diastolic murmur. Patient B is a 78-yr-old woman with a brief diastolic murmur at the left sternal border and mild fatigue. Patient C is a 48-yr-old man with fever, a diastolic murmur and dyspnea at rest. Femoral artery and left ventricular pressures were obtained in all 3 patients (Figs. 1–3, not in order of patients described) through fluid-filled systems using an 8F sheath and 7F pigtail catheter. Compare the pressure tracings and address the following: Which tracing is associated with the most decompensated patient? Which is most compensated? Which has the longest murmur? Which has the loudest and softest? Which tracing likely has the greatest degree of associated angiographic aortic insufficiency and which has the least? And finally, in which tracing would the patient most likely have peripheral vascular disease?

Examine Figure 1. The femoral arterial pressure is 140/45 mm Hg with the left ventricular pressure 118/39 mm Hg. The pulse pressure is nearly 100 mm Hg (normally 40 mm Hg) and the end-diastolic difference between aortic diastolic and left ventricular pressure is about 5–6 mm Hg (normally about 70 mm Hg [normally 80-10 mm Hg]). The wide pulse pressure, rapidly rising slope and elevation of left ventricular diastolic pressure and near end-diastolic equilibration between aortic and left ventricular pressures with the left sternal border diastolic murmur as classic findings for aortic insufficiency. The marked elevation of end-diastolic pressure (40 mm Hg) suggests a poorly compensated left ventricle and probably recent acute onset of aortic regurgitation associated with severe symptoms.

Examine Figure 2. The femoral artery pressure tracing also demonstrates a widened pulse pressure (122-40 mm Hg = 83 mm Hg), but with less approximation of the aortic-ventricular pressures (40-24 = 16 mm Hg) than in Figure 1. The left ventricular diastolic pressure slope also exhibits a more gradual increase over the course of diastole with a less prominent A wave before an end-diastolic pressure of only 24 mm Hg. The hemodynamics demonstrated in this patient are also compatible with

TABLE I. Mechanisms and Etiologies of Aortic Regurgitation

Mechanism	Etiology
Cusp abnormality or perforation	Endocarditis
	Rheumatic or rheumatoid disease
	Ankylosing spondylitis
Aortic root dilatation with malcoaptation of aortic cusps	Ankylosing spondylitis
	Aortitis
	Rheumatoid disease
	Syphilis
	Familial, idiopathic or Ehlers-Danlos, Pseudoxanthomas elasticum
Lack of commissural support with malcoaptation of aortic cusps	Tetralogy of Fallot
	Ventricular septal defect
	Aortic dissection
	Aortitis
	Trauma

severe aortic regurgitation, but more compensated than in Figure 1 with a lower left ventricular end-diastolic pressure and slower left ventricular diastolic pressure rise. One other major difference is the systolic gradient. Note the higher left ventricular systolic pressure (138 mm Hg) compared to aortic pressure (122 mm Hg). This tracing suggests combined mild aortic stenosis and moderate to severe regurgitation.

Finally, consider Figure 3. Aortic pressure is 180/48 mm Hg with left ventricular pressure 180/20 mm Hg. The pulse pressure is 132 mm Hg with a 28 mm Hg difference between aortic and left ventricular end-diastolic pressures. Note the exact matching of femoral artery and left ventricular systolic pressures, flat left ventricular diastolic pressure slope and prominent early A wave. From this tracing one might conclude that if aortic regurgitation was present at all, it would be hemodynamically compensated, probably chronic and not associated with significant left ventricular dysfunction. A brief diastolic murmur and symptoms of fatigue due to hypertension might be a logical association. The prominent A wave, which is completed before left ventricular ejection, is a clue to first degree AV block which is generally of no clinical significance.

Peripheral Pressure Amplification in Aortic Regurgitation

Before matching the pressure tracings to the three patients, recall that the common clinical manifestations of severe isolated aortic regurgitation, which one or more of our patients may have demonstrated, include the striking increase in pulse pressure with an accelerated velocity of ventricular ejection which may cause head bobbing with each heart beat (DeMusset's sign), a collapsing type pulse with abrupt distension and quick collapse (Corigan's pulse), booming systolic and diastolic sounds over the femoral artery (Tralp's sign) or systolic pulsations of the uvula (Müller's sign). A systolic murmur heard over the femoral artery with proximal compression and diastolic murmur when the compression is released (Duroziez's sign), as well as capillary pulsations (Quincke's pulse) can be detected in some patients. These signs are the result of the hyperdynamic state of the arterial pressure wave which is manifested more in the peripheral circulation rather than the proximal larger vessels, producing findings of peripheral arterial pressure amplification hemodynamically observed as the overshoot in femoral artery sheath pressure [6].

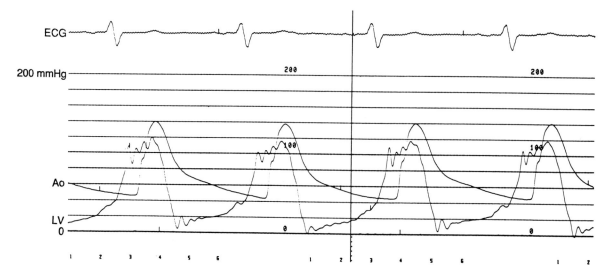

Fig. 1. Left ventricular (LV) and aortic (Ao) pressures using an 8 French femoral sheath and 7 French pigtail catheter with fluid-filled transducers in a patient with a diastolic murmur. See text for details.

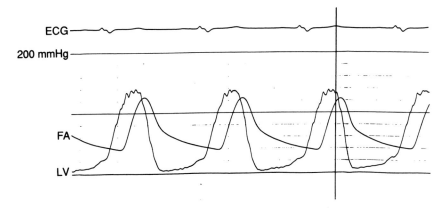

Fig. 2. Femoral artery (FA) and left ventricular (LV) pressures in a patient with systolic and diastolic murmurs. See text for details.

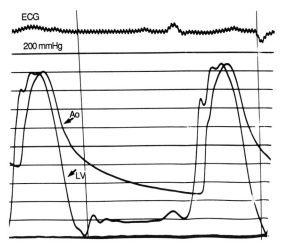

Fig. 3. Hemodynamics in a patient with hypertension. LV = left ventricular pressure; Ao = aortic pressure. See text for details.

Peripheral arterial systolic pressure amplification may occur in any patient with high left ventricular ejection velocities. In aortic regurgitation, peak femoral artery systolic pressure may exceed central aortic pressure by 20 mm Hg to 50 mm Hg. The mechanisms of the arterial pressure amplification has been previously described as the result of summation of pressure wave reflections returning from smaller peripheral arteries [6]. The use of central aortic pressure measurement for accurate computation of the hemodynamic findings, especially in combined aortic regurgitation and stenosis, is optimal. The femoral arterial pressure may be used if previously matched to central aortic pressure as shown on Figure 4A. Peripheral (femoral) pressure shows the normal delay in pressure upstroke with a 15 mm Hg pressure overshoot compared to central aortic pressure (note the well defined dicrotic notch and anacrotic shoulder of the central pressure). These pressures are considered matched and the overshoot can be excluded from calculations af-

ter the central catheter is positioned in the left ventricle (Fig. 4B,4C). Central aortic pressure in patients with peripheral vascular disease or a damped pressure in the femoral sheath will equal or exceed the pressure measured in the femoral artery. Aortic stenosis will result in a higher left ventricular systolic compared to femoral pressure as in Figure 2.

Returning to the descriptions of the pressure waveforms on Figures 1–3, match the tracings with the patients A, B, and C. Figure 1 was obtained in patient C with recent acute bacterial endocarditis and decompensated congestive heart failure from severe aortic insufficiency. This patient had the longest and loudest murmur and the most severe degree of angiographic aortic regurgitation. Figure 2 was obtained in patient A with moderately severe aortic insufficiency, mild aortic stenosis and compensated congestive heart failure. The matching of central aortic and femoral pressures would permit discrimination between the stenotic gradient and reduced femoral arterial pressure due to peripheral vascular disease. Figure 3 was obtained in patient B with hypertension, minimal aortic insufficiency (the least by angiography) and no signs of congestive heart failure. This tracing is also consistent with bradycardia alone, which can produce an exaggerated pulse pressure, as well as a diastolic pressure plateau.

Pathophysiology of Aortic Regurgitation

The pathophysiology of aortic regurgitation hinges on complete systolic left ventricular emptying with an increase in left ventricular end-diastolic volume providing the major hemodynamic compensatory mechanism [7]. To better appreciate the flow dynamics of aortic valvular disease, combined Doppler echocardiographic and hemodynamic data were obtained in a 72-yr-old woman with mixed aortic stenosis and regurgitation (Fig. 5). Simultaneous femoral artery and left ventricular pres-

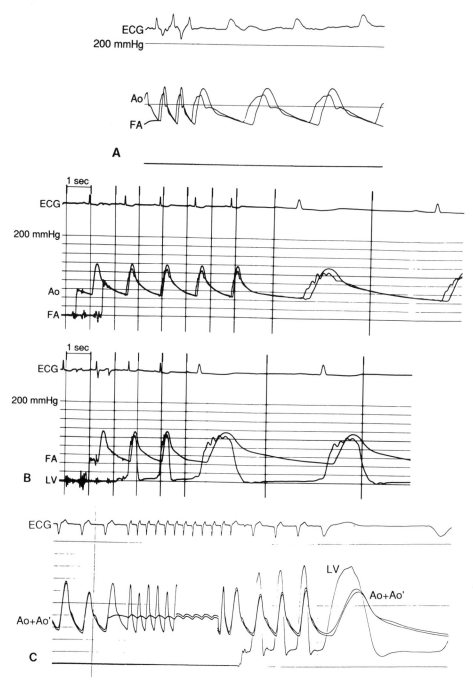

Fig. 4A: Central aortic (Ao) and femoral artery (FA) pressures in a normal subject. A 15 mm Hg femoral pressure overshoot is acceptable. See text for details.

Fig. 4B: Central aortic (Ao) and peripheral (FA) pressures are matched before recording left ventricular (LV)-aortic pressures. See text for details.

Fig. 4C: Systemic hemodynamics obtained with 2 catheters, one in the central aortic position (Ao) and a second through the arterial sheath (Ao'). These pressures match with no signs of peripheral pressure amplification. The left ventricular (LV) pressure was obtained via a transseptal catheter. See text for details.

sures were patched into the Doppler echocardiographic recorder. Flow velocity signals were recorded at the left ventricular outflow tract from the suprasternal notch. Aortic pressure is 130/50 mm Hg and left ventricular pressure 190/40 mm Hg. A significant 50 mm Hg aortic gradient remains when a 10 mm Hg femoral pressure overshoot (not shown) is considered. High systolic aortic flow (area marked by **) with peak velocities of 3.5m/

0.2 sec

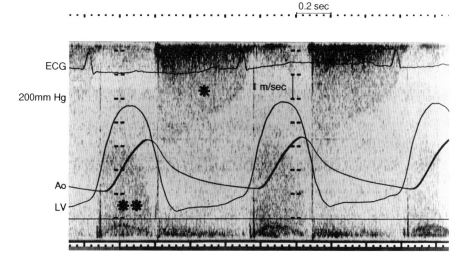

Fig. 5. Combined echo-Doppler and hemodynamic study in a patient with mixed aortic valve disease. Aortic (Ao) and left ventricular (LV) pressures measured as in figure 1. Flow velocities were obtained with continuous mode Doppler from the left ven- **tricular outflow tract. Scale marks for Doppler are 1m/second. Scale marks for pressure are 40 mm Hg per division. (*) diastolic velocity integral; (**) systolic velocity intregral. See text for details.**

sec yielding a pressure gradient from Doppler calculations of 49 mm Hg [5], correspond to the systolic aortic-left ventricular gradient. Equally striking are the continuous diastolic flow velocities (area marked by *) corresponding to the left ventricular-aortic diastolic gradient. The velocity slope (from the initial elevated peak diastolic velocity of 4m/sec which rapidly tapers to 1.5m/sec at end-diastole) parallels the severity of the left ventricular-aortic gradient. The more rapid (>2m/sec) the downslope of the diastolic flow velocity, the more severe the aortic regurgitation [4].

Severe aortic regurgitation can occur with normal effective forward flow and a normal ejection fraction coupled with elevated end-diastolic pressure and volume. With time, left ventricular dilation increases. The left ventricular systolic tension required to maintain the same pressure (or stress) also increases as determined by Laplace's law. The clinical course is then dependent on compensated left ventricular wall stress with replication of sarcomeres in series, stretching of myocardial fibers and wall thickening sufficient to maintain systolic wall stress at a normal level [2,7]. The ventricular thickness to cavity ratio remains normal (e.g., eccentric hypertropy). This process occurs in distinction to that developing in aortic stenosis in which replication of myocardial sarcomeres occurs in parallel with an increased ratio of wall thickness to cavity radius (e.g., concentric hypertrophy). Left ventricular mass in patients with aortic regurgitation is usually greatly elevated, exceeding values reported in isolated aortic stenosis [7].

The clinical course of aortic regurgitation involves left ventricular deterioration when the left ventricular end-

diastolic volume increases without further elevation of left ventricular ejection volume. The left ventricular end-diastolic radius to wall thickness ratio increases with increasing systolic tension and often with afterload mismatch producing a decline in ejection fraction for any additional level of ventricular stress. Ultimately, left ventricular ejection fraction and forward stroke volume diminish producing congestive symptomatology. The advance stages of decompensation of aortic regurgitation involve elevation of left atrial, pulmonary artery wedge, pulmonary arterial, right ventricular, and right atrial pressures with reduction of cardiac output. A proposed physiologic scheme for chronic aortic regurgitation as conceptualized by Borow and Marcus [7] is depicted on Figure 6.

Acute Aortic Regurgitation

Acute aortic regurgitation exposes the unconditioned left ventricle to large diastolic volumes. The immediate and rapid increase in diastolic pressure in the left ventricle with or without a wide aortic pulse pressure is one of several findings which distinguishes acute from chronic aortic regurgitation (see Table II). Early closure of the mitral valve with rapid left ventricular filling limits the increase in pulmonary capillary wedge pressure substantially below left ventricular end-diastolic pressure [8]. The hemodynamic tracings obtained during aortic balloon valvuloplasty, at times, demonstrate the immediate and dramatic results of acute aortic regurgitation [9]. A 78-yr-old woman with critical aortic stenosis required urgent abdominal surgery for a complication of carci-

AORTIC REGURGITATION

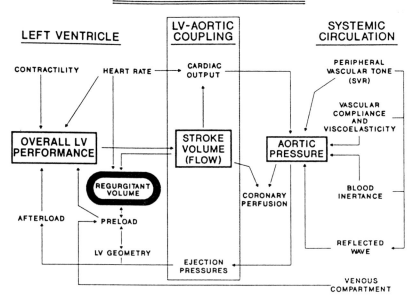

Fig. 6. Physiologic scheme for chronic aortic regurgitation. LV = left ventricle; SVR = systemic vascular resistance. With permission from Borow KM, Marcus RH: Aortic regurgitation: The need for an integrated physiologic approach. J Am Coll Cardiol 17:898–900, 1991.

TABLE II. Major Hemodynamic Features of Severe Aortic Regurgitation

	Acute	Chronic[a]
Left ventricular (LV) compliance	Not increased	Increased
Regurgitant volume	Increased	Increased
LV end-diastolic pressure	Markedly increased	May be normal
LV ejection velocity (dp/dt)	Not significantly increased	Markedly increased
Aortic systolic pressure	Not increased	Increased
Aortic diastolic pressure	Normal to decreased	Markedly decreased
Systemic arterial pulse pressure	Slightly to moderately increased	Markedly increased
Ejection fraction	Not increased	Increased
Effective stroke volume	Decreased	Normal
Effective cardiac output	Decreased	Normal
Heart rate	Increased	Normal
Peripheral vascular resistance	Increased	Not increased

[a]Without left ventricular failure.
With permission from Morganroth J et al. Acute severe aortic regurgitation: Pathophysiology, clinical recognition, and management. Ann Intern Med 1977;87:223–232.

noma of the colon. Aortic valvuloplasty with a single 23mm balloon was performed. The left ventricular and aortic pressures before and after valvuloplasty (Fig. 7) demonstrated a systolic aortic-left ventricular gradient of 90 mm Hg before balloon inflation with left ventricular end-diastolic pressure of 22 mm Hg. Aortic pressure was 140/65 mm Hg with the classic features of aortic stenosis and no aortic regurgitation. Balloon valvuloplasty produced a significant reduction in the stenotic gradient, but also severe acute aortic regurgitation due to an annular tear. Left ventricular pressure was now 150/45 mm Hg with aortic pressure of 125/45 mm Hg. Note the reduced systolic gradient area but the marked increase in minimal

(from 8 to 16 mm Hg) and end-diastolic (40 mm Hg) left ventricular pressure, and rapid diastolic pressure slope increase, equilibrating by mid diastole with aortic pressure. The aortic pulse pressure has increased slightly (from 75 to 80 mm Hg). The complications of aortic valvuloplasty have also been presented in an earlier rounds [9].

Transient Acute Aortic Regurgitation

The hemodynamics of acute aortic insufficiency can also be observed temporarily if the aortic valve leaflets (or a prosthetic valve occluder) are kept open by a catheter or guidewire. With mechanical prosthetic valves,

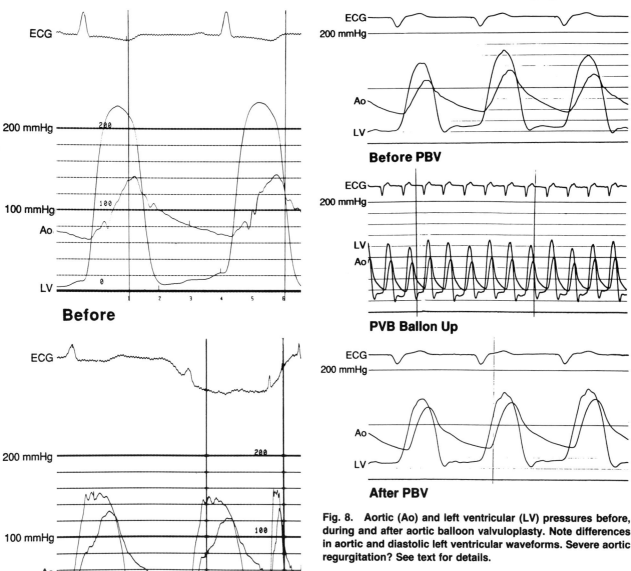

Before

After

Before PBV

PVB Ballon Up

After PBV

Fig. 7. Aortic (Ao) and left ventricular (LV) pressures before and after aortic balloon valvuloplasty. Note differences in diastolic left ventricular waveforms. Severe aortic regurgitation? See text for details.

Fig. 8. Aortic (Ao) and left ventricular (LV) pressures before, during and after aortic balloon valvuloplasty. Note differences in aortic and diastolic left ventricular waveforms. Severe aortic regurgitation? See text for details.

retrograde left ventricular catheterization may force ball valve or disk occluder to remain partially open producing general mild aortic regurgitation, but this technique has been used to estimate systolic aortic valve gradients. The practice of retrograde crossing a disk valve with a catheter should be discouraged since severe aortic regurgitation or death has been reported when the catheter becomes entrapped in the minor valve orifice [10,11].

During aortic valvuloplasty, artificial and transient aortic regurgitation may occur with the balloon catheter or extra-stiff guidewire propping the calcified valve leaflets open. This phenomenon is illustrated on figure 8. Before percutaneous balloon valvuloplasty (PBV), aortic stenosis (0.6cm^2 valve area) with left ventricular dysfunction (left ventricular end-diastolic pressure 35 mm Hg) is associated with slow aortic upstroke and normal pulse pressure. With the balloon catheter inflated, both left ventricular and aortic systolic pressures are reduced, but aortic pulse pressure widens with near end-diastolic aortic-left ventricular pressure equilibration. These waveform abnormalities also persisted with only the guidewire across the valve, but were eliminated on guidewire removal (Fig. 8, lower panel).

Angiographic Determination of Aortic Regurgitation

Despite good quantitation by echocardiography of the amount of regurgitant flow, angiographic regurgitation, at times, differs and is dependent on a variety of factors [12–14]. In general, the severity of the angiographic aortic regurgitation correlates with the regurgitant volume index [12]. However, only the mean values of the mild and moderate (1+ and 2+) groups can be distinguished from the severe (3+ and 4+). Distinction between minimal and mild (1+ and 2+) and moderate and severe (3+ and 4+) was not possible [10]. The qualitative angiographic system in grading a particular degree of regurgitation is influenced by the volume of the chamber into which the contrast is injected, volume of chamber that receives regurgitant flow (aorta), pressure gradients across regurgitant valves, heart rate, cardiac output, angiographic injector rates, as well as factors related to subjective angiographic image interpretation.

Because no practical way exists to measure regurgitant volume directly, indirect measurements are used in the cardiac catheterization laboratory. Specialized studies involving flow velocity transducers and aortic cross-sectional area are not practical for routine clinical purposes. Use of quantitative angiography to measure the total strike volume and net forward stroke volume computed by cardiac output (either by the Fick or indicator dilution methods) yield the regurgitant volume calculated as the difference between stroke volume by angiography and stroke volume by cardiac output. Dividing the regurgitant volume by the body surface area produces the regurgitant volume index (in milliliters/minute/m^2). Regurgitant volume indexes of <700ml/min/m^2 are mild, 700–1700ml/min/m^2 moderate and 1700–3000ml/min/m^2 severe, >3000ml/min/m^2 represents very severe valvular insufficiency. The regurgitant fraction is the regurgitant volume divided by the stroke volume obtained by angiography as a percent (0–20% mild, 20–40% moderate, 40–60% moderately severe and >60% severe insufficiency). Regurgitant fraction calculations are not widely used in routine clinical studies because of the complexity of making accurate measurements. Sources of error include independent and accurate determination of cardiac output and stroke volume simultaneously. Left ventricular volume is dependent on optimal radiographic image, chamber opacification, chamber border identification, normal geometry and stable cardiac cycle with an accurate correction for image magnification and validation within the laboratory obtaining the ventriculogram. Many of these above conditions are not satisfactory in clinical laboratories and thus the computation of regurgitant volume and regurgitation fraction remains elusive.

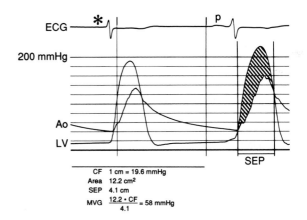

Fig. 9. **Factors used in computing aortic valve area. CF= correction factor for pressure scale; Shaded area = systolic gradient; SEP = systolic ejection period; MVG = mean valve gradient. How does one compensate for mild aortic regurgitation? See text for details. (Reproduced from MJ Kern, ed., "The Cardiac Catheterization Handbook," with permission of the publisher.)**

Calculation of Aortic Valve Area in Patients With Aortic Regurgitation

The Gorlin formula for aortic valve area [15], systolic flow/$\sqrt{}$ gradient, uses the systolic ejection period (SEP) to obtain mean valve gradient (MVG, Fig. 9) without a correction factor for aortic or mitral regurgitation. However, since aortic regurgitation occurs only in diastole, how should we account for the regurgitant lesion in aortic stenosis? Aortic regurgitation increases left-sided forward flow which is underestimated by both Fick and Thermodilution cardiac output methods. A recent survey (by MJK) of knowledgeable catheterization physicians provides no consensus on this problem. In our laboratory, aortic valve area is computed in the traditional manner and reported as the worst case with liberalization of valve area 20% for each degree of angiographic regurgitation.

CONCLUSIONS

The hemodynamics of aortic regurgitation are related to the chronicity and severity of the regurgitant volume. Characteristic waveforms of aortic regurgitation can be used to differentiate acute from chronic aortic regurgitation in the appropriate clinical settings. Currently, there is no consensus on how best to report aortic valve area in patients with mixed valvular lesions.

ACKNOWLEDGMENTS

The authors thank the J.G. Mudd Cardiac Catheterization Laboratory team and Donna Sander for manuscript preparation.

REFERENCES

1. Morganroth J, Perloff JK, Zeldis SM, Dunkman WB: Acute severe aortic regurgitation: Pathophysiology, clinical recognition, and management. Ann Intern Med 87:223–232, 1977.
2. Gaasch WH, Andrias CW, Levine HJ: Chronic aortic regurgitation: the effect of aortic valve replacement on left ventricular volume, mass and function. Circulation 58:825–836, 1978.
3. Abdulla AM, Frank MJ, Erdin RA Jr, Canedo MI: Clinical significance and hemodynamic correlates of the third heart sound gallop in aortic regurgitation: A guide to optimal timing of cardiac catheterization. Circulation 64:464–471, 1981.
4. Labovitz AJ, Ferrara RP, Kern MJ, Bryg RJ, Mrosek DG, Williams DA: Quantitative evaluation of aortic insufficiency by continuous wave Doppler echocardiography. J Am Coll Cardiol 8:1341–1347, 1986.
5. Hatle L, Angelsen B: "Doppler Ultrasound in Cardiology: Physical Principles and Clinical Applications. Philadelphia: Lea & Febiger, 188–205, 1985.
6. Nichols WW, O'Rourke MF: "McDonald's Blood Flow in Arteries: Theoretical, Experimental and Clinical Principles." 3rd edition. Philadelphia: Lea & Febiger, 421–432, 1990.
7. Borow KM, Marcus RH: Aortic regurgitation: The need for an integrated physiologic approach. J Am Coll Cardiol 17:898–900, 1991.
8. Mann T, McLaurin LP, Grossman W, Craige E: Assessing the hemodynamic severity of acute aortic regurgitation due to infective endocarditis. N Engl J Med 293:108, 1975.
9. Deligonul U, Kern MJ: Hemodynamic rounds: Interpretation of cardiac pathophysiology from pressure waveform analysis: Percutaneous balloon valvuloplasty. Cathet Cardiovasc Diagn, in press, 1991.
10. Rigaud M et al.: Retrograde catheterization of left ventricle through mechanical aortic prostheses. Eur Heart J 8:689, 1987.
11. Kober G, Hilgermann R: Catheter entrapment in a Bjork-Shiley prosthesis in aortic position. Cathet Cardiovasc Diagn 13:262, 1987.
12. Croft CH, Lipscomb K, Mathis K, et al.: Limitations of qualitative grading in aortic or mitral regurgitation. Am J Cardiol 53:1593–1598, 1984.
13. Sandler H, Dodge HT, Hay RE, Rackley CE: Quantitation of valvular insufficiency in man by angiocardiography. Am Heart J 65:501–513, 1963.
14. Bolger AF, Eigler NL, Maurer G: Quantifying valvular regurgitation: limitations and inherent assumptions of Doppler techniques. Circulation 78:1316–1318, 1988.
15. Gorlin R, Gorlin SG: Hydraulic formula for calculation of stenotic mitral valve, other cardiac valves, and central circulatory shunts. Am Heart J 41:1–29, 1951.

Chapter 6

Abnormal Hemodynamics After Prosthetic Aortic Root Reconstruction: Aortic Stenosis or Insufficiency?

Morton J. Kern, MD, Frank V. Aguirre, MD, and Marco Guerrero, MD

INTRODUCTION

The hemodynamics associated with aortic root disease mostly involves induction of severe valvular incompetence. Replacement of the aortic root often cures the abnormality at hand. The restored hemodynamics after treating aortic insufficiency with prosthetic aortic root replacement may deteriorate over time and present with unusual findings. We present the case of a patient who developed a new onset of aortic stenosis and insufficiency after aortic root replacement.

CASE REPORT

A 38-year-old man had proximal aortic dissection and underwent aortic repair in January 1997. There was no prior history of aortic valvular disease, connective tissue disease, or trauma before the surgery. In the postoperative recovery he had been symptom-free with rare episodes of palpitations but denied dyspnea on exertion or chest discomfort. The aortic root was replaced with a #32 replacement Dacron graft. As part of routine follow-up 6 months after surgery, echocardiography demonstrated marked aortic dilatation with a question of aortic pseudoaneurysm and severe aortic insufficiency. A chest CT scan demonstrated possible aortic root aneurysm. The patient was asymptomatic.

The blood pressure was 120/60 mm Hg in both arms, pulse 60/min, respirations 14/min. There was 6–7 cm of jugular venous distension. There were no carotid bruits. The heart sounds (both S_1 and S_2) were normal. There was a thrill along the left sternal border with a III/VI mid-peaking holosystolic murmur and a III/VI early to mid-diastolic murmur along the left sternal border. The peripheral pulses were bounding and bilaterally symmetric. There was no peripheral edema or peripheral arterial bruits. The electrocardiogram showed a normal sinus rhythm with non-specific intraventricular conduction defect. Cardiac catheterization was performed.

The right heart hemodynamics showed mildly elevated right atrial pressure with a mean of 8 mm Hg, a right ventricular pressure of 50/10 mm Hg, pulmonary artery pressure of 50/25 mm Hg, a mean pulmonary capillary wedge pressure of 28 mm Hg (Fig. 1). The "A" and "V" waves are well demarcated on both the right atrial and pulmonary capillary wedge pressures. Of interest, this tracing illustrates the classically described relationship that the "A" wave is greater in the right (atrial) compared to the pulmonary capillary wedge pressure, where the "V" wave is usually predominant.

The left ventricular and aortic pressures initially demonstrated aortic stenosis with an aortic pressure of 130/60 mm Hg and a left ventricular pressure of 150/40 mm Hg (Fig. 2). The pulse pressure is 70 mm Hg. The high LVEDP and the rapid rise of the left ventricular end-diastolic pressure suggested only moderately decompensated aortic insufficiency.

However, during pullback of the left ventricular catheter to the aorta, the presumed aortic valve stenosis was, in reality, a supravalvular narrowing. The pressure gradient between the left ventricular and femoral artery persisted when the catheter was positioned in the central aorta (Fig. 2, middle panel). On further retraction of the pigtail catheter from the central aortic position to the lower abdominal aorta, the gradient disappeared and was

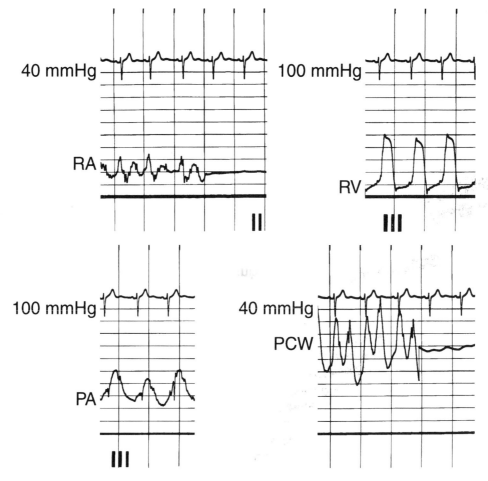

Fig. 1. Right heart hemodynamics showing the right atrial (RA), right ventricular (RV), pulmonary artery (PA), and pulmonary capillary wedge (PCW) pressures. The RA and PCW pressures are on a 0–40 mm Hg scale. The RV and PA pressures are on a 0–100 mm Hg scale. Note the well-defined "A" and "V" waves in the RA and PCW pressure tracings.

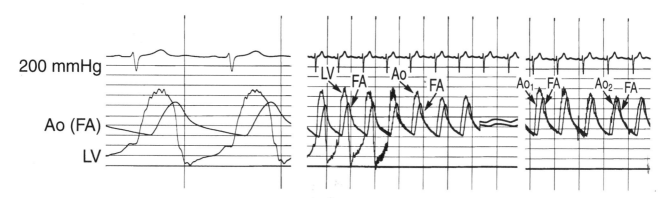

Fig. 2. Left panel: Simultaneous femoral artery (FA) and left ventricular (LV) pressure (0–200 mm Hg scale). Middle panel: Pseudoaortic stenosis on pullback of the left ventricular pressure to the central aortic position. The transprosthetic gradient can be detected, and on further pullback (far right panel) the prosthetic graft gradient (Ao_1-FA) disappears as the pigtail catheter is positioned in the lower abdominal aorta (Ao_2-FA).

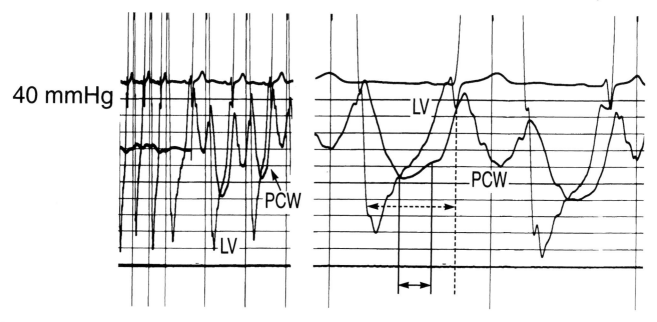

Fig. 3. Simultaneous left ventricular (LV) and pulmonary capillary wedge (PCW) pressures (0–40 mm Hg scale). The PCW pressure falls beneath the LV pressure at the first third of the diastolic period. It is more common to have the left ventricular/pulmonary capillary wedge crossover point occur after the mid-point of the diastolic period. This configuration suggests premature closure of the mitral valve, which was confirmed by two-dimensional echocardiography.

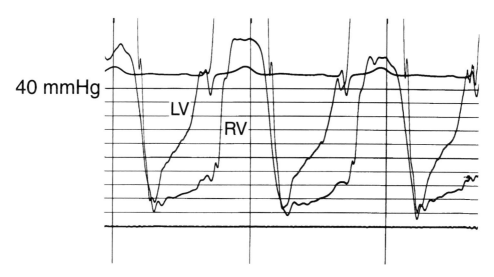

Fig. 4. Simultaneous left (LV) and right ventricular (RV) pressure tracings (0–40 mm Hg scale) demonstrating rapid filling of the left ventricle compared to the right ventricle and the reduced compliance of the left ventricular pressure with the large "A" wave having an end-diastolic pressure of approximately 40 mm Hg.

appreciated only in the grafted region of the prosthetic conduit (Fig. 2, right panel). There was no mitral valve gradient and no significant mitral regurgitation. When comparing the pulmonary capillary wedge pressure to left ventricular pressure (Fig. 3), it can be appreciated that the pressure crossover between the pulmonary capillary

wedge and the left ventricular diastolic pressure occurs in the first one-third of diastole, consistent with premature closure of the mitral valve associated with severe aortic insufficiency.

To assess the compliance differences between the left and right ventricles, a simultaneous measurement of left

LAO

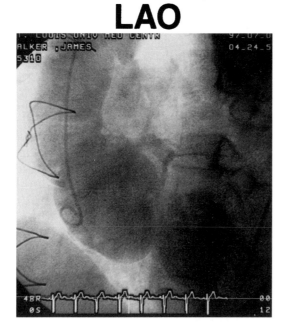

RAO

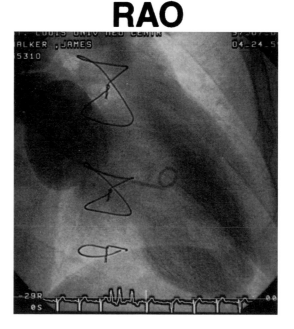

Fig. 5. Cineangiographic frames of aortography performed in the left anterior oblique (LAO, left panel) and left ventriculography performed in the right anterior oblique (RAO, right panel) projection. There is marked dilatation of the aortic root with an indentation noted above the globular configuration of the aneurysm.

and right ventricular pressures was made (Fig. 4) demonstrating a marked increase in the end-diastolic pressure slope of the left ventricle relative to that of the right ventricle. The conduction delay in the excitation and relaxation timing of ventricular contraction can also be appreciated by the position of the right ventricular pressure beneath the left ventricular pressure curve.

On completion of the hemodynamics, left ventriculography and aortography were performed in the right and left anterior oblique projections, respectively. The left ventricle had mild anterior hypokinesis with an ejection fraction of 59%. There was no mitral regurgitation. The unusual configuration and dilated aortic root can be appreciated from the ventriculogram (Fig. 5). Aortography (Fig. 5, left panel) also demonstrated the marked enlargement of the aortic root and an aneurysmal formation near the origin of the coronary ostia. A kink and linear lucency at the insertion of the prosthetic conduit into the native aorta is likely the site of the intragraft stenosis and pressure gradient. There was 4+ aortic insufficiency by contrast angiography.

DISCUSSION

This case demonstrates unusual hemodynamics associated with prosthetic aortic root replacement. The dilatation of the basal part of the native aortic root resulted in aortic insufficiency and, in conjunction with a kink and bend in the elongated graft portion, produced an intragraft

gradient initially mistakenly identified as aortic stenosis. Graft deformation was likely associated with the continuous alterations of the native ungrafted aorta. The abnormal connective tissue of the great vessels requiring the initial repair suggests a Forme Fruste of Marfan's syndrome [1].

The chronic nature of this insidious change in aortic geometry can be contrasted against the presentation of acute aortic insufficiency. Acute aortic regurgitation often precludes necessary myocardial adaptation and, thus, pressure in the left ventricle rises rapidly producing a steep diastolic pressure–volume relationship, a marked elevation of left ventricular end-diastolic pressure, and often premature closure of the mitral valve [2,3]. There is minimal increase in left ventricular end-diastolic volume. The left ventricular stroke volume cannot increase sufficiently to compensate for the regurgitant volume, and, thus, stroke volume and cardiac output may be diminished. The high left ventricular end-diastolic pressure minimizes left ventricular run-off, and diastolic pressure in the aorta may remain near normal despite having severe aortic insufficiency. This physiologic response contrasts with that of chronic aortic regurgitation, wherein the left ventricle adapts to the extensive volume experienced by the left ventricle [4]. Left ventricular end-diastolic pressure does not rise rapidly as the left ventricle can expand to accommodate the volume, and, thus, the slope of the left ventricular end-diastolic pressure has a gradual incline. The aortic pulse pressure continues to be wide, however, since compensation and run-off permit the fall of the aortic pressure to decrease both in the peripheral circulation and back into the left ventricle.

It is interesting to note that the right heart pressures were also elevated in this individual despite minimal congestive symptoms. Although left ventricular hemodynamics suggested only moderately or minimally compensated aortic insufficiency, the elevated pulmonary artery pressure (50 mm Hg) and pulmonary capillary wedge pressure (28 mm Hg) suggested the effects of adverse compensatory left ventricular hemodynamics on right ventricular function. It is interesting to note that Friedberg in his classic text entitled "Diseases of the Heart" in 1958 reports that "The symptoms of left-sided heart failure and aortic insufficiency are eventually combined with or overshadowed by those of failure of the right ventricle" [5]. As the right ventricle dilates, tricuspid regurgitation, right atrial enlargement with reflux, and an increase of vena caval pressure are evident. The degree of decompensation of the ventricle precedes that of the clinical complaints as evident in the right heart hemodynamics as measured in this individual [6].

Premature closure of the mitral valve may effect the extreme of left ventricular end-diastolic pressure increases and may be associated with the presence of an Austin-Flint murmur [7]. Recall that a low, rumbling late diastolic or pre-systolic apical murmur in patients with aortic insufficiency may be indistinguishable from the characteristic murmur of mitral stenosis. In those patients without organic mitral stenosis, such a murmur has been termed an Austin-Flint murmur [7]. This murmur may be associated with a diastolic thrill which was identifiable in this case. This murmur is generally associated with left ventricular failure, evident by hemodynamics but not symptoms in our patient. The frequency of the murmur has been variously estimated but in routine clinical practice appears rare. Although the etiology of the Austin-Flint murmur is disputed, the mechanism is that of the mitral leaflet nearest the aortic valve being forced toward the closing position, producing a functional mitral stenosis impeding inflow to the left ventricle. The disappearance of the Austin-Flint murmur after relief of cardiac failure suggests that the mechanism of ventricular volume and chamber size relates to the degree of insufficiency. In this individual, no Austin-Flint murmur was reported despite the fact that a diastolic thrill was palpable.

Despite the angiographic and hemodynamic degree of aortic regurgitation, the peripheral signs of aortic insufficiency, including low diastolic and high pulse pressure, the Corrigan or radial pulse (water hammer sign), capillary pulsations disproportionate to femoral systolic hypertension (Hill sign), and sharp femoral murmur (pistol shot), were lacking, which is possibly attributable to the stenotic component of the prosthetic graft blunting the

rate of left ventricular ejection or to the relative lack of chronicity of the disease process.

The determination of premature mitral valve closure from hemodynamics in patients with aortic insufficiency may be difficult. However, as suggested in Figure 3, the "crossover point" of the pulmonary capillary wedge pressure and left ventricular end-diastolic pressure occurs within the first one-third to one-half diastole. It can be noted that the crossover of the pulmonary capillary wedge pressure occurs at the first third of diastole, and a continued rapid rise of left ventricular end-diastolic pressure occurs to the point of left ventricular ejection. There is evidence of a lower pulmonary capillary wedge "A" wave pressure than the left ventricular "A" wave. The expected crossover point of these two pressures is normally in the last one-third of diastole. The association of the early crossover of pulmonary capillary wedge pressure and left ventricular pressure likely reflects the premature closure of the mitral valve which was easily demonstrated by two-dimensional echocardiography.

SUMMARY

This unusual hemodynamic presentation emphasizes the continued requirement for excellent hemodynamic evaluation to differentiate disparate clinical findings. Hemodynamic abnormalities can assist or refute clinical information facilitating decisions with regard to repair, replacement, or medical therapy for patients with aortic insufficiency.

ACKNOWLEDGMENTS

The authors thank the J.G. Mudd Cardiac Catheterization Laboratory Team and Donna Sander for manuscript preparation.

REFERENCES

1. Gott VL, Pyeritz RE, Magovern GJ, Jr, Cameron DE, McKusick VA: Surgical treatment of aneurysm of the ascending aorta in the Marfan syndrome: results of composite-graft repair in 50 patients. N Engl J Med 314:1070–1074, 1986.
2. Goldschlager N, Pfeifer J, Cohn K, Popper R, Selzer A: The natural history of aortic regurgitation: a clinical and hemodynamic study. Am J Med 54:577–588, 1973.
3. Osbakken M, Bove AA, Spann JR: Left ventricular function in chronic aortic regurgitation with reference to end-systolic pressure, volume and stress relations. Am J Cardiol 47:193–198, 1981.
4. Borow KM, Marcus RH: Aortic regurgitation: the need for an integrated physiologic approach. J Am Coll Cardiol 17:898–900, 1991.
5. Friedberg CK: Diseases of the Heart. W.B. Saunders, Philadelphia, 1958 pp 684–692.
6. Mann T, McLaurin LP, Grossman W, Craige E: Assessing the hemodynamic severity of acute aortic regurgitation due to infective endocarditis. N Engl J Med 293:108, 1975.
7. Flint A: Am J Med Sci 44:29, 1962.

Chapter 7

Acute Aortic Insufficiency

Krystof J. Godlewski, MD, J. David Talley, MD, and Glenn T. Morris, MD

INTRODUCTION

This chapter will review the hemodynamic findings of acute aortic insufficiency (AI). We present a patient with acute AI and a-waves in the aortic pressure tracing, a highly specific finding which has been rarely described [1]. We will also discuss the features of chronic AI which may aid in diagnosis of acute AI.

PATIENT PRESENTATION

A 59-yr-old morbidly obese male presented with 9 hours of abdominal and chest pain. The pain was severe, non-radiating and associated with shortness of breath. He had systemic arterial hypertension, type II diabetes mellitus, alcoholism, hepatitis, and a history of medical non-compliance. He was diaphoretic, awake with waning consciousness. The blood pressure was 76/26 mmHg and bounding pulses were felt in all extremities. There were diffuse crackles in both lungs and heart sounds were not audible. There was no edema or cyanosis.

A central venous catheter with a side port extension (Arrow International Corp., Reading, PA) was placed in the right internal jugular vein and intravenous Lactated Ringers, dobutamine, and dopamine were begun. The central venous pressure was 30 mmHg. The patient was intubated. Chest X-ray revealed mediastinal dilatation, cardiomegaly, and pulmonary edema. An echocardiogram was technically difficult with only non-diagnostic limited views obtained. An ECG showed sinus tachycardia at 104 beats/min and diffuse ST segment depression of 2–4 mm (Fig. 1a). An ECG from one year earlier was normal (Fig. 1b).

With the differential diagnosis of acute myocardial infarction or acute AI, cardiac catheterization was performed using standard Judkins technique. A 6 French (F) sheath (Cordis Corp., Miami, FL) was inserted in the right femoral artery and a 6 F angled pigtail (Cordis Corp., Miami, FL) placed in the ascending aorta. The aortic pressure was 200/60. This rapid rise in blood pressure was primarily attributed to volume repletion or to preexistent "pseudohypotension" [4,8] and represented the pharmacological response to the intravenous fluids and inotropes begun in the emergency department. Treatment with intravenous nitroglycerin at an initial rate of 10 μg/min was started to achieve pre- and afterload reduction while sodium nitroprusside was being prepared [9]. An ascending aortogram was performed with a total of 40 ml (20 ml/sec for 2 sec) of Optiray (Mallinckrodt Medical Inc., St. Louis, MO), and it demonstrated aortic root dilatation (5 cm) and 4+ AI (Fig. 2). The left ventricular-aorta "pullback" pressure tracing showed a-waves preceding the anacrotic limb of the pressure curve (Fig. 3). Coronary angiography was attempted but the ostia could not be engaged due to catheter "whip."

While awaiting transfer to the surgical suite, the patient suddenly became hypotensive and expired despite resuscitative efforts. Post-mortem examination revealed dissection involving the entire length of the aorta (DeBakey class I) with an intimal flap 3 cm distally from the aortic valve. Dissection extended retrogradely and caused a 3 cm hematoma surrounding the left anterior descending artery (LAD) with 200 ml of pericardial hemorrhage. There was no evidence of LAD, circumflex, or right coronary artery compression. The aortic valve was structurally normal and did not appear to prolapse or to be weakened. Coronary vessels were free of atheroscle rosis. The left ventricle was hypertrophied with no evi-

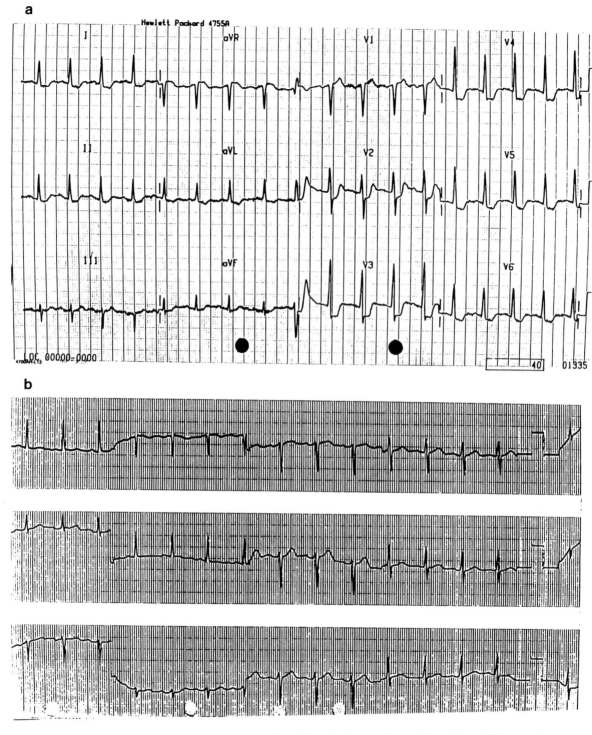

Fig. 1. a. EKG at the time of presentation. There is sinus tachycardia and deep ST segment depressions in anterolateral leads. The patient had no evidence of coronary artery disease on post-mortem examination and the changes were related only to presence of acute AI. b. EKG one year prior to the presentation, with no evidence of myocardial ischemia.

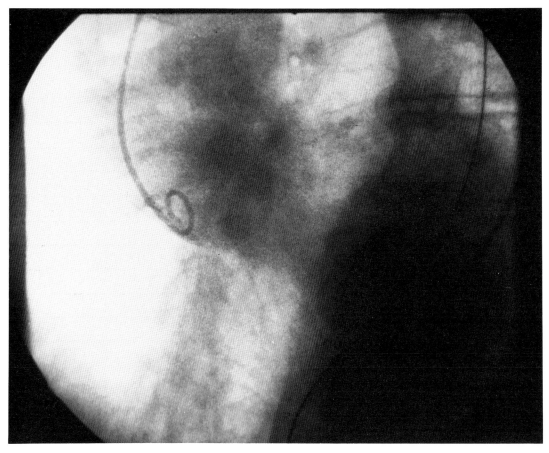

Fig. 2. Ascending aortogram in the left anterior oblique position revealing 4+ aortic insufficiency.

dence of recent or remote myocardial infarction. The cause of death was cardiac tamponade.

DISCUSSION

This patient's presentation illustrates 3 important, but seldom appreciated features of acute AI: 1) the physical findings of acute AI may mimic chronic AI; 2) the endocardial injury pattern on the ECG may have several potential etiologies, and 3) the a-wave in the aortic tracing is highly specific for acute AI.

Chronic AI is characterized by bounding pulses and a wide arterial pulse pressure. These findings are seldom seen with acute AI, especially when it co-exists with left ventricular hypertrophy due to poor left ventricular compliance and the rapid rise of the left ventricular end diastolic pressure [2,3]. Our patient demonstrates that there are exceptions to this rule. The bounding pulses of chronic AI were clearly present and pressure recording from the left ventricular-aorta pull-back demonstrates pulse pressure of 140 mmHg (Fig. 3). The ascending aorta was dilated and the left ventricle hypertrophied

probably related to longstanding systemic arterial hypertension. There was no evidence, either by history or physical examination, to suggest preexisting chronic AI. Therefore, signs of chronic AI may be present in the most severe cases of acute AI, which is precisely where they may be of the greatest diagnostic value [4].

The electrocardiogram in acute AI is frequently described as showing nonspecific changes [2]. The ST segment depressions in Figure 1a are profound and were noted to have occurred within the last year when compared to the previous tracing (Fig. 1b). The mechanism responsible for these changes in our patient was the sudden increase in left ventricular end diastolic pressure producing subendocardial ischemia. Other mechanisms postulated to produce ischemia which were not present in our patient include: 1) an epicardial hematoma surrounding the coronary arteries compressing the vessels leading to the impaired coronary flow; 2) the coincidental presence of coronary atherosclerotic lesions leading to decreased perfusion; 3) impaired systolic performance, leading to decreased coronary perfusion gradient; and 4) experimental data suggest that acute AI caused by an

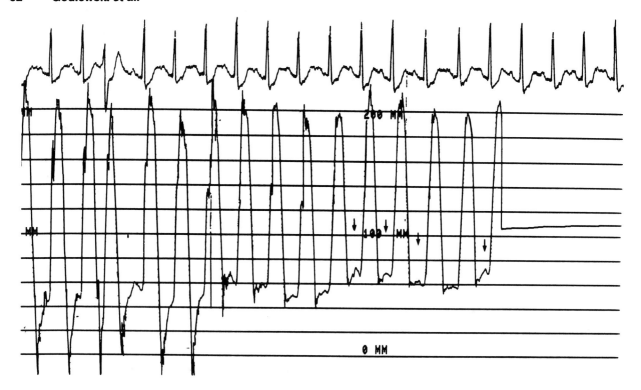

Fig. 3. Pressure recording from the LV pullback to ascending Ao. The pulse pressure is 140 mmHg and the Ao diastolic pressure is approximately equal to LV end diastolic pressure. Preceding the anacrotic limb of the Ao pressure tracing there are positive deflections correlating with the P waves on the EKG (arrow). These a-waves are due to premature opening of the Ao valve in acute AI. (Recording speed = 25 mm/sec.) Abbreviations: LV = left ventricle, Ao = aorta, AI = aortic insufficiency.

incompetent left coronary cusp is associated with more severe hemodynamic consequences and worse LV dysfunction than when other cusps are involved [5]. It can be postulated that the regurgitant flow caused by the failure of the left coronary cusp causes a Venturi effect at the left coronary artery ostium and decreases or reverses the normal antegrade coronary flow. Therefore, while acute ST segment abnormalities may represent a subendocardial injury pattern due to epicardial coronary artery lesions, they may have many other potential mechanisms.

The presence of an a-wave in the aortic pressure tracing has been reported in a patient with acute AI complicating balloon aortic valvuloplasty [1]. Figure 3 shows presystolic waves which coincide with P waves of the EKG. Echocardiographic studies have shown that in the setting of the acute but not chronic AI, the rapid rise in the left ventricular end diastolic pressure causes diastolic mitral regurgitation, premature closure of the mitral valve, and premature opening of the aortic valve [6,7]. The premature opening of the aortic valve allows for the atrial impulse to be transmitted to the aorta. Therefore, this finding has high specificity for acute AI, although its sensitivity is unclear. This finding can be expected only when sinus rhythm is present.

CONCLUSION

Acute AI is a relatively rare event and requires expedient diagnosis and treatment. We have presented a patient who illustrates several salient points to consider in the diagnosis of acute AI. First, the classical physical findings of chronic AI, wide pulse pressure and bounding pulses, may help in identification of the acute AI, especially in severe cases. Second, the ECG may be misleading, suggesting anatomically significant coronary artery lesions when other mechanisms are operative, such as: dramatic elevation of the left ventricular end diastolic pressure, vessel compression by an epicardial hematoma, and decreased or reversed flow in the coronary artery due to Venturi effect caused by regurgitant flow at the left coronary ostium. Lastly, the presence of the a-waves in the aortic pressure tracing is virtually diagnostic of acute AI.

ACKNOWLEDGMENTS

The authors appreciate the secretarial assistance of Carole Clark and Barbara Newlin in the preparation of this manuscript.

REFERENCES

1. Alexopulos D, Sherman W: Unusual hemodynamic presentation of acute aortic regurgitation following percutaneous balloon valvuloplasty. Am Heart J 116:1622–1623, 1988.
2. Kereiakes DJ, Ports TA: Emergencies in valvular heart disease. In: Greenberg BH (ed): "Valvular Heart Disease," Littleton, Ma: PSG Publishing Co., 1987: 215–233.
3. Dalen JE, Pape LA, Conn LH, Koster JK, Jr. Collins JJ, Jr.: Dissection of the aorta: Pathogenesis and treatment. Prog Cardiovasc Dis 23:237–245, 1980.
4. Eagle KA, DeSanctis RW: Diseases of aorta. In: Braunwald E (ed): "Heart disease: A Textbook of Cardiovascular Medicine," Philadelphia: W.B. Saunders, 1988: 1554–1562.
5. Nakao S, Nagatomo T, Kiyonaga K, Kashima T, Tanaka H: Influence of localized aortic valve damage on coronary artery blood flow in acute aortic regurgitation: An experimental study. Circulation 76:201–207, 1987.
6. Meyer T, Sareli P, Pocock WA, Dean H, Epstein M, Barlow J: Echocardiographic and hemodynamic correlates of diastolic closure of mitral valve and diastolic opening of aortic valve in severe aortic regurgitation. Am J Cardiol 559:1144–1148, 1987.
7. Downes TR, Nomeir AM, Hackshaw BT, Kellam LJ, Watts LE, Little WC: Diastolic mitral regurgitation in acute but not chronic aortic regurgitation: Implications regarding the mechanism of mitral closure. Am Heart J 117:1106–1112, 1989.
8. Wheat MW: Acute dissecting aneurysms of aorta. In: Goldberger E, Wheat MW (eds): "Treatment of Cardiac Emergencies," St. Louis: C.V. Mosby Co, 1990: 221–236.
9. Klepzig HH, Warner KG, Siouffi SY, Saad AJ, Hayes A, Kaltenbach M, Khuri SF: Hemodynamic effects of nitroglycerin in an experimental model of acute aortic insufficiency. J Am Coll Cardiol 13:27–935, 1989.

Commentary

Morton J. Kern, MD

Drs. Godlewski, Talley, and Morris present an interesting and uncommon hemodynamic finding in a patient who developed acute aortic insufficiency secondary to aortic dissection. The demonstration of an A wave on the arterial pulse transmitted from the left ventricular end diastolic pressure into the aorta is specific for an acute decompensation with markedly increased left ventricular filling pressures. The normal valvular chamber separation between the left ventricle and aorta is virtually eliminated. Although only a single pressure tracing is available the matching of aortic and left ventricular end diastolic pressures is easily appreciated. Features which usually differentiate acute from chronic aortic insufficiency [1] are somewhat mixed, confounding interpretation of the pressure waveform. Acute aortic insufficiency is characterized by tachycardia, lower end diastolic, end systolic, and total stroke volume, as well as markedly reduced systolic, diastolic, and mean arterial pressures. This patient had tachycardia but high pressure on vasopressors. The pulse pressure in acute aortic insufficiency is usually significantly less than that with chronic aortic insufficiency. This patient's pulse pressure was 140 mmHg. Systemic vascular resistance may be the same in both presentations. One of the findings not shown in the current hemodynamic rounds is that of the left ventricular and pulmonary capillary wedge pressures, indicating premature mitral valve closure. The massive reflux of blood from the aorta enters the left ventricle in diastole and rapidly increases end diastolic volume and pressure

closing the mitral valve prematurely. An unusually steep increase on the left ventricular diastolic pressure with loss of a clear A wave and a markedly elevated left ventricular end diastolic pressure is suggestive. The wedge pressure is consistently lower than left ventricular end diastolic pressure for nearly half of the diastolic interval in this setting [2].

Other hemodynamic findings which may differentiate acute from chronic aortic regurgitation include the presence of a single contour of the arterial pressure in acute aortic regurgitation compared to a bisferiens pulse seen in chronic aortic insufficiency. Pulsus alternans is also more common in acute aortic insufficiency and rare in chronic aortic insufficiency. The hyperdynamic nature of the left ventricular apical impulse and pressure rise is also less striking in acute compared to chronic aortic insufficiency[3].

The striking findings of acute aortic insufficiency with wide pulse pressure and transmitted A wave into the arterial pressure as described by Godlewski and colleagues should be considered as an important, although infrequent, marker of acute decompensation of aortic insufficiency.

REFERENCES

1. Mann T, et al: Assessing the hemodynamic severity of acute aortic regurgitation due to infective endocarditis. N Engl J Med 293:108, 1975.
2. Grossman W: Profiles in valvular heart disease. In Grossman W and Baim DS (eds): "Cardiac Catheterization, Angiography and

54 **Godlewski et al.**

Intervention,'' 4th edition. Philadelphia: Lea & Febiger, 1991, pp 557–581.

3. Benotti JR: Acute aortic insufficiency: In Dalen JE (ed): ''Valvular Heart Disease,'' 2nd edition. Boston: Little & Brown, Co., 1987, pp 331–337.

Chapter 8

Multivalvular Regurgitant Lesions

Morton J. Kern, MD, Frank V. Aguirre, MD, Thomas J. Donohue, MD, and
Richard G. Bach, MD

INTRODUCTION

The majority of classic hemodynamic descriptions for
valvular lesions have characteristics which are unique for
that lesion as a single or isolated entity. Although significant multivalvular disease is infrequent, many patients may have mild to moderate impairment of one
valve while an associated severe valve lesion appears to
be responsible for the major clinical symptomatology.
The clinical severity of the presentation depends on the
severity of each individual lesion [1]. However, the characteristic and ''classical'' findings may thus be modified
when accompanied by lesions in other valves, producing
changes in blood flow which may act synergistically
with or nullify the usual perturbations of hemodynamic
waveforms. In general, the clinical manifestations are
produced by the more upstream or proximal lesion [2].
Characteristic hemodynamic waveforms of isolated lesions of the aortic, mitral, tricuspid and pulmonary
valves have been discussed in earlier rounds [3–8]. This
rounds will review the hemodynamic findings in a patient who has severe multivalvular regurgitant lesions
and emphasizes the consideration of such hemodynamics
when more than one valve may be affected.

MULTIPLE HEART MURMURS AFTER MITRAL VALVE REPLACEMENT

A 63-yr-old woman had a history of porcine mitral
valve replacement 15 years ago for mitral stenosis. In the
last 3 years the patient reported increasing exertional
dyspnea. In the last 6 months, progressive orthopnea and
paroxysmal nocturnal dyspnea were noted. There has
been no history of chest pain or myocardial infarction.
Medications at the time of the current evaluation included Lasix and digoxin. Physical examination revealed
a blood pressure of 130/80mmHg and a pulse of 75 beats
per minute. There were no carotid bruits. The examination of the lungs was clear. S_1 and S_2 were diminished
with an associated S_3 gallop. There was a grade III/VI
holosystolic murmur at the left sternal border radiating to
the axilla with a grade II/VI left-sided diastolic murmur
and a variable diastolic murmur over the right sternal
border. Echocardiographic (transesophageal) examination revealed mild to moderate mitral regurgitation
(among other regurgitant valve lesions to be discussed)
and an enlarged left atrium.

Because of the suspected progression of prosthetic mitral valve dysfunction, cardiac catheterization was performed using routine fluid-filled catheters from the femoral approach. An 8 French arterial sheath, a 7 French
pigtail catheter and an 8 French balloon-tipped flotation
catheter were initially used for the right and left heart
catheterizations.

Hemodynamic data were obtained prior to angiography and are summarized on table I. These data were
obtained before changes due to contrast ventriculographic alterations of myocardial function and peripheral
vasodilation. However, the angiogram in this patient offers insight into the abnormal hemodynamic findings. A
frame from the cineangiogram of the left ventriculogram

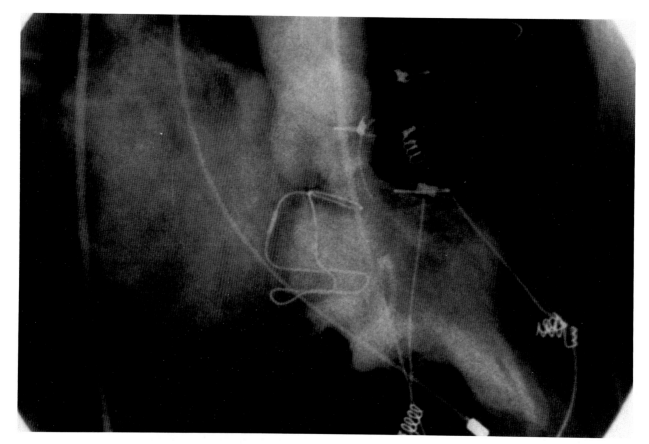

Fig. 1. A still frame from cine left ventriculogram showing end systolic contraction of the left ventricle and large left atrium well opacified. The left atrial appendage is not seen. Multiple metal roentgenographic shadows can be identified showing the bioprosthetic struts and pacemaker wires of the epicardial and endocardial leads.

(Fig. 1) has been selected to show the characteristic bioprosthetic struts which can be clearly seen in the mitral position. Multiple metal roentgenographic shadows of wires and pacemakers further demonstrated the extensive prior surgical procedures. On the single frame angiogram, motion of this strut cannot be appreciated but a rocking motion suggested a perivalvular leak, often coexistent with prosthetic leaflet degeneration. The left atrium is larger than the ventricle and is well opacified due to severe angiographic mitral regurgitation. Although not seen on this angiogram, left atrial appendage filling during left ventriculography is an additional indicator of severe mitral regurgitation. The left ventricular function appeared normal despite the severe angiographic regurgitation.

THE TRICUSPID VALVE

Consider the abnormal right atrial pressure waveforms (Fig. 2). The elevated pressure, large systolic fused V wave and absent A wave occur during the VVI pace-

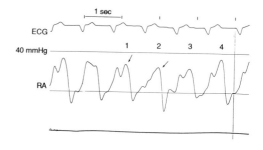

Fig. 2. Right atrial (RA) pressure (0–40mmHg scale) demonstrating altering waveforms during paced rhythm. Arrow is large 'V'? See text for details.

maker rhythm and complete heart block. (Note the P wave after the T wave on beat #3.) The abnormally large V wave without a clear A wave with a mean pressure exceeding 20mmHg varies with inspiration. The waveform abruptly and consistently increases during systolic contraction (immediately after or at the R wave) in this paced rhythm. Occasional P waves appear to deform the right atrial pressure waveform. There are no consistent A

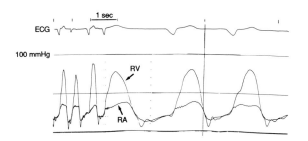

Fig. 3. Simultaneous right ventricular (RV) and right atrial (RA) pressures (0–100mmHg scale). Note systolic upstroke of right atrial pressure and matching of pressures in diastole. See text for details.

waves because of the dissociated rhythm. The V wave is combined with the 'S' wave producing the characteristic pattern of severe tricuspid regurgitation. To confirm the severity of tricuspid regurgitation, simultaneous right ventricular and atrial pressures were recorded (0–100mmHg scale) using a 2 catheter technique (Fig. 3). The degree of tricuspid regurgitation is demonstrated by the height of right atrial pressure rise under the enclosure of the right ventricular systolic waveform [7]. There is no tricuspid stenosis as evident by matching of the diastolic pressure waveforms of both tracings. Systolic pulmonary artery pressure was equal to right ventricular systolic pressure (Table I).

Tricuspid regurgitation in the setting of clinical mitral regurgitation with severe pulmonary hypertension is not an uncommon combination of valvular lesions. Long standing mitral regurgitation produces left ventricular dysfunction with elevated left atrial and ultimately pulmonary artery pressures. Mitral regurgitation begets functional tricuspid regurgitation with right ventricular pressure overload. The interaction of high right ventricular pressures on left ventricular septal wall motion is probably the only significant interaction between the two hemodynamic presentations. The tricuspid valve generally has no influence on left-sided valvular function.

THE AORTIC VALVE

The aortic pressure tracings, obtained from a 7 French pigtail catheter in the left ventricle and the side arm of the 8 French femoral artery sheath with fluid-filled transducers, were matched. Prior to crossing the aortic valve, there was a 10mmHg overshoot of the femoral artery pressure. With consideration of the normal phase delay of the femoral artery pressure, peak systolic left ventricular pressure exceeds femoral artery pressure by approximately 20–25mmHg (Fig. 4). Although Doppler echocardiography suggested moderate mixed aortic valve disease hemodynamically, the left ventricular-

TABLE I. Hemodynamic Data

	Pressure (mmHg)	Oxygen saturation (%)
Right atrial pressure mean	14	46
Superior vena cava	—	48
Inferior vena cava	—	48
Right ventricular pressure	85/8	—
Pulmonary artery pressure (mean)	85/25 (45)	48
Arterial pressure (mean)	145/76 (92)	87
Left ventricular pressure	140/20	—
Left atrial pressure (mean)	40/20 (26)	—

Body surface area	1.54m^2
Heart rate (beats/minute)	70
Oxygen consumption (ml/minute)	256
Cardiac ouput-thermodilution (L/min)	3.2
Cardiac output-Fick (L/min)	4.0
Cardiac index-thermodilution (L/min/m^2)	2.0
Cardiac index-Fick (L/min/m^2)	2.6
Systemic vascular resistance (dynes.sec.cm^{-5})	1560
Pulmonary vascular resistance (dynes.sec.cm^{-5})	380
Mitral valve gradient (mmHg)	16
Mitral valve area (cm^2)	0.9

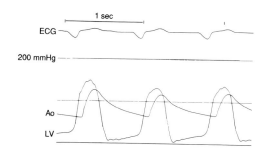

Fig. 4. Simultaneous aortic (Ao) and left ventricular (LV) pressures (0–200mmHg scale) in a patient with diastolic murmur.

aortic gradient demonstrated only minimal aortic obstructive narrowing, a finding further supported when consideration of femoral overshoot has been made. From this tracing, is significant aortic regurgitation present?

Based on our previous demonstrations of the spectrum of insufficient aortic valve hemodynamics [4], the aortic pressure decline and left ventricular diastolic pressure rise do not suggest aortic insufficiency. The features suggesting severe aortic insufficiency of wide pulse pressure, rapidly rising left ventricular end diastolic pressure and significant overshoot of the femoral artery are missing. However, mild aortic regurgitation would not be unexpected in a patient such as this with a sclerotic aortic valve and prior mitral valve replacement.

As indicated by Doppler echocardiography and later angiography, mild aortic insufficiency was present. Does the mild degree of aortic insufficiency in this patient

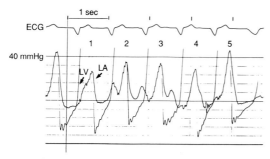

Fig. 5. Simultaneous left atrial (LA) and left ventricular (LV) pressures (0–40mmHg scale) with transseptal technique. Note changing A waves during paced rhythm. See text for details.

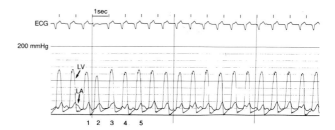

Fig. 6. Left atrial (LA) and left ventricular (LV) pressures (0–200mmHg scale) as in Figure 5. Note repetitive pattern of atrial waveform in a patient with paced rhythm.

contribute to the severity of mitral regurgitation? Reflux of blood into the left ventricle from the insufficient aortic valve produces extra left ventricular end diastolic volume enlarging the left ventricle. One could postulate that over time, mild mitral regurgitation would more rapidly become severe with the extra load produced by chronic aortic insufficiency. The increased left ventricular end diastolic volume would increase the regurgitant volume prior to left ventricular decompensation. After left ventricular decompensation, the aortic insufficiency might appear to reduce mitral regurgitation backflow velocity compared to a prior echocardiographic study. Unfortunately, these considerations remain unproven observations since serial studies in such patients are generally unavailable.

THE MITRAL VALVE

In this patient, regurgitant lesions of the tricuspid and aortic valves, identified by clinical, echocardiographic and hemodynamic examination, appear with the findings of the predominant mitral valve lesion. To identify the abnormal hemodynamics of the prosthetic mitral valve, and because a pulmonary capillary wedge would not be reliably obtained (due to severe pulmonary hypertension), direct measurement of left atrial pressure was obtained with a transseptal puncture. Crossing the prosthetic mitral valve into the left ventricle was not necessary with the pigtail catheter in the left ventricle. Figure 5 shows simultaneous left atrial and left ventricular pressures during the paced cardiac rhythm. Note the variable but consistent pattern of atrial contraction. There is a large V wave to 40mmHg and rapid Y descent characteristic of mitral regurgitation. The left atrial pressure, however, does not decline to match the left ventricular diastolic pressure. Also, the changing position of the A wave reflects the dissociated sinus mechanism more clearly than the electrocardiogram as previously described [9]. On beat #1 (Figure 5), the left atrial pres-

sure shows no A wave, but a fused A and systolic regurgitant V waveform differentiated from separated waves on the following beats. On beat #2, the A wave appears to fall just inside the left ventricular upstroke. On beat #3, the A wave precedes left ventricular upstroke. A small P wave can be appreciated on the electrocardiogram and appears in mid diastolic cycle. Beat #5 has minimal A wave and the largest V wave. This cycle repeats itself every fifth beat and demonstrates the dissociated atrial and ventricular rhythms (Fig. 6). The mitral valve gradient is approximately 16mmHg with a cardiac output of 3.2L/min, yielding a valve area of 0.9cm². In the setting of 4 + angiographic mitral regurgitation, this calculation is an estimate of only the minimal valve area.

Of special interest is the comparison of the simultaneous left and right atrial pressures measured after pullback of the pulmonary artery catheter. The matching left and right atrial pressures (Fig. 7) demonstrates slight differences in A and V wave activity with the large, broad tricuspid regurgitant waves maintained on the right atrial pressure with less striking mitral regurgitant V waves of the left atrial pressure. Left atrial pressure more clearly demonstrates the intermittent activity of A waves better than right atrial pressure waveforms (Fig. 8). Equivalency of the left and right atrial pressure transducers is appreciated on transseptal catheter pullback from the left to right atrium as shown on the far right side of Figure 8.

POST-SURGICAL HEMODYNAMICS

Although several years after open heart surgery, evidence of constrictive or restrictive physiology should be checked by comparing the simultaneously recorded right and left ventricular diastolic pressures (Fig. 9). The ventricular waveforms clearly show normal filling patterns with separation in diastole. Of note is the delay in right ventricular upstroke and fall in right ventricular pressure consistent with pulmonary hypertension and bundle branch block activity discussed in previous rounds [8].

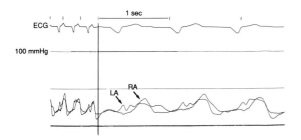

Fig. 7. Simultaneous left atrial (LA) and right atrial (RA) pressures (0–100mmHg scale) prior to transseptal catheter pullback.

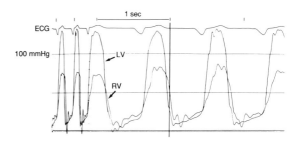

Fig. 9. Simultaneous left (LV) and right ventricular (RV) pressure tracings (0–100mmHg scale). Note the delay in upstroke and downstroke of right ventricular pressure under left ventricular pressure envelope in paced rhythm with bundle branch block pattern. See text for details.

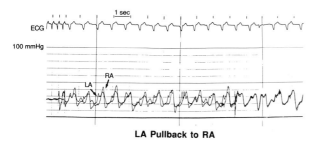

LA Pullback to RA

Fig. 8. Simultaneous left (LA) and right atrial (RA) pressures (0–100mmHg scale) showing matching of pressure waveforms on pullback to the right atrium.

Pulmonary hypertension, as well as the abnormal conduction delay, produces this unusual waveform where the right ventricular downstroke is delayed 40–120msec and falls outside the left ventricular pressure downstroke. Normally the right ventricular waveform is completely contained inside the left ventricular tracing.

Recognition of multivalvular lesions preoperatively is important since failure to correct these lesions at the time of surgery increases surgical mortality. In such patients the relative severity of each lesion may be difficult to estimate by clinical and non-invasive techniques alone since one lesion may mask the manifestations of another. Complete clinical and hemodynamic evaluation with right and left heart catheterization and angiography is often mandatory. At times, questions concerning the presence of significant aortic stenosis in patients with mitral valve disease requires direct valve inspection. Palpation of the tricuspid valve at the time of mitral valve replacement may also identify significant, previously unappreciated valvular disease [2]. The frequency of concomitant paired valve lesions is hard to estimate. Two-thirds of patients with severe mitral stenosis may have mitral regurgitation. This degree of regurgitation is usually clinically insignificant. However, in 10% of patients with rheumatic mitral stenosis, rheumatic aortic regurgitation has been recognized [10]. Mitral stenosis masks

the hemodynamic detection of left ventricular volume overload which is characteristic of aortic insufficiency [11]. The combination of mitral stenosis and aortic insufficiency is slightly greater than the 8% incidence of combined aortic and mitral valve disease with pure stenosis of both valves [1]. Aortic and mitral regurgitation are more frequently combined [12] than other lesions since rheumatic disease may often affect both valves. In some patients, connective tissue disorders may be an apparent cause of multivalvular regurgitation. In combined mitral and aortic regurgitation, the clinical features of aortic regurgitation may predominate and it is difficult to determine whether mitral regurgitation is secondary to ventricular dilatation or a primary organic lesion. With combined regurgitant lesions, regardless of the etiology, reflux of blood from the aorta into both left ventricle and left atrium produce high pulmonary venous pressures. When mitral regurgitation occurs secondary to the left ventricular dilatation of deteriorating aortic regurgitation, mitral regurgitation may be diminished following aortic valve replacement. Severe mitral regurgitation may require annuloplasty at the time of aortic valve replacement [2].

The surgical outcome for treatment of multivalvular disease has been reviewed by Kirklin et al. [13] who report a 5 year survival rate of 70% after double valve replacement compared to 80% for single valve replacement. Long-term survival is dependent on the ventricular functional status prior to surgery. Patients who had combined aortic and mitral insufficiency had poorer outcome than those receiving valves for other multilesion combinations. Triple valve replacement is a complex procedure associated with a mortality of at least 18% for patients in functional class III and 40% in patients in functional class IV [14]. Substantial clinical improvement has been demonstrated to occur in these patients in the early postoperative period with arrhythmias and congestive heart failure complicating the late postoperative course.

SUMMARY

Multivalvular regurgitant lesions may have a common etiology, such as an underlying connective tissue disorder, Marfan's disease or cardiomyopathy. Careful collection of routine simultaneous left and right heart hemodynamics will document the individual valvular lesions. Combined echocardiography and angiographic data will further support the interpretation of the hemodynamic waveforms. Clinical decisions for valve repair or replacement will be based on the severity of associated lesions, myocardial function and other patient specific characteristics [9] indicating the acceptable limits of surgical risk.

ACKNOWLEDGMENTS

The authors thank the J.G. Mudd Cardiac Catheterization Laboratory Team and Donna Sander for manuscript preparation.

REFERENCES

1. Paraskos JA. Combined valvular disease. In Dalen JE and Alpert JS (eds): "Valvular Heart Disease." 2nd ed. Boston, Little, Brown and Company, 1987, pp 439–508.
2. Braunwald E (ed). Valvular heart disease. In "Heart Disease: A Textbook of Cardiovascular Medicine." Philadelphia, W. B. Saunders Co., 1988, pp 1023–1992.
3. Kern MJ, Deligonul U. Hemodynamic rounds: Interpretation of cardiac pathophysiology from pressure waveform analysis. I. The stenotic aortic valve. Cathet Cardiovasc Diagn 21:112–120, 1990.
4. Kern MJ, Aguirre FV. Hemodynamic rounds: interpretation of cardiac pathophysiology from pressure waveform analysis. Aortic regurgitation. Cathet Cardiovasc Diagn 26:232–240, 1992.
5. Kern MJ, Aguirre F. Hemodynamic rounds: Interpretation of cardiac pathophysiology from pressure waveform analysis. Mitral valve gradients, Part I. Cathet Cardiovasc Diagn (In press).
6. Kern MJ, Aguirre F. Hemodynamic rounds: Interpretation of cardiac pathophysiology from pressure waveform analysis. Mitral valve gradients, Part II. Cathet Cardiovasc Diagn (In press).
7. Kern MJ, Deligonul U. Hemodynamic rounds: Interpretation of cardiac pathophysiology from pressure waveform analysis. II. The tricuspid valve. Cathet Cardiovasc Diagn 21:278–286, 1990.
8. Kern MJ. Hemodynamic rounds: Interpretation of cardiac pathophysiology from pressure waveform analysis. The pulmonary valve. Cathet Cardiovasc Diagn 24:290–213, 1991.
9. Kern MJ, Deligonul U. Hemodynamic rounds: Interpretation of cardiac pathophysiology from pressure waveform analysis. Pacemaker hemodynamics. Cathet Cardiovasc Diagn 24:22–27, 1991.
10. Segal J, Harvey WP, Hufnagel CA. Clinical study of one hundred cases of severe aortic insufficiency. Am J Med 21:200, 1956.
11. Gash AK, Carabello BA, Kent RL, Frazier JA, Spann JF. Left ventricular performance in patients with coexistent mitral stenosis and aortic insufficiency. J Am Coll Cardiol 3:703, 1984.
12. Melvin DB, Tecklenberg PL, Hollingsworth JF, Levine FH, Glancy DL, Epstein SE, Morrow AG. Computer-based analysis of preoperative and postoperative factors in 100 patients with combined aortic and mitral valve replacement. Circulation 48(suppl III): 58, 1973.
13. Kirklin JW, Barratt-Boyes BG. Combined aortic and mitral valve disease with or without tricuspid valve disease. In: Cardiac Surgery. New York, John Wiley and Sons, 1986, pp 431–446.
14. Stephenson LW, Kouchoukos NT, Kirklin JW. Triple valve replacement: an analysis of eight years' experience. Ann Thorac Surg 23:327, 1977.

Chapter 9

Mitral Valve Gradients—Section I

Morton J. Kern, MD, and Frank V. Aguirre, MD

INTRODUCTION

The prevalence of rheumatic mitral disease is declining in the industrial world while increasing in Latin America, Asia, Africa, and the Middle East. Patients with the classic findings of severe mitral stenosis, likely to be encountered in both urban and rural medical centers in North America, are usually older (>45 yr) with calcified annular and subvalvular structures. In distinction to younger patients, the poorly mobile valve leaflets and heavy calcification make these older individuals at higher risk for complications of mitral valve balloon catheter commissurotomy [1–3]. Regardless of the clinical presentation, the determination of the mitral valve gradient with its characteristic atrial and (consequently altered) pulmonary and ventricular pressure waveforms is critical to both diagnostic and therapeutic considerations.

The use of echo-Doppler and flow velocity in determination of the mitral valve area has been widely accepted and compared to various hemodynamic methods calculating valve area [4,5]. Because of changes in the pressure-volume relationship, computation of the valve area after mitral balloon valvuloplasty based on hemodynamics, as well as echocardiographic techniques, has been questioned [6]. Discrepancies among these results are due to differences in atrial and ventricular chamber volume and flow characteristics (compliance) in a setting of a changing valve orifice area. This hemodynamic rounds will examine examples of mitral valve gradients and discuss features of the pressure waveforms and factors which influence the determination of mitral valve area for clinical decision making.

MITRAL STENOSIS WITH LARGE V WAVES

A 47-yr-old woman with progressive exertional dyspnea and fatigue has a diastolic murmur of a low rumbling quality with a narrow opening snap and a brief systolic murmur. The patient reported a history of rheumatic fever as a child but physicians did not diagnose the heart murmur until 4 yr prior to this examination. Echocardiography confirmed that severe mitral stenosis was present. The patient underwent cardiac catheterization using fluid-filled catheters prior to consideration for definitive valve repair. The right atrial pressure, measured with a balloon flotation catheter, was 6 mm Hg, right ventricular pressure 45/6 mm Hg, pulmonary artery pressure 45/25 mm Hg. The pulmonary capillary wedge pressure was elevated and equal to the left atrial pressure obtained with a transseptal puncture. The mitral valve gradient was obtained from the simultaneously recorded left ventricular and left atrial pressures obtained through 7 French pigtail and Brockenbrough catheters, respectively (Fig. 1). The cardiac output, measured by both Fick and thermodilution techniques, was 3.5 L/min. From the brief clinical data and pressure waveforms, address the following: Does the patient have long-standing mitral stenosis? Is there coexistent mitral regurgitation? Identify the A, C and V waves on left atrial pressure tracing. What is the valve area from available data?

In the examination of every pressure tracing, review the cardiac rhythm. Atrial fibrillation is the underlying rhythm, often associated with long-standing and severe mitral stenosis. This rhythm is also associated with loss of the A wave on both left atrial and left ventricular pressure tracings. The V waves are large. However, the

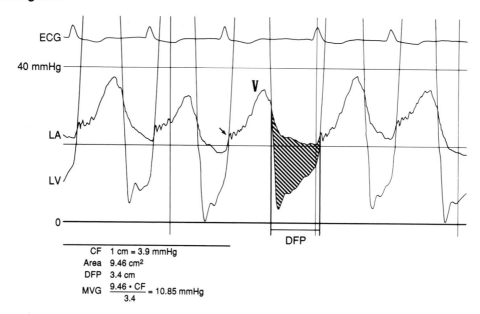

Fig. 1. Left atrial (LA) and left ventricular (LV) pressures (0–40 mm Hg scale) in a patient with dyspnea on minimal exertion. Shaded area is mitral valve gradient (MVG). CF = correction factor to convert paper distance to pressure value. DPF = diastolic filling period. "Notch" at arrow. See text for details. With permission from *The Cardiac Catheterization Handbook,* Kern (ed), p 116, 1991, Mosby-Year Book, Inc.

presence of large V waves in mitral stenosis is common, often reflecting a low compliance (stiff) chamber, and does not necessarily indicate clinically significant mitral regurgitation. Recall large V waves result from factors altering chamber compliance with pressure changes occurring due to flow volume and chamber dimensions acting together as discussed in earlier rounds [7]. Mitral regurgitation is determined by clinical examination, angiography, and echo-Doppler studies. This patient's systolic murmur was due to aortic ejection and not mitral regurgitation.

TECHNICAL NOTES FOR MITRAL VALVE AREA CALCULATION

For the most accurate results, use the waveforms of directly measured chamber pressures. Although technically more difficult to obtain, the left atrial pressure by transseptal puncture resolves any doubt about small but significant mitral gradients. The left atrial and pulmonary capillary wedge pressures are usually matched in a majority of cases [8]. In patient #1 (Fig. 1), the left atrial pressure is differentiated from a pulmonary capillary wedge pressure by the abrupt pressure notch at the C wave with left ventricular ejection and continued pressure rise (left atrial filling) across systole with the peak V wave occurring within the left ventricular pressure downstroke. The pulmonary capillary wedge tracing, although equal to the left atrial pressure in many patients, will

always be delayed by 40–120 msec (Fig. 2) with the peak V wave being inscribed after the left ventricular pressure downslope (Fig. 3).

In patients in whom the pulmonary capillary wedge pressure is used to measure mitral valve gradients, phase shift of the peak of the V wave to the downslope of the left ventricular pressure before planimetering the gradient area. Note that when phase shifting the pulmonary capillary wedge tracing to the left ventricular pressure on Figure 3, the gradient becomes even smaller. The pulmonary capillary wedge pressure should not be used when there is an unreliable tracing, when there are known causes of abnormally high pulmonary capillary wedge pressure, or when there is a mitral valve prosthesis. However, in most cases, the pulmonary capillary wedge pressure can be used to measure mitral valve gradients [8]. The correspondence of typical left atrial and pulmonary capillary wedge pressures in a patient without mitral stenosis (Fig. 2) also shows the slightly higher left atrial (2–4 mm Hg) pressure difference which can normally be expected.

To calculate mitral valve gradient, average 10 consecutive mitral valve gradient areas (Fig. 1, shaded area) when data is obtained from patients in atrial fibrillation or 5 gradient areas from sinus rhythm. The fastest paper recording speed (usually 100 mm/sec) with the pressure gradient displayed on the largest scale possible (usually a 0–40 mm Hg scale) is optimal.

In the patient in Figure 1, assuming the cardiac output

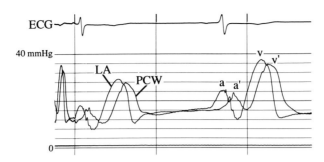

Fig. 2. Simultaneous pulmonary capillary wedge (PCW) and left atrial (LA) pressures in a patient in sinus rhythm. Pressure transmission from the left atrial to pulmonary capillary wedge is delayed 40–120 msec and reduced 2–4 mm Hg. a', v' = pulmonary capillary wedge pressure waves. See text for details. With permission from *The Cardiac Catheterization Handbook*, Kern (ed), p 150, 1991, Mosby-Year Book, Inc.

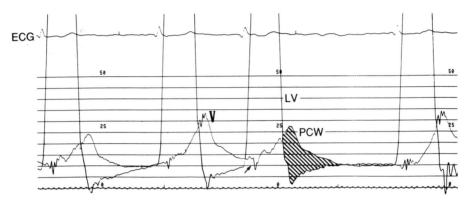

Fig. 3. Pulmonary capillary wedge (PCW) and left ventricular (LV) pressures in a patient with mild mitral stenosis/regurgitation in atrial fibrillation. Note the position of the C and V waves relative to left ventricular pressure and the equilibration of pulmonary capillary wedge-left ventricular pressures by the first 1/2 of diastole on long RR intervals. Cardiac output = 4.5 L/min; Mitral Valve Gradient = 8.4 mm Hg; Mitral Valve Area = 1.1 cm^2. See text for details.

is 3.5 L/min and heart rate 80 beats/min, the valve area by available data could be estimated as transvalvular flow/$\sqrt{\text{gradient}}$ (CO/$\sqrt{\text{gradient}}$ [Hakki "Quick" formula for aortic stenosis [9] as 3.5/$\sqrt{11}$ = 3.5/3.3 = 1.1 cm^2). The computation of valve area by the Gorlin formula is:

$$MVA = \frac{CO/DFP * HR}{K\sqrt{MVG}}$$

where CO = cardiac output (mL/minute); DFP = diastolic filling period (sec); MVA = mitral valve area; MVG = mean valve gradient (mm Hg); K = constant from Gorlin's empiric data [10] for mitral values (44.3*0.8 = 38).

$$MVA = \frac{\dfrac{3,500}{0.34} * 80}{38\sqrt{10.85}} = \frac{129}{38*3.3} = \frac{129}{125} = 1.0 \text{ cm}^2$$

In mitral stenosis, the "quick" valve area estimate should be used with caution, if at all, especially in patients with tachycardia [11].

PATHOPHYSIOLOGY OF MITRAL STENOSIS

The fundamental hemodynamic lesion of mitral stenosis is the increased left atrial pressure due to restriction of normal outflow. Normal mitral valve flow patterns can be precisely described by Doppler-echocardiography (Fig. 4A). In sinus rhythm, mitral flow velocity has an initial peak filling wave occurring in early diastole (PE = peak early filling wave). This flow pattern is the result of passive filling from left ventricular relaxation and a "negative" left atrial-left ventricular gradient in early diastole [12]. Passive left atrial filling slows until atrial contraction produces the active flow velocity (peak A, PA). The PA wave corresponds to the left atrial and left ventricular A wave pressure.

In patients with mitral stenosis, the normal flow velocity pattern is dramatically altered. (Fig. 4B,C). The

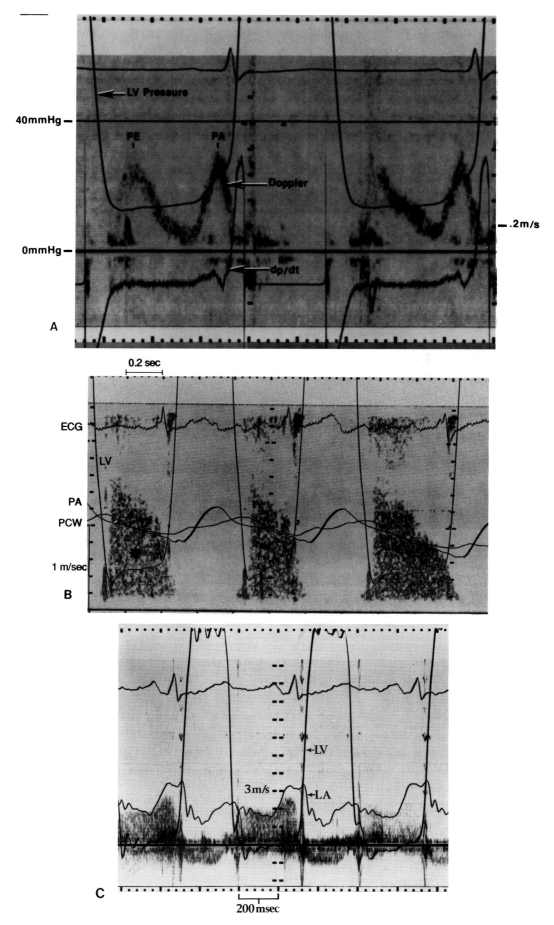

Fig. 4.

mitral flow velocity pattern parallels the left atrial-left ventricular gradient with a sustained increase in flow velocity occurring across all of diastole. The peak early velocity occurs earlier than the normal PE at the highest gradient point. The decline of flow velocity (and pressure) creates a characteristic velocity envelope with a flattened slope. The slope of diastolic flow is proportional to the severity of the stenosis [4]. In some patients with mitral stenosis in sinus rhythm, mitral flow velocity may increase with contractions, producing acceleration of blood at the wave (Fig. 4C). In other patients, the atrial flow wave is often abolished due to high pressure or atrial fibrillation. The mitral valve gradient (15 mm Hg, F.g 4B, asterisk) shows the characteristic diastolic velocity envelope with a maximal flow velocity of 1.8m/sec. The diastolic slope of flow velocity is used to compute mitral valve area by the left atrial pressure half-time method as described elsewhere [4,5]. The shape of mitral velocity envelope and the absolute flow velocity values are influenced by both the pressures in the left atrium and in the receiving left ventricular chamber and the net compliance of the individual chambers [6].

MITRAL STENOSIS AND REGURGITATION

In patients with concomitant mitral regurgitation, reversed high velocity flow can be identified occurring in under the systolic ejection period (Fig. 4C). The highest left atrial-left ventricular pressure gradient and flow velocity occurred at end diastole after atrial systole (Fig. 4C) with a regurgitant mitral flow velocity jet in a reversed direction seen immediately at the initiation of systole. Although the Gorlin method of calculating mitral valve area in patients with pure mitral stenosis is universally accepted, in patients with coexisting valvular regurgitation, the formula underestimates the true valve area. Forward cardiac output is used in the numerator of

Fig. 4. A: Combined hemodynamic and Doppler flow velocity signals demonstrating normal mitral flow physiology. PA = peak atrial filling wave; PE = peak early filling wave velocity. (Velocity scale is 0.2m/sec per division.) With permission from *The Cardiac Catheterization Handbook,* Kern (ed), p 333, 1991, Mosby-Year Book, Inc. B: Combined hemodynamic and Doppler echocardiographic data demonstrating severe mitral stenosis. LV = left ventricular pressure; PA = pulmonary artery pressure; PCW = pulmonary capillary wedge (pressure scale 0–40 mm Hg). * denotes mitral flow velocity envelope with classical appearance of mitral stenosis. The highest flow velocity (approximately 1.8m/sec) corresponds to the largest left ventricular-pulmonary capillary wedge gradient in early diastole. With permission from *The Cardiac Catheterization Handbook,* Kern (ed), p 335, 1991, Mosby-Year Book, Inc. C: Left atrial (LA) and left ventricular (LV) pressures in a patient with mitral stenosis and regurgitation. Note reversal of flow velocity during systole (arrow) due to mitral regurgitation. With permission from reference 15.

the formula and does not account for the regurgitant fraction contributing to the total transmitral diastolic flow. Qualitative correction for angiographic degree of valvular regurgitation has significant limitations and, therefore, is not generally used. Quantitative cineangiographic left ventricular stroke volume provides a more precise value in the numerator of flow in the Gorlin formula and has improved the accuracy of valve area calculation [13], but requires meticulous technique. Left ventricular volume calculations may be distorted in patients with atrial fibrillation or extra systoles during ventriculography.

ALTERNATIVE METHODS FOR VALVE AREA CALCULATIONS

Three alternative methods, the pressure half-time method of Libanoff and Rodbard [14], the Doppler mitral velocity half-time method, and two-dimensional echo planimetry, are currently available for computing mitral valve area (Fig. 5A).

Pressure Half-Time Methods

Using the simultaneous left atrial and left ventricular diastolic pressures in patients with combined mitral stenosis and regurgitation, the maximal transmitral valve gradient occurring during the 120 msec of diastolic filling period is measured (Fig. 5B). From this point (marked zero time), the diastolic pressure gradient is measured in 20 msec intervals until the onset of ventricular systole. The logrhythm of each transmitral diastolic pressure difference measured at 20 msec intervals is plotted against time. Using a linear extrapolation to the Y axis, the time required for pressure difference to decrease from the extrapolated maximal gradient to one-half that value is the hemodynamic pressure half-time. Pressure half-time in mild mitral stenosis is 100–200 msec, moderate 200–300 msec, and severe >300 msec. Normal valves have a pressure half-time of <25 msec [14]. In patients with combined mitral stenosis and regurgitation, the mitral valve area by the hemodynamic pressure half-time method correlated closely with valve areas determined by Doppler echocardiography (r = 0.90) [15].

Doppler Method

Doppler methodology employs a slightly different technique where the flow velocity is substituted for pressure [16]. The pressure half-time from Doppler is computed as $220/T_{1/2}$, where $T_{1/2}$ is the time from peak to one-half of peak (peak$_{1/2}$) velocity. Peak$_{1/2}$ velocity is the peak mitral velocity divided by 1.4, representing the velocity at which the diastolic transvalvular pressure gradient has fallen by one-half. The Doppler pressure half-

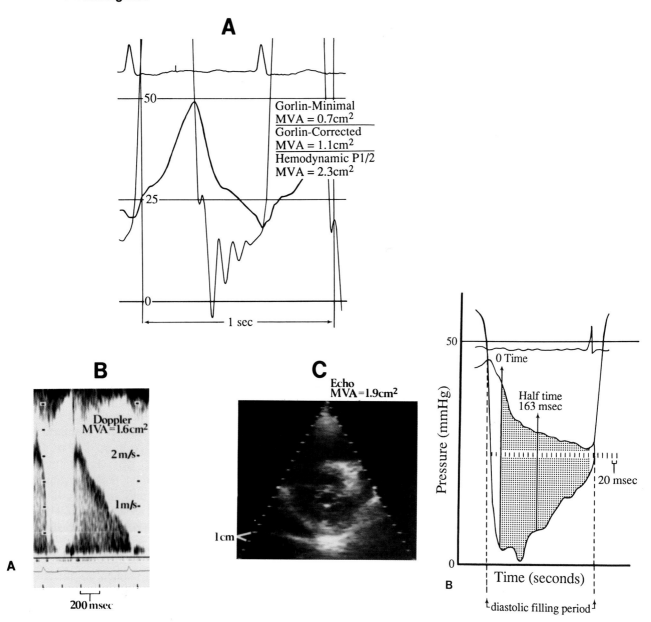

Fig. 5. A: Hemodynamic, Doppler, and two-dimensional echocardiographic data from a single patient with mitral stenosis and 4+ mitral regurgitation. (A) Simultaneous left atrial and left ventricular pressures showing diastolic transmitral pressure gradient. The mitral valve areas (MVA) calculated by the Gorlin formula, Gorlin formula corrected for mitral regurgitation, and the hemodynamic pressure half-time ($P_{1/2}$) method are shown. (B) Doppler velocity tracings of transmitral flow. The mitral valve area calculated by the Doppler half-time method is shown. (C) Parasternal short-axis view of the mitral valve orifice frozen during diastole. The mitral valve area determined by planimetry is shown. With permission from reference 15. B: Simultaneous left atrial and left ventricular diastolic pressures in a patient with combined mitral stenosis and regurgitation. The maximal transmitral gradient occurring during the initial 120 msec of the diastolic filling period is measured. From this point, marked "0 time," the diastolic pressure gradient is measured at 20 msec intervals until the onset of ventricular systole. Shaded area shows the diastolic transmitral pressure gradient diminishing with time from the initial peak level. The pressure half-time for this diastolic period is shown. With permission from reference 15.

time value has been shown to correlate well with the severity of mitral stenosis at catheterization [15,16]. A modification of this technique has been proposed by Halbe et al. [5] with an equally reliable determination for Doppler derived mitral valve area. The Gorlin formula with and without correction for mitral regurgitation did not correlate as well with the Doppler estimated valve areas (r = 0.47 and r = 0.56, respectively) [15].

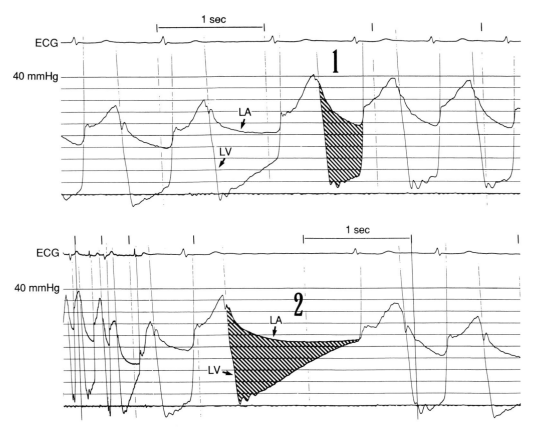

Fig. 6. Top: Left atrial (LA) and left ventricular (LV) pressures in a patient with atrial fibrillation. Beat #1 with short RR interval produces large gradient (mitral valve gradient = 22 mm Hg) with reduced mitral valve area. Bottom: Beat #2 with long RR interval (mitral valve gradient = 29 mm Hg) demonstrates left atrial-left ventricular pressure equilibration at end diastole. See text for details.

Two-Dimensional Echocardiographic Planimetry

Correlation between Doppler-derived mitral valve area and planimetered valve area from two-dimensional echocardiography was satisfactory (r = 0.84) compared to the hemodynamic pressure half-time method with planimetry (r = 0.78) [15]. The Gorlin formula, even with correction for mitral regurgitation, did not correlate well with two-dimensional echocardiographic planimetered valve areas (r = 0.30 and r = 0.35, respectively). These comparisons indicated that in patients with combined mitral valve disease, the hemodynamic pressure half-time method was more accurate than the Gorlin formula and should be considered for hemodynamic assessment of mitral valve area orifice in patients with mixed mitral valve disease given the limitations of the method [14–16].

INFLUENCE OF HEART RATE ON DETERMINATION OF VALVE AREA

The Gorlin formula works best in patients in sinus rhythm with no mitral regurgitation, normal left ventric-ular function, and no other valve lesions. Mitral valve area calculation using hemodynamic parameters may be especially difficult in patients with atrial fibrillation, tachycardia, mitral regurgitation, or low cardiac output states. In these patients, numerous studies [16,17] indicate that clinical correlation with Doppler echocardiography will provide additional information enhancing clinical decision making.

The effect of heart rate on the mitral valve gradient is evident from the hemodynamic data obtained in a 39 yr old woman with systolic and diastolic murmurs (Fig. 6). Echocardiography confirmed moderate-severe mitral stenosis with mild regurgitation. Note the dramatic difference in gradient areas between the short and long RR intervals. In Figure 6, end-diastolic equilibration of left atrial and left ventricular pressure occurs only during the longest RR interval. Compare this gradient to that in Figure 3 which achieves equilibration by mid diastole in a patient with only mild mitral stenosis and moderate regurgitation. The gradient at mid point in the longest diastolic cycle of Figure 6 is 12 mm Hg compared to 0 mm Hg in the longest cycle in Figure 3. The pressure gradient areas between beats may differ by >30% depending on the RR interval. Since the square root of the mean valve gradient is used in the calculation, these differences have less effect on valve area, but for increased accuracy, the average of >5 consecutive beats is used.

SUMMARY

The mitral valve gradient is dependent on the precise measurement of left atrial (or pulmonary capillary wedge) and left ventricular pressures. Artifacts involving either pressure measurement will produce inaccuracies which may have clinical significance. Several methods and formulas using both invasive and noninvasive techniques should verify clinical findings and confirm the severity of mitral valve disease prior to definite therapy. The changes in mitral valve gradients after balloon catheter valvuloplasty will be discussed in part II of this hemodynamic rounds.

ACKNOWLEDGMENTS

The authors thank the J.G. Mudd Cardiac Catheterization Laboratory Team and Donna Sander for manuscript preparation.

REFERENCES

1. McKay CR, Kawanishi DT, Kotlewski A, Parise K, Odom-Maryon T, Gonzales A, Reid CL, Rahimtoola SH: Improvement in exercise capacity and exercise hemodynamics 3 months after double-balloon catheter balloon valvuloplasty treatment of patients with symptomatic mitral stenosis. Circulation 77: 1013–1021, 1988.
2. Palacios IF, Block PC, Wilkins GT, Weyman AE: Follow-up of patients undergoing percutaneous mitral balloon valvotomy. Circulation 79:573–579, 1989.
3. Turi ZG, Reyes VP, Raju S, Raju AR, Kumar DN, Rajagopal P, Sathyanarayana PV, Rao DP, Srinath K, Peters P, Connors B, Fromm B, Farkas P, Wynne J: Percutaneous balloon versus surgical closed commissurotomy for mitral stenosis: a prospective, randomized trial. Circulation 83:1179–1185, 1991.
4. Hatle L, Angelsen B, Tromsdal A: Noninvasive assessment of atrioventricular pressure half-time by Doppler ultrasound. Circulation 60:1096–1104, 1979.
5. Halbe D, Bryg RJ, Labovitz AJ: A simplified method for calculating mitral valve area using Doppler echocardiography. Am Heart J 116:877–879, 1988.
6. Thomas JD, Wilkins GT, Choong CYP, Abascal VM, Palacios IF, Block PC, Weyman AE: Inaccuracy of mitral pressure half-time immediately after percutaneous mitral valvotomy: dependence on transmitral gradient and left atrial and ventricular compliance. Circulation 78:980–993, 1988.
7. Kern MJ: Hemodynamic rounds: interpretation of cardiac pathophysiology from pressure waveform analysis. The left-sided V wave. Cathet Cardiovasc Diagn 23:211–218, 1991.
8. Lange RA, Moore DM, Cigarroa RG, Hillis LD: Use of pulmonary capillary wedge pressure to assess severity of mitral stenosis: is true left atrial pressure needed in this condition? J Am Coll Cardiol 13:825–829, 1989.
9. Hakki AH, Iskandrian AS, Bemis CE, Kimbiris D, Mintz GS, Segal BL, Brice C: A simplified valve formula for the calculation of stenotic cardiac valve areas. Circulation 63:1050–1055, 1981.
10. Gorlin R, Gorlin G: Hydraulic formula for calculation of the area of the stenotic mitral valve, other cardiac valves, and central circulatory shunts. Am Heart J 41:1–29, 1951.
11. Brogan WC III, Lange RA, Hillis LD: Simplified formula for the calculation of mitral valve area: potential inaccuracies in patients with tachycardia. Cathet Cardiovasc Diagn 23:81–83, 1991.
12. Courtois M, Kovâcs SJ, Jr., Ludbrook PA: The transmitral pressure-flow velocity relationship: the importance of regional pressure gradients in the left ventricle. Circulation 78:661–671, 1988.
13. Grossman W: Profiles in valvular heart disease. In Grossman W (ed): "Cardiac Catheterization and Angiography, 4th Ed." Philadelphia: Lea & Febiger, 1991, pp 565–566.
14. Libanoff AJ, Rodbard S: Atrioventricular pressure half-time: measure of mitral valve orifice area. Circulation 38:144–150, 1968.
15. Fredman CS, Pearson AC, Labovitz AJ, Kern MJ: Comparison of hemodynamic pressure half-time method and Gorlin formula with Doppler and echocardiographic determinations of mitral valve area in patients with combined mitral stenosis and regurgitation. Am Heart J 119:121–129, 1990.
16. Smith MD, Wisenbaugh T, Grayburn PA, Gurley JC, Spain MG, DeMaria AN: Value and limitations of Doppler pressure half-time in quantifying mitral stenosis: a comparison with micromanometer catheter recordings. Am Heart J 121:480–488 ,1991.
17. Bryg RJ, Williams GA, Labovitz AJ, Aker U, Kennedy HL: Effect of atrial fibrillation and mitral regurgitation on calculated mitral valve area in mitral stenosis. Am J Cardiol 57:634–638, 1986.

Chapter 10

Mitral Valve Gradients—Section II

Morton J. Kern, MD, and Frank V. Aguirre, MD

INTRODUCTION

The effect of valvuloplasty on pressure gradients and valve area calculations is often dramatic and has been discussed in previous rounds [1]. Balloon catheter valvuloplasty is now commonly performed in patients with mitral stenosis, including patients with heavily calcific and deformed mitral valve apparatus [2–4]. A recently reported randomized prospective trial comparing balloon catheter commissurotomy with surgical closed commissurotomy in 40 patients with severe rheumatic mitral stenosis revealed that comparable hemodynamic improvement is achieved and sustained through 8 mo of follow-up at a 50% reduction in the cost of the procedure [4]. This rounds will present hemodynamics of mitral valvuloplasty and its effects on the mitral gradient and pressure waveforms.

Examine the hemodynamic data obtained in a 52-yr-old woman with mitral stenosis and class III symptoms (Fig. 1, upper panel). The tracings show atrial fibrillation with well demarcated left atrial C waves and large V waves (up to 55 mm Hg). The mitral gradient was 16 mm Hg before valvuloplasty with a cardiac output of 4.1 L/min, yielding a calculated mitral valve area of 1.0 cm². There was no angiographic mitral regurgitation, also confirmed by transesophageal echocardiography which is now performed in all our patients to document the absence of left atrial thrombus prior to mitral valvuloplasty. Mitral balloon valvuloplasty using standard 2-balloon technique [3,4] produced a marked reduction in the left atrial pressure and mitral valve gradient (Fig. 1, lower panel). After valvuloplasty, the mean gradient was 5 mm Hg, cardiac output was unchanged (4.2 L/min), and the calculated mitral valve area increased to 2.1 cm²

with new but mild (1 +) mitral regurgitation. Note the differences in the left atrial pressure waveform after valvuloplasty. Sinus rhythm with first degree AV block produced an A wave. Both the C and V waves are markedly reduced. The atrial pressure waveform after balloon mitral valve commissurotomy is the result of multiple factors relating to improved flow and mostly likely a concomitant shift in the left atrial compliance [5,6]. The hemodynamic factors influencing the atrial pressure are strongly dependent on chamber compliance and peak transmitral pressure gradient, two variables which change dramatically with valvuloplasty, rendering the pressure half-time method unreliable in the setting of rapidly changing mitral valve function after balloon valvular dilatation and commissurotomy [5,7].

Mitral valve gradients may be completely eliminated in some patients with balloon valvuloplasty. Compare the hemodynamics of the mitral valve in a 29-yr-old woman with mitral stenosis and regurgitation (Fig. 2) to the previous patient. Before valvuloplasty (Fig. 2, upper panel), large left atrial V waves (to 50 mm Hg) and 2 + mitral regurgitation on ventriculography were present. The left atrial pressure wave is damped (compared to Fig. 1) with slightly delayed and rounded C and V wave peaks. The left ventricular pressure was underdamped with a "ringing" artifact. The mean mitral gradient was 14 mm Hg. Atrial fibrillation produced marked differences among valve gradients, evident when comparing beat #1 and #3 (the shaded beat). Cardiac output was 5.6 L/min, yielding a calculated mitral valve area of 1.2 cm². After mitral valvuloplasty (Fig. 2, lower panel), left atrial and ventricular catheters (and pressure manifolds) were flushed. The left atrial pressure corresponds closely to left ventricular pressure throughout diastole. There is

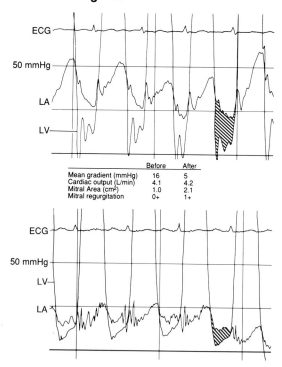

	Before	After
Mean gradient (mmHg)	16	5
Cardiac output (L/min)	4.1	4.2
Mitral Area (cm²)	1.0	2.1
Mitral regurgitation	0+	1+

Fig. 1. Left atrial (LA) and left ventricular (LV) pressures before (top) and after (bottom) balloon catheter mitral commissurotomy. See text for discussion. With permission from *The Cardiac Catheterization Handbook,* Kern (ed), p 166, 1991, Mosby-Year Book, Inc.

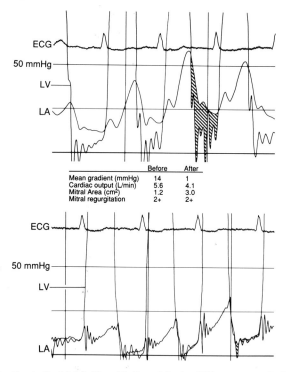

	Before	After
Mean gradient (mmHg)	14	1
Cardiac output (L/min)	5.6	4.1
Mitral Area (cm²)	1.2	3.0
Mitral regurgitation	2+	2+

Fig. 2. Left atrial (LA) and left ventricular (LV) pressures before (top) and after (bottom) balloon catheter mitral commissurotomy. See text for discussion. With permission from *The Cardiac Catheterization Handbook,* Kern (ed), p 167, 1991, Mosby-Year Book, Inc.

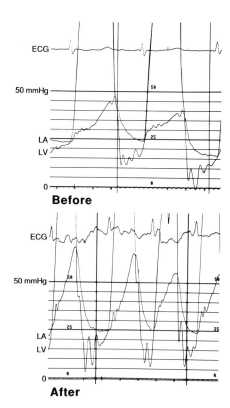

Before

After

Fig. 3. Left atrial (LA) and left ventricular (LV) pressures in a patient with mitral stenosis before (top) and after (bottom) balloon catheter mitral valvuloplasty. Note larger V waves after the procedure. See text for details.

virtually no mitral valve gradient. The cardiac output, although decreased to 4.1 L/min, yields a mitral valve area of 3.0 cm². There was no change in the angiographic degree of mitral regurgitation. The diminution of left atrial V waves again indicates improved left atrial chamber compliance without change in valvular regurgitation.

Fig. 4. A: Pulmonary capillary wedge (PCW) and left ventricular (LV) pressures in a patient with mitral stenosis before valvuloplasty. From the pressure tracings, what is the rhythm? Should this tracing be used to compute mitral valve area? See text for details. B: Left atrial (LA) and left ventricular (LV) pressures in the patient in Figure 4A. From this pressure tracing, what is the rhythm? Should this tracing be used to compute mitral valve area? See text for details. C: Simultaneous pulmonary capillary wedge (PCW) and left atrial (LA) pressures in a patient with mitral stenosis. Is pulmonary capillary wedge satisfactory for gradient determination in this case? See text for details. D: Pulmonary capillary wedge (PCW) and left ventricular (LV) pressures after mitral valvuloplasty. A successful procedure? E: Left atrial (LA) and left ventricular (LV) pressures after mitral valvuloplasty obtained at the same time as pressures in D. Explain the large C wave on the last beat. See text for details.

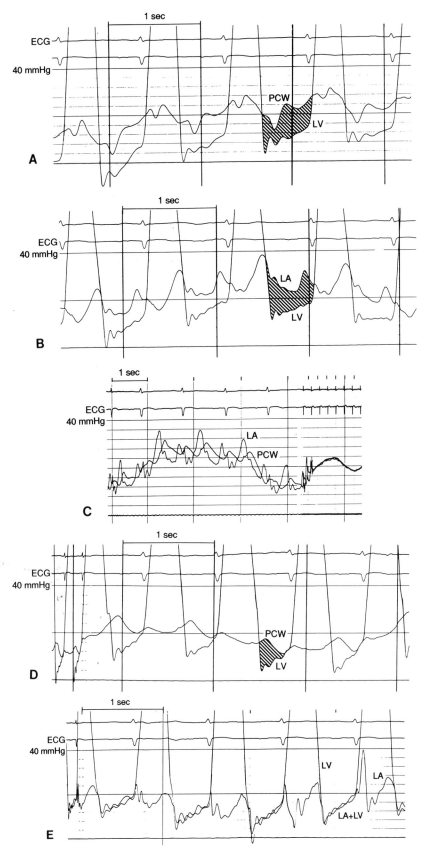

Fig. 4A–E

MITRAL REGURGITATION AFTER BALLOON VALVULOPLASTY

Inherent to mitral balloon valvuloplasty or surgical commissurotomy is excessive valvular dilatation or leaflet tearing resulting in malcoaptation of the leaflets with valvular regurgitation. Fortunately, mitral regurgitation is an infrequent complication [1–4]. Of 40 patients undergoing mitral commissurotomy randomized to the balloon catheter or surgical approach, only 2 had severe mitral regurgitation at the completion of either procedure [4].

Consider the hemodynamic tracings obtained in a 56-yr-old woman with severe mitral stenosis undergoing balloon catheter mitral valvuloplasty (Fig. 3, upper panel). Before valvuloplasty, the left atrial pressure mean was 23 mm Hg with V waves to 45 mm Hg and an evident absence of atrial activity (atrial fibrillation). The downslope of the V wave was moderately delayed consistent with severe mitral stenosis. Angiographic mitral regurgitation was minimal. The corresponding left ventricular end-diastolic pressure was approximately 20 mm Hg. The mitral valve gradient of 12 mm Hg yielded a valve area of calculation of 0.95 cm^2.

After valvuloplasty (Fig. 3, lower panel), large V waves (twice the mean pressure) to 70 mm Hg are seen and are associated with the new severe angiographic mitral regurgitation. The V waves now have a steep downslope (Y descent) with only a modest reduction in the mean left atrial-ventricular gradient (approximately 8 mm Hg with an increased heart rate). The left atrial-left ventricular end-diastolic gradient is still evident. Although valve area was enlarged (1.6 cm^2), severe mitral regurgitation produced congestive heart failure requiring mitral valve replacement 2 d after the procedure.

USE OF THE PULMONARY CAPILLARY WEDGE DURING VALVULOPLASTY

Mitral valve area calculations using pulmonary capillary wedge pressure tracings can be misleading [8], an especially critical issue when using the pulmonary capillary wedge pressure for monitoring the progress of valve dilation during valvuloplasty. A 31-yr-old woman with rheumatic mitral stenosis had class III congestive heart failure 4 mo post-partum. Fatigue and shortness of breath occurred with minimal activity during the course of routine newborn child care. Non-invasive evaluation confirmed mitral stenosis. Balloon catheter mitral valve commissurotomy was requested. Left ventricular and pulmonary capillary wedge pressures were measured simultaneously using fluid-filled systems (Fig. 4A). Despite attention to manifold and catheter flushing, and catheter positioning, the pulmonary capillary wedge trac-

ing shown was the best that could be obtained with the balloon-tipped thermodilution catheter. Are the pressure tracings satisfactory for mitral valve area assessment? Based on the pressures, is the patient in sinus rhythm?

The pulmonary capillary wedge tracing is of poor quality. A poor waveform may be due to improper positioning (over-wedging), damping due to a bubble, catheter or pressure line kink, or inadequate flushing of the fluid path. The placement of a balloon-tipped catheter in this patient was difficult. Repositioning of the catheter and flushing did not produce a much better tracing. Left atrial pressure was then obtained with transseptal technique (Fig. 4B). One can appreciate the distinct A and V waves and elevated left atrial-left ventricular enddiastolic pressure with a mean gradient of 14 mm Hg. The more precise atrial pressure wave with a distinct A wave emphasizes the limitation of using the pulmonary capillary wedge in this case and easily confirms sinus rhythm.

The pulmonary capillary wedge pressure can be improved by checking four steps: 1) repositioning the catheter; 2) flushing the entire fluid to transducer path; 3) checking for catheter kinks; and 4) using a stiffer endhold catheter. Confirm pulmonary capillary wedge pressure by pulmonary capillary wedge saturation (>95%).

Before mitral valvuloplasty, the matching of left atrial and pulmonary capillary wedge pressures permits the operator to use (or exclude) a pulmonary capillary wedge pressure during intraprocedural monitoring periods when left atrial pressure is unobtainable. Compare the left atrial and pulmonary capillary wedge pressures in this patient (Fig. 4C). Although the 2 pressure means track together, phasic responses are not well matched.

During and after balloon valvuloplasty, the hemodynamic result was initially assessed by pulmonary capillary wedge and left ventricular pressures (Fig. 4D) (a 5 French pigtail catheter is positioned in the left ventricle for the duration of the entire procedure). A lower but persistent mitral gradient can be appreciated. Is the valve dilation satisfactory? Since the pulmonary capillary wedge tracing was suboptimal, the success of the procedure must be confirmed by direct measurement of the simultaneous left atrial and left ventricular pressures. Figure 4E shows that there is no residual mitral valve gradient with matching of left ventricular-left atrial diastolic pressures. One interesting feature of the left atrial pressure wave is the sharp C wave (Fig. 4E, last beat from right) produced by catheter migration into the left ventricular cavity in early systole. Repositioning of the left atrial catheter eliminated this waveform artifact.

SUMMARY

Balloon mitral commissurotomy in many patients will be as satisfactory as closed surgical commissurotomy.

Data from combined hemodynamic and echocardiographic techniques elegantly elucidate the mechanisms of mitral valve flow and pathophysiology of disturbed pressure relationships between the left atrial and left ventricular chambers, both before and after balloon valvuloplasty. The pulmonary capillary wedge pressure may not be satisfactory to assess the success of gradient reduction after mitral valvuloplasty.

ACKNOWLEDGMENTS

The authors thank the J.G. Mudd Cardiac Catheterization Laboratory Team and Donna Sander for manuscript preparation.

REFERENCES

1. Deligonul U, Kern MJ: Hemodynamic rounds: interpretation of cardiac pathophysiology from pressure waveform analysis. Percutaneous balloon valvuloplasty. Cathet Cardiovasc Diagn (in press), 1991.
2. McKay CR, Kawanishi DT, Kotlewski A, Parise K, Odom-Maryon T, Gonzales A, Reid CL, Rahimtoola SH: Improvement in exercise capacity and exercise hemodynamics 3 months after double-balloon catheter balloon valvuloplasty treatment of patients with symptomatic mitral stenosis. Circulation 77:1013–1021, 1988.
3. Palacios IF, Block PC, Wilkins GT, Weyman AE: Follow-up of patients undergoing percutaneous mitral balloon valvotomy. Circulation 79:573–579, 1989.
4. Turi ZG, Reyes VP, Raju S, Raju AR, Kumar DN, Rajagopal P, Sathyanarayana PV, Rao DP, Srinath K, Peters P, Connors B, Fromm B, Farkas P, Wynne J: Percutaneous balloon versus surgical closed commissurotomy for mitral stenosis: a prospective, randomized trial. Circulation 83:1179–1185, 1991.
5. Thomas JD, Wilkins GT, Choong CYP, Abascal VM, Palacios IF, Block PC, Weyman AE: Inaccuracy of mitral pressure half-time immediately after percutaneous mitral valvotomy: dependence on transmitral gradient and left atrial and ventricular compliance. Circulation 78:980–993, 1988.
6. Kern MJ: Hemodynamic rounds: interpretation of cardiac pathophysiology from pressure waveform analysis. The left-sided V wave. Cathet Cardiovasc Diagn (in press), 1991.
7. Hatle L, Angelsen B, Tromsdal A: Noninvasive assessment of atrioventricular pressure half-time by Doppler ultrasound. Circulation 60:1096–1104, 1979.
8. Lange RA, Moore DM, Cigarroa RG, Hillis LD: Use of pulmonary capillary wedge pressure to assess severity of mitral stenosis: is true left atrial pressure needed in this condition? J Am Coll Cardiol 13:825–829, 1989.

Chapter 11

Mitral Valve Gradients—Section III:
Mitral Stenosis and Pulsus Alternans

Morton J. Kern, MD

INTRODUCTION

For interested individuals, the classic article by Dr. Paul Wood [1] provides a most comprehensive and interesting background on the clinical and basic hemodynamic aspects of mitral stenosis. Paul Wood, as physician in charge of the Cardiac Department at the Brompton Hospital and as physician to the National Heart Hospital and Director of Studies at the Institute of Cardiology in London, personally characterized the clinical presentations, hemodynamic findings, electrocardiographic manifestations, and outcomes for 350 patients with mitral valve disease. The lecture, entitled "An Appreciation of Mitral Stenosis (Part I): Clinical Features," was delivered before the San Francisco Heart Association on October 29, 1953, and has stood the test of time, characterizing what we continue to understand as the most important aspects of mitral valve pathophysiology. This hemodynamic rounds discusses an unusual case of mitral stenosis and reviews the findings in the context of those observations of Dr. Wood.

CASE REPORT

A 73-year-old woman with dyspnea on exertion presented with complaints of progressive fatigue, breathlessness, weakness, and pedal edema over the last several months. She had known heart murmurs since childhood and had avoided medical attention for many years. She had had cardiac valve replacements for aortic stenosis 12 years ago and mitral stenosis 9 years ago, both with porcine valves. Physical examination demonstrated neck vein distension with prominent A waves and sinus tachycardia. Blood pressure was 123/77 mm Hg. There

was a diastolic murmur of mitral stenosis and II/VI murmur at the upper left sternal border. There was a short S_1-OS interval. There was no S_4 gallop. The abdomen was benign and the peripheral pulses were normal, without evidence of edema in the extremities.

Doppler echocardiography identified moderate prosthetic mitral stenosis without significant aortic stenosis or insufficiency. Hemodynamic evaluation was performed for continued dyspnea prior to consideration of a second mitral valve replacement. Left ventriculography showed mild (1+) mitral regurgitation with a normal ejection fraction (75%) and calcification of one mitral valve leaflet. Coronary angiography was normal. The mean right atrial pressure was 8 mm Hg with large "V" waves and prominent "Y" descents (Fig. 1, left). The right ventricular and pulmonary artery pressures were elevated, with a peak systolic pulmonary pressure of 70 mm Hg. Interestingly, there was pulmonary systolic pressure wave alternans (Fig. 1, middle and right). Pulsus alternans was also observed in the initial aortic (Fig. 2, left) and pulmonary capillary wedge pressure tracings (Fig. 3, top). The systolic right ventricular pressure (70 mm Hg) alternated with 50 mm Hg, despite evident respiratory variation (Fig. 1, middle). Similarly, the pulmonary artery pressure alternans (Fig. 1, right) could be seen within the normal cycle of respiration. Arterial and left ventricular pressures also demonstrated pulsus alternans with a systolic pressure of 180 mm Hg and a left ventricular end-diastolic pressure of 12 mm Hg, alternating with systolic pressures <140 mm Hg (Fig. 2, left). In reviewing the left ventricular hemodynamics, there was a 20 mm Hg peak-to-peak aortic valve gradient which is consistent with a 12-year-old calcified valve prosthesis.

In assessing the mitral valve hemodynamics, the pulmonary capillary wedge pressure was measured simulta-

G.S.

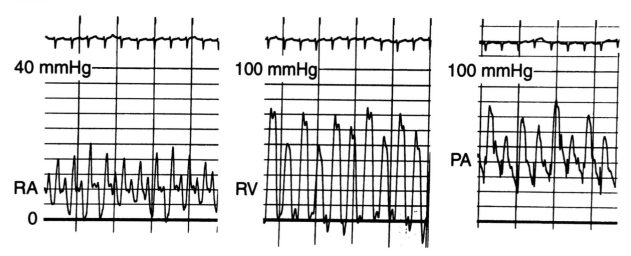

Fig. 1.   Right atrial (RA), right ventricular (RV), and pulmonary artery (PA) pressures on a 0–40 mm Hg scale and 0–100 mm Hg scale. RV pressure mean is approximately 8 mm Hg, with large "V" waves. PA and RV pressures demonstrate alternating systolic pressures.

G.S.

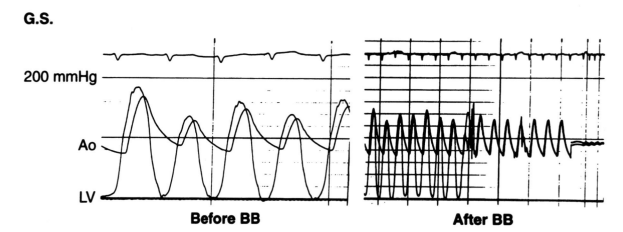

Fig. 2.   Aortic (Ao) pressure before and after beta blockade (BB) on a 0–200 mm Hg scale. Before beta blockade, hemodynamic tracings were recorded at a paper speed of 100 mm. After beta blockade, hemodynamic tracings are shown at a 25-mm paper speed. Note the attenuation of alternans after beta blockade.

neously with left ventricular end-diastolic pressure (Fig. 3). The mean pulmonary capillary wedge pressure was 34 mm Hg with "V" waves to 50 mm Hg. The pulmonary capillary wedge pressure, in addition to demonstrating alternans of the large "V" wave, produced a mean transmitral gradient of 22 mm Hg. To assess the effect of heart rate reduction, hemodynamics, including the mitral valve gradient, were measured before and again after intravenous esmolol (Fig. 3, bottom). Beta blockade slowed the heart rate from 120 to approximately 70 beats/min and reduced the mean pulmonary capillary wedge pressure from 32 mm Hg to 24 mm Hg and the

transmitral gradient from 22 mm Hg to 9 mm Hg. It is also noteworthy that in addition to reducing heart rate and mitral gradient, beta blockade abolished the pulsus alternans in the left ventricular and pulmonary capillary wedge pressures. The hemodynamic data are summarized in Table I.

To confirm the accuracy of the initial gradient using the pulmonary capillary wedge pressure, direct left atrial pressure measurements were made using the standard transseptal technique (Fig. 4). Compare the left atrial and pulmonary capillary wedge pressures (Fig. 4, right). After the administration of beta blockade, the mean mitral

G.S.

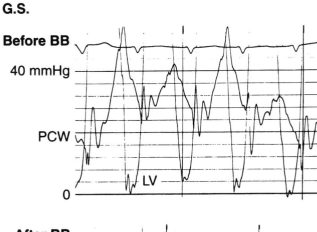

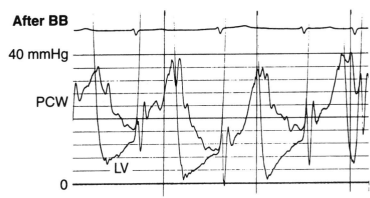

Fig. 3. Pulmonary capillary wedge (PCW) and left ventricular (LV) pressures on a 0–40 mm Hg scale before and after beta blockade (BB).

TABLE I. Hemodynamic Data

	Heart rate (bpm)	Right atrial (mm Hg)	Right ventricular (mm Hg)	Pulmonary artery (mm Hg)	Pulmonary capillary wedge (mm Hg)	Left atrial (mm Hg)	Left ventricular (mm Hg)	Aortic (mm Hg)	Cardiac output (l/min)	Mean gradient (mm Hg)	Mitral valve area (cm²)
Baseline	120	8	70/8	70/35	32	–	150/14	144/80	3.3	22	0.93
After beta blockade	70	–	–	–	24	22	140/10	132/78	4.0	9	1.50

gradient was calculated (using the left ventricular and direct left atrial pressure measurement) as 8 mm Hg. With a cardiac output of 4 l/min, the mitral valve area was calculated at 1.3–1.5 cm². The normalization of the arterial pulse (without alternans) and reduction of the pulmonary capillary wedge pressure, an unusual response, suggested improved cardiac function. The patient was treated medically.

DISCUSSION

This case is interesting in several respects: 1) in the setting of mitral stenosis, the presence of pressure alternans and its elimination with beta blockade; 2) the improvement in mitral valve gradient after beta blockade; and 3) the confirmatory gradient measurement with the transseptal approach.

When compared to the typical case described by Dr. Wood [1], the early clinical similarities remain striking, with a history of rheumatic fever in childhood, symptoms of dyspnea, a history of pulmonary edema, and paroxysmal nocturnal dyspnea. Most mitral stenosis cases [1] have elevations of the left atrial pressure (22–23 mm Hg) with cardiac outputs ranging from 3.5–4.6 l/min. The most common level of pulmonary resistance units is usually <4 Wood units with an average of 2.9 for patients with a history of pulmonary edema, of 4.7 with paroxysmal nocturnal dyspnea, and of 9.2 in patients without such symptoms.

To my knowledge, pulsus alternans is an unusual phenomenon in mitral valve disease and especially in mitral stenosis [2–5]. Pulsus alternans is most commonly associated with decreased left ventricular function, a condition not present by ventriculography or echocardiog-

G.S.

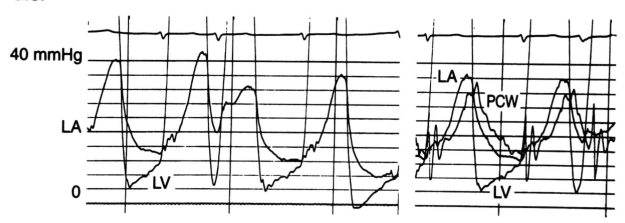

Fig. 4. Left: Left atrial (LA) and left ventricular (LV) pressures on a 0–40 mm Hg scale after beta blockade. Right: LA, pulmonary capillary wedge (PCW), and LV pressures on a 0–40 mm Hg scale simultaneously recorded.

raphy. More interesting is the abolition of pulsus alternans after beta blockade, which suggests a heart rate-related phenomenon and/or an improvement in ventricular function perhaps related to right ventricular contractility. We can only speculate on the mechanisms resulting in this unusual hemodynamic response. The reduced heart rate without pulsus alternans also permitted a more accurate calculation of mitral valve gradients [6–8].

The atrial waveforms are also interesting when compared to indirect left atrial tracings reported by Dr. Wood, who noted "A" waves higher than "V" waves in one third of patients, "A" and "V" waves of equal amplitude in 39%, and with "V" waves greater than "A" waves in 29%. Giant "A" waves, considered more than 5 mm Hg above the "V" wave, were a rare occurrence. The difference between the "A" and "V" is one of Wood's initial observations that we continue to discuss when presenting hemodynamics. He remarked that the difference between left and right atrial hemodynamics pertained principally to the height of the "A" and "V" waves [6]. The "A" wave was greater in the right than in the left atrium. Wood also noted considerable overlap between the size of "V" waves and stated, "It is fair to say that a "V" wave over 15 mm Hg in amplitude nearly always meant mitral incompetence and a "V" wave under 5 mm Hg nearly always excluded it." The "V" wave in the case example was 40 mm Hg with only mild mitral regurgitation. Certainly, postoperative chamber compliance can account for large "V" waves in the absence of significant valvular regurgitation [6], and such is the case in the patient example.

Left Atrial vs. Pulmonary Capillary Wedge Pressure

None will dispute that the most precise way to assess the mitral gradient is by the left atrial vs. left ventricular

pressures via the transseptal approach. However, when pulmonary capillary wedge pressure is low and normal, the clinical difference obtained using left atrial pressure to diagnose significant mitral stenosis is negligible. For several practical reasons, the pulmonary capillary wedge pressure remains a first-line tool for hemodynamic evaluation of mitral valve gradients. However, for patients with elevated pulmonary capillary wedge pressures or those with marginal pulmonary capillary wedge pressure waveforms, transseptal left atrial pressure will increase clinical confidence in the accuracy of measurements [9,10]

It is interesting to note that the pulmonary capillary wedge and left atrial pressures, although different in magnitude by 4 mm Hg, yielded nearly identical gradient measurements because the left atrial "V" wave peak, although higher than that of the pulmonary capillary wedge pressure, had a more rapid "V" wave decline. Thus, the area under the two pressure curves is similar [7,8].

CONCLUSIONS

The hemodynamics of mitral stenosis continue to provide interesting material on the subject of valvular heart disease. Careful inspection of the pressure waves will confirm previous observations and lead to insights into the pathophysiologic aspects of each individual patient.

ACKNOWLEDGMENTS

The author thanks the J.G. Mudd Cardiac Catheterization Laboratory for technical support and Donna Sander for manuscript preparation.

REFERENCES

1. Wood P: An appreciation of mitral stenosis: Part I. Clinical features. Brit Med J 1:1051–1064, 1954.
2. Laskey WK, St. John Sutton M, Unterecker WJ, Martin JL, Hirschfield JW: Mechanics of pulsus alternans in aortic valve stenosis. Am J Cardiol 52:809–812, 1983.
3. Hess OM, Surber EP, Ritter M, Krayenbuehl HP: Pulsus alternans: Its influence on systolic and diastolic function in aortic valve disease. J Am Coll Cardiol 4:1–7, 1984.
4. Gleason WL, Braunwald E: Studies on Starling's law of the heart. VI. Relationship between left ventricular end-diastolic volume and stroke volume in man with observations on the mechanism of pulsus alternans. Circulation 25:841–847, 1962.
5. Ryan JM, Schieve FJ, Hull HB, Osner BM: The influence of advanced congestive heart failure on pulsus alternans. Circulation 12:60–63, 1955.
6. Thomas JD, Wilkins GT, Choong CYP, Abascal VM, Palacios IF, Block PC, Weyman AE: Inaccuracy of mitral pressure half-time immediately after percutaneous mitral valvotomy: Dependence on transmitral gradient and left atrial and ventricular compliance. Circulation 78:980–988, 1988.
7. Bryg RJ, Williams GA, Labovitz AJ, Aker U, Kennedy HL: Effect of atrial fibrillation and mitral regurgitation on calculated mitral valve area in mitral stenosis. Am J Cardiol 57:634–638, 1986.
8. Brogan WC III, Lange RA, Hillis LD: Simplified formula for the calculation of mitral valve area: Potential inaccuracies in patients with tachycardia. Cathet Cardiovasc Diagn 23:81–83, 1991.
9. Lange RA, Moore DM, Cigarroa RG, Hillis LD: Use of pulmonary capillary wedge pressure to assess severity of mitral stenosis: Is true left atrial pressure needed in this condition? J Am Coll Cardiol 13:825–829, 1989.
10. Kern MJ, Aguirre FV: Mitral valve gradients: Part II. In Kern MJ (ed): "Hemodynamic Rounds: The Interpretation of Cardiac Pathophysiology From Pressure Waveform Analysis." New York: Wiley-Liss, 1993, pp 43–47.

Chapter 12

Mitral Valve Gradients—Section IV: Hemodynamic Evaluation of a Stenotic Bioprosthetic Mitral Valve

Elie Azrak, MD, Morton J. Kern, MD, Richard G. Bach, MD, and Thomas J. Donohue, MD

INTRODUCTION

The evaluation of the severity of prosthetic valve stenosis may be complicated by differences between hemodynamic and Doppler estimates of the degree of obstruction to flow [1,2]. Since postoperative and recuperative changes alter myocardial function and compliance, left atrial pressure-volume curves, and responses to exercise status, a precise determination of both resting and exercise-induced hemodynamic function requires careful examination. To illustrate the difficulty of assessing valve function based on hemodynamic and Doppler data, we present the hemodynamic data from a patient with prosthetic mitral valve stenosis evaluated several years after valve implantation.

CASE EXAMPLE

A 74-year-old woman reported progressive symptoms of dyspnea on exertion and decreasing exercise tolerance for the past year. She had a history of rheumatic mitral stenosis and two porcine mitral valve replacements, the first 20 yr earlier, and the second valve replacement 12 yr earlier. She had chronic atrial fibrillation but denied orthopnea or paroxysmal nocturnal dyspnea. A two-dimensional echocardiogram revealed thickened bioprosthetic mitral valve leaflets and moderate-to-severe mitral stenosis with an estimated valve area of 1.3 cm^2 without valvular regurgitation. Doppler flow velocity data suggested mild mitral stenosis with a peak velocity of 2 m/sec. Estimated pulmonary artery pressure of 30 mm Hg was also reported.

To evaluate the coronary artery disease and progres-

sion of hemodynamic valvular dysfunction, a right- and left-heart cardiac catheterization (including a transseptal approach) using fluid-filled catheters was performed. Right-heart hemodynamics demonstrated a mean right atrial pressure of 12 mm Hg with prominent "Y" descent (Fig. 1, top left), with an absent "A" wave or "X" descent due to the atrial fibrillation. The right ventricular pressure was 48/12 mm Hg (Fig. 1, middle top), pulmonary artery pressure was 48/16 mm Hg, and mean pulmonary capillary wedge pressure was 16 mm Hg, with prominent "V" waves (Fig. 1, bottom middle). A transseptal puncture using the Brockenbrough technique provided left atrial pressure averaging 16 mm Hg, with prominent "V" waves to 22 mm Hg (Fig. 1, top right and bottom left). Simultaneously recorded pulmonary artery and left atrial pressures (Fig. 1, top right) and left atrial and left ventricular pressures (Fig. 1, bottom left) are shown. Simultaneous aortic and left ventricular pressures (Fig. 1, bottom right) showed an aortic pressure of 125/70 mm Hg and left ventricular pressure of 125/18 mm Hg. There was no aortic valve gradient.

The mitral-valve pressure gradient was obtained from simultaneous recordings of left ventricular pressure using a 7F pigtail catheter and left atrial pressure using an 8F Brockenbrough catheter. For comparison, pulmonary capillary wedge pressure was also recorded (Fig. 1, bottom left).

After recording hemodynamics and thermodilution cardiac output at rest, data were then obtained during symptom-limited dynamic arm exercise. During exercise, heart rate increased from 55 to 65 beats/min with a moderate increase in pulmonary artery pressure (48/18 mm Hg to 60/30 mm Hg) and left ventricular end-diastolic pressure (16 mm Hg to 24 mm Hg) (Fig. 2).

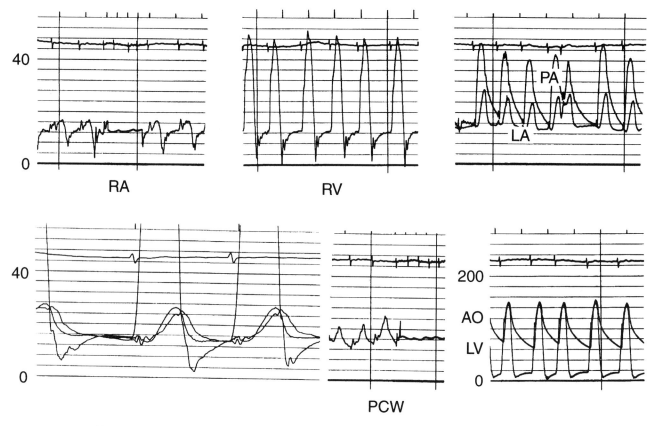

Fig. 1. Right and left heart hemodynamics at rest, demonstrating right atrial (RA, top left), right ventricular (RV, top right), and pulmonary artery (PA, top middle) pressures on a 0–40 mm Hg scale. Also shown are left atrial (LA), pulmonary capillary wedge (PCW), and left ventricular (LV) pressures on a 0–40 mm Hg scale (bottom left), and pulmonary capillary wedge (bottom middle, PCW) and aortic (Ao) and left ventricular (LV) pressures on a 0–200 mm Hg scale (bottom right).

There was no significant change in the mean mitral valve gradient (6 mm Hg to 8 mm Hg) (Fig. 3) or in the calculated prosthetic mitral valve area (1.30 cm²). The left ventricular, left atrial, and pulmonary artery pressures at rest and at peak dynamic arm exercise are compared in Figures 2 and 3. The hemodynamic data are summarized in Table I.

Based on the above findings, it was suspected that left ventricular dysfunction (evidenced by exercise-induced increased left ventricular end-diastolic pressure without significant decrease in mitral valve area or increase in mitral valve gradient) was, in part, responsible for the patient's symptoms. The patient was started on oral afterload reduction therapy. Repeat two-dimensional echocardiography was planned in 3–6 mo.

DISCUSSION

Assessment of prosthetic valves is a common clinical problem, with more than 60,000 valve replacements performed annually in the United States [1]. This patient example illustrates typical hemodynamics frequently re-

quired in the assessment of prosthetic mitral valve dysfunction, and highlights several potential limitations of conclusions based on the data.

Prosthetic Valves: Natural History

Prosthetic valves have different natural histories due to characteristics of durability, thrombogenicity, and hemodynamics. Prosthetic valves are classified as either bioprosthetic or mechanical. Mechanical valves are composed of metal or carbon alloys and have mechanisms described as caged-ball, single-tilting disks, or bileaflet tilting disks. Bioprosthetic valves may be manufactured from heterografts, composed of porcine or bovine tissue (either pericardial or valvular) which is supported by metal struts. Homograft bioprostheses are preserved human aortic valves. Mechanical valves have been documented to last 20–30 yr. In contrast, 10–20% of homograft bioprostheses fail within 10–15 yr. For heterograft bioprosthesis, 30% may fail within the same time period [2–4]. It is well-known that patients under age 40 yr have a high incidence of premature heterograft bioprosthetic valve failure. Bioprosthetic valves are preferred in patients who

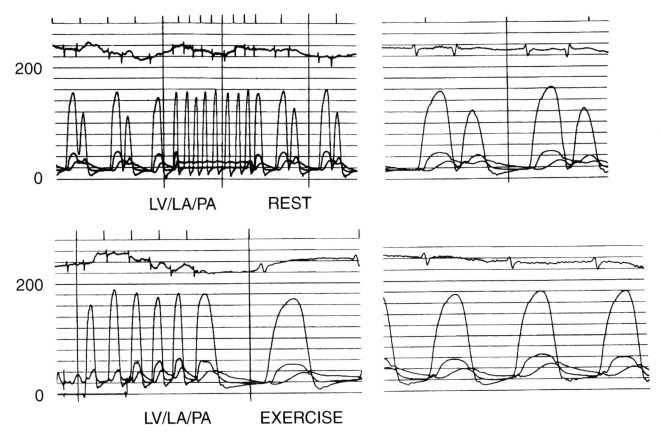

Fig. 2. Left ventricular (LV), left atrial (LA), and pulmonary artery (PA) pressures at rest and during exercise on a 0–200 mm Hg scale.

are elderly, have a life expectancy <10–15 yr, or who cannot take anticoagulants.

Valve Areas

For any given valve size, the heterograft bioprosthesis and caged-ball mechanical valves have the smallest effective orifice areas, whereas homograft bioprostheses have valve areas similar to those of native valves [5,6]. The data in the current case suggest a moderately narrowed mitral valve (1.3 cm²). This valve area may be compared to caged-ball valve areas for mitral prostheses ranging from 1.4–3.1 cm², for single-tilting discs ranging from 1.9–3.2 cm², and for heterograft bioprostheses ranging from 1.3–2.7 cm² [5,6].

Mechanisms of Prosthetic Valve Failure

The symptom complex associated with bioprosthetic valve failure usually involves the gradual onset of dyspnea and symptoms of heart failure as noted in the case example. The structural failure of bioprosthetic valve material may occur in 30% of heterografts within 10–15 yr of replacement [12,13]. The incidence of bioprosthetic valve failure is particularly high in younger patients, as previously noted. The most common mecha-

nism of bioprosthetic valve failure appears to be a tear or rupture of one or more valve cusps, resulting in severe regurgitation. Calcification and increased rigidity promote the destruction of the valve. Few patients develop severe valvular stenosis [14]. Bioprosthetic valve stenosis is initially detected by auscultation. The magnitude of valve dysfunction is principally assessed by echocardiography and cardiac catheterization before consideration of valve replacement.

Methods to Assess Valve Dysfunction

Several nonhemodynamic methods complement the assessment of prosthetic valve dysfunction. Cinefluoroscopy is a rapid, inexpensive, and often overlooked technique. Although the leaflets of a bioprosthetic valve cannot be visualized, the structural integrity of a mechanical valve, especially the motion of the disk ring or poppet, can indicate dysfunction due to tissue ingrowth or thrombus. Excessive rocking of the base ring may suggest partial dehiscence [7,8]. Cinefluoroscopy has been used to detect the separation of the outlet strut of a Bjork-Shiley tilting disk valve before complete strut fracture occurs [9].

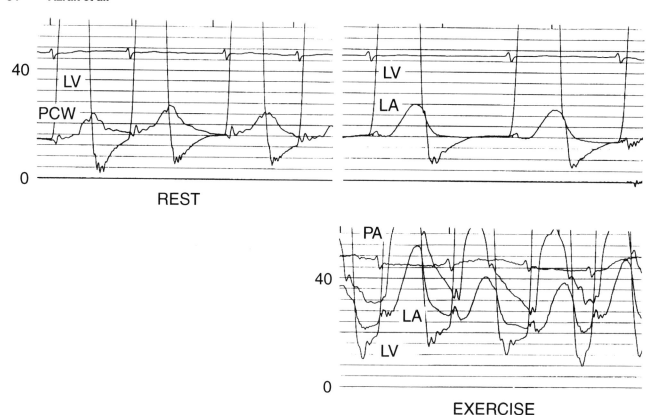

Fig. 3. Left ventricular (LV), pulmonary capillary wedge (PCW), left atrial (LA), and pulmonary artery (PA) pressures on a 0–40 mm Hg scale at rest and during exercise.

TABLE I. Hemodynamic Data

	Rest	Exercise
Heart rate (beats/min)	55	64
Right atrial mean pressure (mm Hg)	12	
Right ventricular pressure (mm Hg)	48/12	
Pulmonary artery pressure (mm Hg)	48/18	60/30
Pulmonary artery mean pressure (mm Hg)	26	40
Pulmonary capillary wedge mean pressure (mm Hg)	18	30
Left ventricular pressure (mm Hg)	150/16	190/24
Aortic pressure (mm Hg)	150/70	
Cardiac output (L/min)	3.2	3.6
Pulmonary vascular resistance (dynes · sec · cm^{-5})	200	222
Mitral valve gradient (mm Hg)	6	8
Mitral valve area (cm^2)	1.30	1.27

Two-dimensional and Doppler transthoracic echocardiography are the most popular modalities to assess sewing-ring stability, leaflet motion, and valve orifice area. In contrast to the transthoracic approach, transesophageal echocardiography (TEE) provides an improved viewing window for atrial and mitral valve planes and higher image resolution. The TEE technique is highly recommended for the assessment of prosthetic mitral valve dysfunction. However, because of flow masking, transesophageal echocardiography is somewhat limited in detecting aortic prosthetic valve obstruction or regurgita-

tion, especially when a concomitant mitral prosthesis is present [10,11]. Doppler echocardiography easily identifies prosthetic valve obstruction and valvular or perivalvular regurgitation and provides vital comparative data for serial evaluations.

Hemodynamic Assessment of Prosthetic Valve Dysfunction

Transvalvular hemodynamic data from catheterization are used as a gold standard in calculating the effective valve orifice area. Although a catheter can be safely passed through a bioprosthetic valve without adverse hemodynamic effects, the most accurate method of obtaining hemodynamic data is that which does not interfere with valvular motion. For tilting disc valves, catheter entrapment in the minor orifice has been associated with complications and, rarely, the requirement of surgical catheter removal. Hemodynamic evaluation of valvular dysfunction is indicated when noninvasive methods remain inconclusive or contradictory, and is confirmatory when performed in the routine course of preoperative coronary angiography.

Despite initial noninvasive evaluation, diagnostic hemodynamics, performed at the time of coronary angiography, add to the considerations for valve replacement. In the case example, the symptoms during initial evaluation were not attributed to the severity of mitral stenosis. However, the Doppler evaluation prompted further investigation. Hemodynamics of mild mitral stenosis of either native or prosthetic valves may not be representative of the conditions during daily activity which produce symptoms. Exercise-induced hemodynamic alterations during cardiac catheterization may be required to associate symptoms with the corresponding hemodynamics. In some cases, exercise hemodynamics may separate valvular from left ventricular dysfunction. In the present case, during exercise, the left ventricular, pulmonary capillary wedge, and pulmonary artery pressures increased substantially with no change in mitral valve gradient or calculated area. The exercise cardiac output failed to increase normally and may explain why the patient reported dyspnea on exertion without alteration in the calculated mitral valve area. It remains unclear whether such a patient may also show improvement after mitral valve replacement.

Pulmonary Capillary Wedge vs. Left Atrial Pressure

When pulmonary capillary wedge pressure is low and normal, transseptal left atrial pressure is generally unnecessary. When abnormal, pulmonary capillary wedge pressure may be erroneously high and elevate the calculation of the mitral gradient [15]. Misinterpretation of the pressure gradient based on an improperly (usually overly damped) wedged or misleading pulmonary artery pressure results in an overestimation of left atrial pressure and higher transmitral gradient. Confirmation of pulmonary capillary wedge pressure may be performed through several different techniques: 1) a stable wedge position occurs with a "fern" pattern on contrast injection seen on fluoroscopy; 2) an accurately timed "V" wave will be related to the "T" wave of the electrocardiogram; 3) the pulmonary capillary wedge blood oxygen saturation is equal to left atrial blood oxygen saturation; and 4) importantly, the pulmonary artery diastolic pressure should be greater than the pulmonary capillary wedge pressure. As in our case example, use of the transseptal technique to measure left atrial pressure directly had significant importance and probably should be considered the technique of choice for prosthetic mitral valve pressure measurements.

Exercise Hemodynamics

The absence of a significant increase in mean mitral valve gradient during dynamic arm exercise argues against the presumption that the patient's progressive dyspnea on exertion is solely attributable to severe mitral stenosis. Constant pulmonary vascular resistance with exercise (Table I) also suggests that the development of a "second stenosis," i.e., organic obliterative changes in the pulmonary vascular bed which are a complication of long-standing severe mitral stenosis, was not advanced.

SUMMARY

The evaluation of prosthetic valves requires accurate and, at times, dynamic hemodynamic measurements. The operator's confidence in the data can be increased by using the transseptal technique for prosthetic valves in both the mitral and aortic positions.

ACKNOWLEDGMENTS

The authors thank the J.G. Mudd Cardiac Catheterization Team (Saint Louis University Health Sciences Center, St. Louis, MO) for technical support and Donna Sander for manuscript preparation.

REFERENCES

1. Vongpatanasin W, Hillis LD, Lange RA: Prosthetic heart valves. N Engl J Med 335:407–416, 1996.
2. Yacoub M, Rasmi NRH, Sundt TM, Lund O, Boyland E, Radley-Smith R, Khaghani A, Mitchell A: Fourteen-year experience with homovital homografts for aortic valve replacement. J Thorac Cardiovasc Surg 110:186–194, 1995.
3. O'Brien MF, Stafford EG, Gardner MA, Pohlner PG, Tesar PJ, Cochrane AD, Mau TK, Gall KL, Smith SE: Allograft aortic valve replacement: Long-term follow-up. Ann Thorac Surg [Suppl 1] 60:65–70, 1995.
4. Bloomfield P, Wheatley DJ, Prescott RJ, Miller HC: Twelve-year comparison of a Bjork-Shiley mechanical heart valve with porcine bioprostheses. N Engl J Med 324:573–579, 1991.
5. Gray RJ, Chaux A, Matloff JM, DeRobertis M, Raymond M, Stewart M, Yoganathan A: Bi-leaflet, tilting disc and porcine aortic valve substitutes: In vivo hydrodynamic characteristics. J Am Coll Cardiol 3:321–327, 1984.
6. McAnulty JH, Morton M, Rahimtoola SH, Kloster FE, Ahuja N, Starr AE: Hemodynamic characteristics of the composite strut ball valve prostheses (Starr-Edwards track valves) in patients on anticoagulation. Circulation [Suppl 1] 58:159–161, 1978.
7. Czer LSC, Matloff J, Chaux A, DeRobertis M, Yoganathan A, Gray RJ: A 6 year experience with the St. Jude medical valve: Hemodynamic performance, surgical results, biocompatibility and follow-up. J Am Coll Cardiol 6:904–912, 1985.
8. Vogel W, Stoll HP, Bay W, Frohlig G, Schieffer H: Cineradiography for determination of normal and abnormal function in mechanical heart valves. Am J Cardiol 71:225–232, 1993.
9. O'Neill WW, Chandler JG, Gordon RE, Bakalyar DM, Abolfathi AH, Castellani MD, Hirsch JL, Wieting DW, Bassett JS, Beatty KC: Radiographic detection of strut separation in Bjork-Shiley convexo-concave mitral valves. N Engl J Med 333:414–419, 1995.

10. Mohr-Kahaly S, Kupferwasser I, Eerbel R, Wittlich N, Iversen S, Oelert H, Meyer J: Valve and limitations of transesophageal echocardiography in the evaluation of aortic prostheses. J Am Soc Echocardiog 6:12–20, 1993.
11. Karalis DG, Chandrasekaran K, Ross JJ Jr, Micklin A, Brown BM, Ren JF, Mintz GS: Single-plane transesophageal echocardiography for assessing function of mechanical or bioprosthetic valves in the aortic valve position. Am J Cardiol 79:1310–1315, 1992.
12. Grunkemeier GL, Jamieson WRE, Miller DC, Starr A: Actuarial versus actual risk of porcine structural valve deterioration. J Thorac Cardiovasc Surg 108:709–718, 1994.
13. Gallo I, Ruiz B, Nistral F, Duran CMG: Degeneration in porcine bioprosthetic cardiac valves: Incidence of primary tissue failures among 938 bioprostheses at risk. Am J Cardiol 53:1061–1065, 1984.
14. Scohen EJ, Hobson CE: Anatomic analysis of removed prosthetic heart valves: Causes of failure of 33 mechanical valve and 58 bioprostheses, 1980 to 1983. Hum Pathol 16:549–559, 1985.
15. Lange RA, Moore DM Jr, Cigarroa RG, Hillis LD: Use of pulmonary capillary wedge pressure to assess severity of mitral stenosis: Is true left atrial pressure needed in this condition? J Am Coll Cardiol 13:825–831, 1989.

Chapter 13

Mitral Valve Gradients—Section V:
Left Ventricular Puncture for Hemodynamic Evaluation of Double Prosthetic Valve Stenosis

Morton J. Kern, MD

INTRODUCTION

Catheter access to the left ventricle is limited by the presence of prosthetic valves in the mitral and aortic positions. Retrograde catheterization of the left ventricle with certain mechanical prosthetic valves may be hazardous [1,2] and has been unsuccessful in some individuals with homograft, xenograft, or severely calcified native aortic valves. Transseptal left atrial access to the left ventricle is similarly inhibited by prosthetic or mechanical mitral valves and, thus, only one approach, direct percutaneous left ventricular puncture, remains to assess cardiac hemodynamics in individuals with both aortic and mitral mechanical prostheses. Although infrequent, critical hemodynamic assessment for the severity of valvular compromise in patients with double-valve prostheses is especially important before interventions. Although the technique and methodology have been well-described [3–5], their infrequent application makes periodic review worthwhile.

We report on a case of a patient who presented with congestive heart failure attributed to a possible stenotic prosthetic mitral valve after replacement of a stenotic prosthetic aortic valve. The approach by direct left ventricular puncture was instrumental in the clinical decision for a second operation.

CASE REPORT

The patient was a 61-year-old woman with rheumatic heart disease who had had aortic and mitral valve replacements in 1977. A pacemaker was inserted for tachy-brady syndrome in 1996. In May 1997, transesopha-geal echocardiography demonstrated a normal mitral valve prosthesis with severe prosthetic aortic stenosis. A second valve replacement (22-mm St. Jude Medical, Minneapolis, MN.) for aortic stenosis was performed, leaving the mitral valve (29-mm Bjork-Shiley, Baxter Co., Los Angeles, CA.) in place based on near-normal echocardiographic data. In the postoperative period the patient had congestive heart failure and was unable to be weaned from mechanical ventilation. She required both vasopressor and vasodilatory support without decreasing the elevated ($>$60 mm Hg systolic) pulmonary artery pressures. Repeat echocardiographic examination did not identify the etiology of pulmonary hypertension and showed only minimal mitral regurgitation with a small transmitral gradient, normal left ventricular function, no pericardial effusion, and a normally functioning aortic valve. There was no left atrial thrombus. Hemodynamic evaluation was requested to assess whether the mitral prosthetic valve function was associated with continued pulmonary hypertension and the failure to resolve the congestive symptoms.

Right- and left-heart catheterization was performed using the right femoral artery and vein access by the standard Seldinger technique. A balloon-tipped pulmonary artery catheter was advanced to the pulmonary artery. A 6F pigtail catheter was positioned in the central aorta above the prosthetic valve. Transseptal catheterization by the standard Brockenbrough technique was performed, placing the catheter in the left atrium.

On completion of the initial catheter placements, the transapical approach to the left ventricle was then undertaken. Two-dimensional echocardiography in the cardiac catheterization laboratory identified the true position of

B.H.

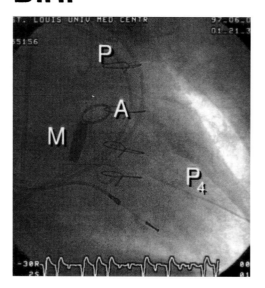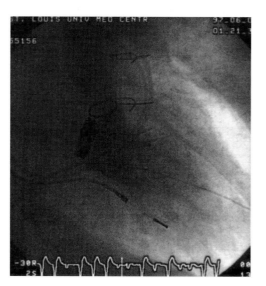

Fig. 1. Cineangiographic frames before (left) and during (right) left ventriculography through the pigtail catheter (P4) positioned from the left ventricular apex. The supervalvular pigtail catheter (P) is positioned above the aortic ring (A), which is adjacent to the mitral ring (M). There are multiple pacing leads and two pulmonary artery catheters positioned near the superaortic pigtail catheter. Contrast injection during ventriculography shows no mitral regurgitation.

the left ventricular apex between the fourth and fifth intercostal space lateral to the midclavicular line. This position was marked with a pen. The area was prepared in a sterile fashion. An 18-gauge pericardial needle was connected to a pressure monitoring line. The needle was advanced in the plane of the echocardiogram and on the line of the left ventricular apex to the aortic outflow. The needle was introduced slowly, with intermittent administration of additional lidocaine. The pulsations of the left ventricle could be felt transmitted through the needle during puncture. Under pressure monitoring, the apex of the ventricle was punctured. After confirmation of left ventricular pressure, a 0.035″ standard J-wire was advanced into the left ventricular cavity and exchanged for a 4F pigtail catheter (Fig. 1). Left- and right-heart hemodynamic data were then acquired in a standard fashion. Following hemodynamic data collection, left ventriculography was performed in the right anterior oblique projection, using 42 cc of contrast at 12 cc/sec.

The left ventriculogram showed only trace mitral regurgitation and an ejection fraction of 50% with normal wall motion (left ventricular score = 5).

The hemodynamic data showed that the right atrial pressure was 22 mm Hg with an "M" configuration (Fig. 2, left). Note the "A" wave on the pressure tracing, without a visible "P" wave in the paced QRS ECG complex. Right ventricular pressure was 75/24 mm Hg, and pulmonary artery pressure was 75/40 mm Hg (Fig. 2,

right). Mean pulmonary capillary wedge pressure was 40 mm Hg, with "V" waves to 50 mm Hg. Mean left atrial pressure was 38–42 mm Hg, with "V" waves to 50 mm Hg (Figs. 2, 3). On matching of the pulmonary capillary wedge and left atrial pressures (Fig. 2), there was good correspondence of the "V" wave peak but slight delay of the pulmonary capillary wedge "V" wave decline, resulting in a higher mean value (and left ventricular-pulmonary capillary wedge gradient). Figure 3 compares the left and right atrial pressures during catheter pullback. Note the large left atrial "V" waves, despite only minimal mitral regurgitation by left ventriculography. As an aside, the initial ventricular systolic pressure was lower than the aortic pressure (Fig. 4). This pressure matched the right ventricular pressure recorded during right-heart catheterization. The needle was then withdrawn and reintroduced at a more posterior angle with immediate achievement of the left ventricular pressure waveform (Fig. 5). The left ventricular pressure was 140/28 mm Hg, and aortic pressure was 120/76 mm Hg. There was a peak-to-peak left ventricular-aortic gradient which varied from 15–30 mm Hg. In addition, there was a left ventricular-mitral gradient which varied from 8–13 mm Hg (Fig. 6). Cardiac output was 4.4 l/min. Note the influence of RR cycle length on the left atrial-left ventricular gradient with equilibration before end-diastole. The reduction of the mitral gradient was followed by an increased aortic-left ventricular gradient following the sinus beat (Fig. 5, third

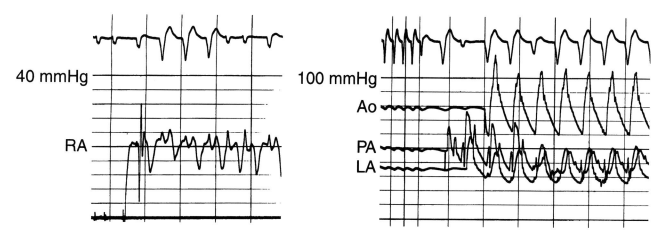

Fig. 2.   Left: Right atrial (RA) pressure wave (0–40 mm Hg) showing a distinct "M" configuration, with an elevated mean pressure of approximately 20 mm Hg. Right: Aortic (Ao), pulmonary artery (PA), and left atrial (LA) pressures (0–100 mm Hg scale). There is fair concordance of the pulmonary capillary wedge (after 3 beats of pulmonary artery pressure) and left atrial pressures.

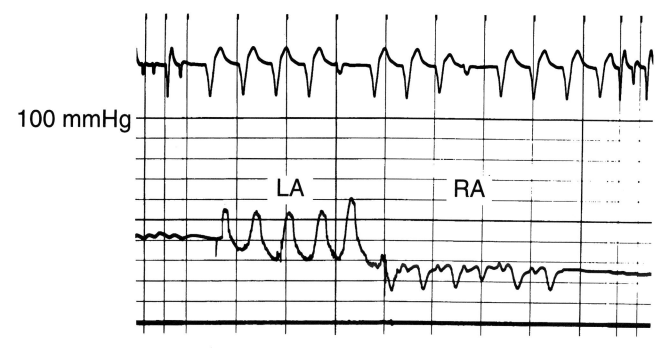

Fig. 3.   Pressure recorded during catheter pullback from the left atrium (LA) to the right atrium (RA). The left atrial mean pressure is approximately 42 mm Hg, with a mean right atrial pressure of 25 mm Hg. The left atrial "V" waves exceed 50 mm Hg. Is this consistent with constrictive physiology? Scale, 0–100 mm Hg.

beat). The aortic valve area thus varied from 0.8 (4.4 l/min/$\sqrt{30}$) to 1.1 cm^2 (4.4 min.$\sqrt{15}$)

The mitral valve area also demonstrated variation from 1.4–2.07 cm^2 (Fig. 6). It is interesting to note the higher left ventricular end-diastolic pressure in Figure 6, far right, which resulted in the lowest mitral gradient. The left atrial pressure was lower during the paced rhythm as compared to sinus beats (Fig. 6, middle).

The right and left ventricular end-diastolic pressures were elevated and identical, suggesting some degree of restrictive physiology (Fig. 7). There was no oximetric or angiographic evidence of intracardiac shunts.

After left ventriculography, the pigtail catheter was withdrawn over a guidewire. The patient was monitored in the laboratory for 20 min. A repeat echocardiogram was performed which showed no pericardial effusion.

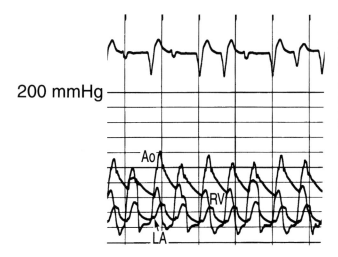

200 mmHg

Fig. 4. Simultaneous aortic (Ao), right ventricular (RV), and left atrial (LA) pressures (0–200 mm Hg scale). The long needle was withdrawn and repositioned.

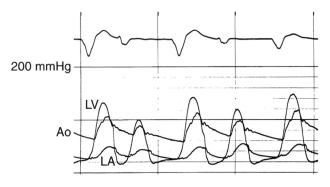

200 mmHg

Fig. 5. Left ventricular (LV), left atrial (LA), and aortic (Ao) pressures (0–200 mm Hg scale), demonstrating the aortic and mitral prosthetic valve gradients. Note the influence of the paced beats on the valve gradients.

Because of the need for continued low-intensity anticoagulation, an Angioseal™ vascular closure device (Sherwood, Davis, Gek Medical Co., St. Louis, Mo.) was used to obtain right femoral artery hemostasis.

The patient underwent reoperation for mitral valve replacement. Recovery was complicated by prolonged ventilatory support, but hemodynamics were improved.

DISCUSSION

This case was interesting for several important clinical reasons. The precise calculation of valve areas remains critically dependent on pressure gradients and cardiac output, both of which are a subject of variation in patients with arrhythmias or fluctuating hemodynamic baseline conditions [6]. Both factors were present in this patient and resulted in variability in the valve area results.

The aortic valve stenosis was thought to be the principal cause of pulmonary hypertension and congestive heart failure. However, after valve replacement, the mitral valve was suspected of being dysfunctional. The aortic outflow obstruction was also considered partly contributory since the intrinsic gradient of a newly positioned 22-mm St. Jude was at least 15–20 mm Hg. The valve size was limited by the aortic root in this small woman.

The changing left atrial and left ventricular pressures (Fig. 6) suggested moderate mitral stenosis and, given the limited options and poor response to aggressive pharmacotherapy, also suggested that mitral valve replacement would be the best therapeutic approach. After mitral valve was replaced, a slow and gradual reduction of pulmonary artery pressures to 45–50 mm Hg systolic and cessation of intermittent hemoptysis was noted.

The simultaneous use of transseptal left atrial and transapical left ventricular hemodynamics was required to identify a hemodynamically compromised mitral valve. This approach has obvious clinical value, although the computation of valve area still remains the parameter with greatest variance. The interesting question of restrictive physiology (Fig. 7) remains unanswered. Cardiac constriction appeared to be excluded by the separation of the left atrial/right atrial pressures (Fig. 3).

Complications

Evaluation of the left ventricular cavity by the direct percutaneous method was first described in 1933 by Reboul and Racine [7] in experimental canines and by Buchbinder and Katz [8] in 1949 in patients. Other investigators [3–5] have provided the cardiology community with clinical examples in larger series involving over 300 patients, and have demonstrated the major complication rates, estimated to be at 3–4%.

The use of a long 18-gauge pericardiocentesis needle to place a guidewire followed by the 4F catheter has been described [4,5,9] and is associated with minimal complications. The reported complications of direct left ventricular puncture have included transient hypotension, vasovagal symptoms, pneumothorax, ventricular arrhythmias, coronary laceration, and postpericardiotomy syndrome. In children, a death was reported with this technique when assessing complex congenital heart disease, including transposition of the great vessels [5]. Death was related to intramural contrast injection. A relatively low incidence of pericardial bleeding is thought to be reduced in patients with myocardial hypertrophy and by the systolic contraction, which is thought to seal the puncture site on removal of catheters. Previous thoracic surgery limits the active pericardial space and often is associated with lung-tissue adhesion to the anterior heart. This technique, described by Semple et al. [9], Wong et al.

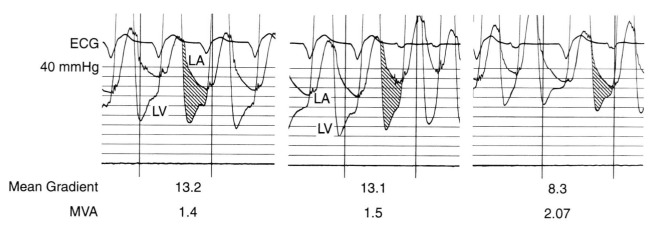

Fig. 6.   Left ventricular (LV) and left atrial (LA) pressure tracings during changing ventricular rhythms. The variation of the mitral valve area (MVA, cm²) is shown. Shaded area represents the diastolic pressure gradient. Elevation of the left ventricular end-diastolic pressure (far right) during the procedure decreases the gradient, despite lack of significant change in the left atrial pressure. Variation of the mitral valve area occurred without change in cardiac output.

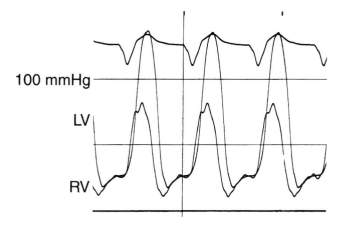

Fig. 7.   Simultaneous left ventricular (LV) and right ventricular (RV) pressure tracings during paced rhythm. The matching and elevation of the diastolic periods suggest some degree of restrictive or constrictive physiology, concomitant with the valvular dysfunction. Note the early rise of right, relative to left, ventricular pressure due to the paced ventricular activation.

[10], and others [3–5], has used even larger catheters with similarly low complication rates.

Placement of catheters across the Bjork-Shiley (Baxter Inc., Los Angeles, CA) or Starr-Edwards valves has been performed safely in some individuals [1,2]. However, retrograde cannulation of tilting mechanical discs may result in potential catheter entrapment. The potential creation of false valvular regurgitation by propping open the prosthetic occluder limits the confidence in some observations. The risk of valve emboli is also increased for the tilting disc valves.

The largest experience of direct left ventricular access was summarized by Morgan et al. [5], who examined the results of the technique in 112 patients from 20,000 catheterizations performed between 1973–1987. Thirty-nine patients had mechanical prosthetic aortic valves, 25 with additional mechanical mitral valves. The remainder of the patients studied had severe native aortic valve stenosis (70 patients), xenograft aortic prosthetic stenosis (1 patient), and homograft aortic valve stenosis (2 patients). Direct left ventricular puncture was used to study mitral valve disease or prosthetic mitral valve dysfunction in 17 (16%) patients. In contrast to more recent studies [4], their most common technique involved fluoroscopic identification of a pical marker placed on the chest at the point of maximal impulse, with subsequent fluoroscopically-guided insertion of a 19-gauge needle connected to pressure tubing [5]. The Seldinger technique for catheter insertion was then performed, using a guidewire and short 6F catheters. In this series [5], there was one death 4 days after direct left ventricular puncture in a patient with severe aortic stenosis. No death was attributed to the direct left ventricular puncture itself. Two patients subsequently died during hospitalization. Two patients had pericardial tamponade, one whose INR (International Normalize Ratio) was >2.1. One patient had pneumothorax, and 2 patients had pericardial effusion which did not cause hemodynamic compromise. Pericardial and pleuritic pain was present in 7 patients, and 5 patients had vagal episodes. Six patients had left ventricular cavities which could not be entered, and the study was terminated uneventfully. Major complications occurred in 3% of patients with a successful direct percutaneous left ventricular puncture (95% of patients). These data are similar to those on transseptal punctures reported by Lew et al. [11] in 207 patients, with morbidity in only 5% and major complications in 1%, with failure to enter the left ventricle in 15%.

CONCLUSIONS

Direct left ventricular puncture is generally a safe and simple method with minimal mortality and morbidity, comparing favorably to the transseptal approach, and it offers unique angiographic and hemodynamic data, especially in the setting of abnormal prosthetic mitral or aortic valve involvement.

ACKNOWLEDGMENTS

The author thanks the J.G. Mudd Cardiac Catheterization Laboratory Team for technical support, and Donna Sander for manuscript preparation.

REFERENCES

1. Rigand M, Dubourg O, Luwaert R, Rocha P, Hamoir V, Bardet J, Bourdarias JP: Retrograde catheterization of the left ventricle through mechanical aortic prosthesis. Eur Heart J 8:689–696, 1987.
2. Karsh DL, Michaelson SP, Langou RA, Cohen LS, Wolfson S: Retrograde left ventricular catheterization in patients with an aortic valve prosthesis. Am J Cardiol 41:893–896, 1978.
3. Levy LJ, Lillehei WC: Percutaneous direct cardiac catheterization. N Engl J Med 271:273–280, 1964.
4. Cata CJ, Grassman ED, Johnson SA: Technique of apical leftventricular puncture revisited: A case report of double-valve prothesis evaluation. J Invas Cardiol 6:251–255, 1994.
5. Morgan JM, Gray HH, Geeder C, Miller GA: Left heart catheterization by direct ventricular puncture: Withstanding the test of time. Cathet Cardiovasc Diagn 16:87–90, 1989.
6. Cannon SR, Richard KL, Crawford M: Hydraulic estimation of stenotic orifice area: A correction of the Gorlin formula. Circulation 71:1170–1178, 1985.
7. Reboul H, Racine M: Ventriculographic cardiaque experimentale. Presse Med 37:763, 1933.
8. Buchbinder WC, Katz LN: Intraventricular pressure curves of the human heart obtained by direct transthoracic puncture. Proc Soc Exp Biology Med 71:673, 1949.
9. Semple T, McGuiness JB, Gardner H: Left heart catheterization by direct ventricular puncture. Br Heart J 30:402–406, 1968.
10. Wong CM, Wong PH, Miller GA: Percutaneous left ventricular angiography. Cathet Cardiovasc Diagn 7:425–432, 1981.
11. Lew AS, Harper RW, Federman J, Anderson ST, Pitt A: Recent experience with transseptal catheterisation. Cathet Cardiovasc Diagn 9:601–609, 1983.

Chapter 14

The Left-Sided V Wave

Morton J. Kern, MD, and Ubeydullah Deligonul, MD

INTRODUCTION

The hemodynamic waveforms obtained with pulmonary capillary wedge pressure tracings in the cardiac catheterization laboratory or during monitoring in the intensive care unit are probably among the most important and practical clinical data. These waveforms indicate filling pressure of the left ventricle, function of the mitral valve, and resistance of the pulmonary circuit. Normally, V waves on the pulmonary capillary wedge tracing reflect left atrial filling during ventricular systole and atrial emptying immediately after ventricular systole and ventricular relaxation. The morphology and magnitude of the V wave is determined principally by the pressure-volume relationship of the left atrium. Large V waves may be due to valvular mitral regurgitation or stenosis, or a number of other non-valvular conditions in which the pressure/volume relationship of the atrial chamber is altered (e.g., high atrial volume due to ventricular septal defect or stiffening of chamber elasticity due to ischemia or hypertrophy) [1,2]. The accurate interpretation of the V wave has clinical importance in a variety of common circumstances and has been the subject of numerous experimental and clinical studies characterizing factors of relevance. In this hemodynamic rounds we will examine several examples of the left-sided V waves and address the physiology and postulated mechanisms altering its waveform.

CASE PRESENTATIONS AND DISCUSSION
V Wave Alternans

A 69-yr-old man was evaluated for advanced congestive heart failure after several prior hospitalizations for atypical chest pain and 2 remote myocardial infarctions. Right and left heart hemodynamics were obtained prior to coronary arteriography (Fig. 1). The hemodynamic tracings of the left ventricular and pulmonary capillary wedge pressures were obtained with a 7 French pigtail catheter and balloon-tipped pulmonary artery catheter through fluid-filled transducers. Consider the following questions: Why are the V waves of different size? Where is the pulmonary capillary wedge A wave? Does the V wave indicate significant mitral regurgitation or is there some degree of mitral stenosis? Besides an elevated mean pulmonary capillary wedge pressure, what other features of either pressure tracing indicate poor left ventricular function?

On examination of the simultaneous pulmonary capillary wedge and left ventricular pressures, beat #1 shows a left ventricular A wave of 28 mm Hg and a pulmonary capillary wedge V wave of 48 mm Hg. On beat #2, the left ventricular end diastolic pressure (taken at the end of the A wave) is 34 mm Hg and the corresponding pulmonary capillary wedge V wave exceeds 60 mm Hg. This alternating pattern repeats on beats #3–5. This unusual example of V wave alternans was produced as a function of a failing left ventricle with pulsus alternans demonstrated in the arterial pressure waveform. As one will see, the function of the left ventricle and its filling pattern (ventricular pressure/volume relationship) has a great influence on the V wave generation [2,3].

Normal A and V Wave Patterns

Before discussing abnormal pulmonary capillary wedge waveforms, review briefly the normal atrial

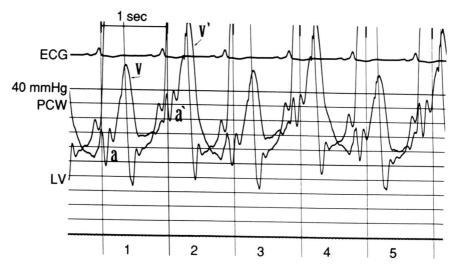

Fig. 1. Simultaneous left ventricular (LV) and pulmonary capillary wedge (PCW) pressure tracings (0–40 mm Hg scale) in a patient with congestive heart failure. See text for details.

waveforms (Fig. 2). The following definitions for atrial or pulmonary capillary wedge waveforms will be used. The A wave is the first positive wave due to contraction of the atria (after the P wave on the electrocardiogram). The second positive wave appearing on the downslope of the A wave is the C wave of ventricular contraction. The C wave may not be visible. The third positive wave, the V wave, is due to atrial filling occurring at the end of ventricular systole. The peak of the V wave usually corresponds to the electrocardiographic T wave. The negative slopes of the A and V waves are termed the X and Y descents. The X descent may be broken into the X and X′ divided by the presence of a C wave. The Y descent occurs on the downslope of the V wave. The minimal X and Y descent pressures are termed the troughs. These points of pressure measurement are thought to be better correlated with left ventricular end diastolic pressure under pathologic conditions than the mean pulmonary capillary wedge pressure [4]. The left ventricular end diastolic pressure is obtained after atrial contraction, which usually produces a visible deformity of the left ventricular pressure (see Fig. 2, LV 'a' wave). The left ventricular end diastolic pressure is measured after the A wave corresponding to the peak of the R wave (on Fig. 2, follow the ventricular time line at the first R wave down to its crossing point on the left ventricular pressure).

The tracings on Figure 2 were obtained in a 59-yr-old woman 10 days after inferior myocardial infarction. The left ventricular pressure A wave (of approximately 22 mm Hg) usually exceeds the pulmonary capillary wedge pressure A waves (of at 18 mm Hg). These particular pulmonary capillary wedge waveforms are elevated, but normal in morphology and timing. The normal delay in

pressure transmission from the atria to the pulmonary capillaries of approximately 140 msec is also demonstrated on this tracing (see small arrows on beat #3, Fig. 2). The peak of both the A and V waves are similarly delayed. When measured directly, the true left atrial V wave peak, as we will see, should occur within the downslope of the left ventricular tracing. In contrast to the right atrial pressure waves, the left-sided V wave is usually greater than the A wave.

Correspondence of Pulmonary Capillary Wedge and Left Ventricular End Diastolic Pressures

The pulmonary capillary wedge pressure is a reliable indicator of left atrial and ventricular end diastolic pressure in most circumstances. Simultaneous pulmonary capillary wedge pressures (8 F balloon-tipped catheter) and left atrial pressure (obtained from the transeptal approach using a Brockenbrough catheter) were measured during assessment of severe aortic stenosis (Fig. 3). The pulmonary capillary wedge pressure is nearly identical in magnitude and duration to left atrial pressure. The largest discrepancy between left atrial and pulmonary capillary wedge A and V wave pressures is usually ≤ 5 mm Hg [6]. In over 700 cardiac catheterizations, left atrial pressures obtained by transeptal and pulmonary artery diastolic pressures were nearly identical [5]. Simultaneous measurements of left atrial and pulmonary capillary wedge pressures measured at the time of surgery were also concordant in 90% of cases by < 1 mm Hg difference with a 95% confidence limit for 2 mm Hg difference between left atrial and pulmonary capillary wedge pressure [5,6]. The timing delay of the pulmonary capillary wedge pressure relative to left atrial pressure ranges from 140 to 200 msec.

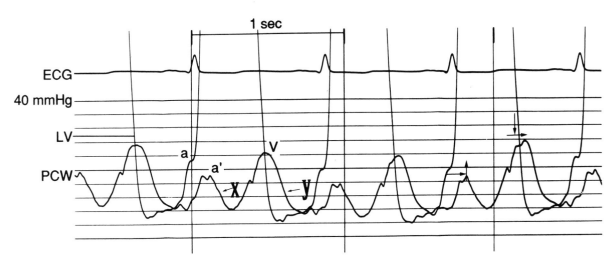

Fig. 2. Simultaneous left ventricular (LV) and pulmonary capillary wedge (PCW) pressure tracing (0–40 mm Hg scale) in a patient after myocardial infarction. See text for details.

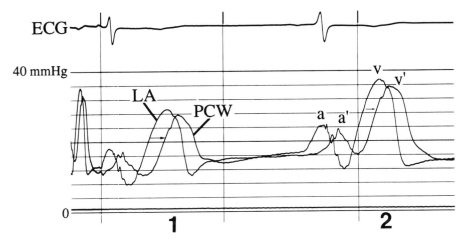

Fig. 3. Simultaneous left atrial (LA) and pulmonary capillary wedge (PCW) pressures measured with fluid-filled catheters. See text for details (A' and V' are PCW waveforms).

However, the pulmonary capillary wedge pressure may not accurately reflect left ventricular end diastolic pressure in the presence of obstructive airway disease and conditions altering intrathoracic pressures, such as assisted mechanical ventilation with positive end expiratory pressure [2,5,6]. Both the pulmonary capillary wedge and left atrial pressure may be disparate with the left ventricular end diastolic pressure in patients with low left ventricular compliance (e.g., acute myocardial infarction, hypertension, hypertrophic or congestive cardiomyopathy) or with valvular mitral stenosis or regurgitation or other conditions in which atrial flow characteristics are highly abnormal [6].

Obtaining an accurate pulmonary capillary wedge pressure may be difficult in patients with pulmonary hypertension, dilated right ventricle, severe tricuspid regurgitation or anatomic deformations due to acquired (post-operative or calcified cardiac annulus) or congenital anomalies. When using a balloon-tipped catheter, an accurate pulmonary capillary wedge pressure is verified by clear A and V waves as described above. Confirmation of catheter position by a small 1–2 cc injection of contrast may produce a characteristic angiographic "fern'" pattern, but is a time consuming maneuver. Beside pressure damping, clearing the catheter after this "test" may cause the catheter tip to migrate. Confirming an arterial oxygen saturation value from the pulmonary capillary wedge location is difficult with an inflated balloon since venous blood trapped by the balloon often mixes with oxygenated pulmonary capillary blood. If the pulmonary capillary wedge is in question, obtain a pressure tracing with the balloon deflated. A satisfactory oxygen saturation ($> 95\%$) may then be obtained. If this is not possible, consider using a stiff, large diameter end holed cath-

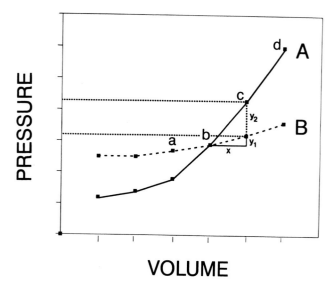

PRESSURE

VOLUME

Fig. 4. Pressure/volume relationship determining the morphology and magnitude of atrial pressure waves.

eter, such as Cournand or Goodale-Lubin catheter or perform a transeptal puncture with left atrial cannulation.

Factors Influencing Size of the V Wave

The compliance of the ventricle and atrium is the major determinant of changes in the atrial and ventricular pressure waves. Figure 4 illustrates a hypothetical left atrial pressure-volume (P-V) relationship. Four principal factors acting on the P-V relationship influence the morphology of the V wave: 1) the volume of blood entering the atrium during ventricular systole, 2) rate of forward flow into the atrium, 3) systemic afterload (influencing emptying) and 4) left ventricular contractile force (affecting left ventricular end diastolic volume and pressure). In a highly compliant left atrium (such as occurring with a P/V curve B, Fig. 4), a known increase in volume (x ml moving up the curve from Point b to c) will produce a small change in pressure (Y_1 mm Hg), generating a small V wave. In contrast, when atrial compliance is reduced, that is the atria becomes stiffer, a new compliance (P-V) curve is formed. The same volume of blood entering the left atrium on P/V curve A and moving from Point b to c will produce a much larger increase in pressure (Y_2 mm Hg) and a large V wave. A change in the shape or location of the P-V curve can occur due to alteration in atrial chamber properties (i.e., post-operative or rheumatic inflammation), fluid mechanics (e.g., regurgitation), as well as alteration of atrial or ventricular musculature (e.g., ischemia). In a poorly compliant, stiff left ventricle, such as occurring in the first patient with a myocardial infarction (Fig. 1), the atrial contraction and contribution to left ventricular filling increases left ventricular end diastolic pressure well

above the mean left atrial pressure and pulmonary capillary wedge pressure. In patients with myocardial infarction, the mean pulmonary capillary wedge pressure often correlates better with the pressure before the A wave at the beginning of atrial systole [7]. Haskel et al. [4] indicate that in patients with large left-sided V waves due to mitral regurgitation the trough of the X descent is the best predictor of left ventricular end diastolic pressure. In contrast, if the V wave is a small wave, the mean pulmonary capillary wedge pressure or direct left atrial pressure is still the more accurate estimate of left ventricular end diastolic pressure despite concurrent mitral regurgitation.

The Large V Wave and Mitral Regurgitation

It is known that the height of the V wave does not accurately reflect the degree of mitral regurgitation. Pichard et al. [8], Fuchs et al. [9] and others [10,11] have shown that a large V wave in the pulmonary capillary wedge pressure tracings is neither sensitive nor specific for severe mitral regurgitation. The use of the X trough [4], the ratio of QT to QV interval and downslope of the V wave [11] have been proposed as reliable signs of significant mitral regurgitation, but the sensitivity and specificity of these signs remains poor. The size of the V wave is determined by the position on the atrial compliance curve during the filling period rather than the degree of filling occurring. Severe mitral regurgitation in a very large and compliant atrium will produce little or no change in atrial pressure and, hence, little or no change in the pulmonary capillary wedge V wave. Giant V waves may be eliminated after changing ventricular afterload with nitroprusside [12]. Conditions other than mitral regurgitation that increase flow or volume in a non-compliant left atrium, such as ventricular septal defect, mitral stenosis, post-operative surgical conditions or rheumatic alterations of the atrial wall can produce large V waves without mitral regurgitation. In addition, tachycardia resulting in a shorter diastolic emptying period from the left atrium may also cause large pulmonary capillary wedge V waves.

Contribution of Atrial Systole to Left-Sided V Waves

A 49-yr-old woman with combined mitral stenosis and regurgitation underwent right and left heart cardiac catheterization prior to consideration of balloon catheter valvuloplasty. Hemodynamics tracings were obtained with fluid-filled catheters in the left ventricular and pulmonary capillary wedge position (Fig. 5). Examine the A and V waves of this tracing and explain the "giant" V wave on beat #2. The cardiac rhythm demonstrates a late P wave on beat #2 (seen in the T wave). Late atrial systole markedly increases atrial volume occurring dur-

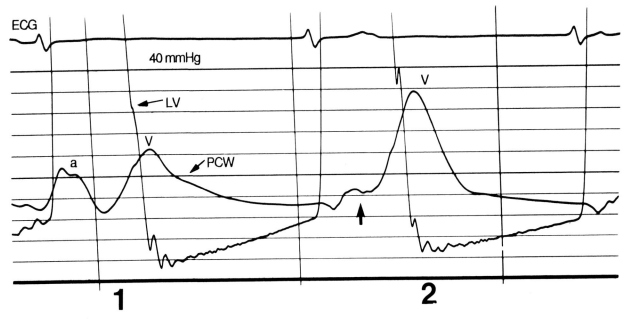

Fig. 5. Simultaneous pulmonary capillary wedge (PCW) and left ventricular (LV) pressure tracings in a patient with mitral stenosis. Is mitral regurgitation present in this individual? See text for details.

ing mid- and late-ventricular systole. Consider now the hemodynamic tracings in Figures 3 and 6. Both left atrial (Fig. 3) and pulmonary capillary wedge pressure (Fig. 6) A and V waves are large on beat #2 compared to beat #1. As in Figure 5, the responsible mechanism for the increase in A and V waves on these tracings is the timing of atrial systole. In Figure 3, the astute observer will appreciate the upright P wave on beat #1 compared to beat #2. Beat #2 has an ectopic atrial focus. The late timing of atrial systole increases both the A wave and the V wave. In Figure 6, the ectopic and delayed A wave on beat #2 did not augment the left ventricular end diastolic pressure (18 vs. 23 mm Hg). The late atrial systole occuring during the left ventricular systolic period markedly increases the V wave. In this patient without clinical or angiographic mitral regurgitation, the larger V wave does not result from increased regurgitant flow. The augmented atrial volume due to delayed atrial systole produces these large V waves.

V Wave Morphology

The morphology, and specifically, the downslope of the V wave in Figure 5 is also characteristic of mixed mitral stenosis and regurgitation. Compare this V wave downslope to that in Figures 1 and 2. The downslope of the V wave in the patient with left ventricular failure in Figure 1 suggests associated mitral regurgitation. However, quantitation of the severity of regurgitation does not correlate with the V wave downslope. The delayed

downslope suggests, but is not directly proportional to the severity (i.e., valve area) of co-existent mitral stenosis. Use of the pressure half-time method appears to be more predictive of true valve area in patients with hemodynamic tracings of combined mitral regurgitation and stenosis [13,14].

Left atrial V waves

A 52-yr-old woman had a prosthetic mitral valve implanted 4 years prior to the recent onset of severe dyspnea and fatigue. A new murmur was appreciated at the clinician's first examination. Because of signs and symptoms of congestive heart failure with new onset of clinical mitral regurgitation, a complete hemodynamic study was performed. Pulmonary hypertension was present (75/30 mm Hg), but a reliable pulmonary capillary wedge pressure could not be obtained. Because of this difficulty, transeptal catheterization was performed from the right femoral vein. The left atrial pressure was obtained with a Brockenbrough catheter. The left ventricular pressure was obtained with a 7 F pigtail catheter (Fig. 7). Examine the hemodynamic tracing and consider the pressure waves numbered 1, 2 and 3 and assign the A, C, V designation. As can be seen from the electrocardiogram, the rhythm is atrial fibrillation. There is no A wave on either the electrocardiogram, or the left ventricular or left atrial pressure tracings. Therefore, the waveform number 1 in the absence of any atrial pressure deformity of left ventricular upstroke is part of the wave-

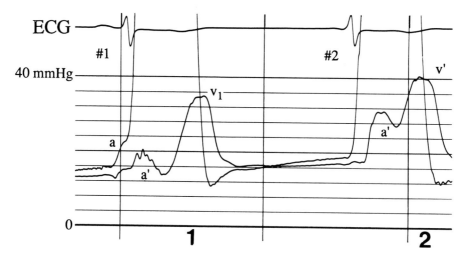

Fig. 6. Pulmonary capillary wedge and left ventricular pressure tracings in a patient with aortic stenosis. a' and v' are the pulmonary capillary wedge pressure waveforms. See text for details.

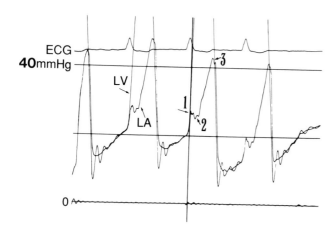

Fig. 7. Simultaneous left atrial (LA) and left ventricular (LV) pressure tracings (0–40 mm Hg scale) in a patient with new systolic murmur. See text for details.

form #2, the C wave. Waveform #3 is obviously the large, steep V wave characteristic of severe mitral regurgitation. The rapid filling occurs early under the left ventricular pressure wave. Also note that the downslope of the V wave is identical to the left ventricular pressure tracing, indicating no resistance to outflow despite marked regurgitation of blood into the left atrium. As discussed earlier, the timing of the peak of the V wave occurs slightly inside the downslope of the left ventricular pressure tracing in distinction to the wedge pressure V wave peak occurring with the characteristic delay on or outside the left ventricular pressure (Fig. 2, 5). Compare the downslope of the V wave in this tracing with that of Figure 5 in which the downslope of the V wave is markedly delayed due to resistance to outflow due to concomitant mitral stenosis. Note also that the left atrial pressure is identical to the diastolic left ventricular pres-

sure and is an accurate reflection of left ventricular filling in patients without mitral outflow restriction.

The Disparate Pulmonary Capillary Wedge and Left Atrial Pressures

A 63-yr-old patient with significant mitral regurgitation following mitral commissurtomy 8 years earlier underwent hemodynamic study for progressive fatigue. Simultaneous left atrial, pulmonary capillary wedge and left ventricular pressures were obtained after transseptal catheterization (Fig. 8). Atrial fibrillation is the underlying rhythm. The differences between left atrial and pulmonary capillary wedge pressure are evident on the upper left panel of Figure 8, showing the higher left atrial pressure and lower pulmonary capillary wedge pressure with its characteristic phase delay and slower V wave downslope. In this patient, use of this pulmonary capillary wedge pressure would have introduced an error with regard to presence of mitral stenosis. After flushing and rechecking zero levels of the pulmonary capillary wedge tracing (Fig. 8, lower panel), the severity of the regurgitant valvular lesion can be better appreciated. The upper right hand panel of Figure 8 shows the left atrial pressure superimposed on left ventricular pressure. The C and V waves evident on left atrial pressure (compare with Fig. 7) are less distinct than seen on the pulmonary capillary wedge. From the shape of the V wave, severe mitral regurgitation would be anticipated. The botton panel of Figure 8 shows the delay in the pulmonary capillary wedge and artifactual gradient of the pulmonary capillary wedge and left ventricular pressure when tracings are used without appropriate phase shifting. In patients with suspected mitral stenosis, a properly obtained and confirmed time adjusted pulmonary capillary wedge pressure accurately reflects left atrial pressure. In most

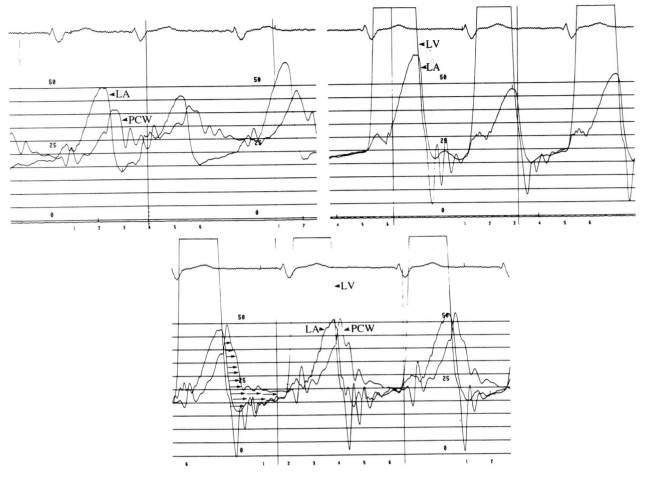

Fig. 8. Simultaneous left atrial (LA) and left ventricular (LV) pressure tracings (0–40 mm Hg scale) in a patient with new onset of fatigue. See text for details.

cases, transseptal left heart catheterization to measure left atrial pressure is not necessary [15]. However, when a diastolic mitral valve gradient is a critical measurement, the left atrial pressure should be measured directly.

SUMMARY

The left-sided V wave is dependent on both left atrial and ventricular pressure/volume filling relationship. The cardiac rhythm and timing of atrial systole also influences the V wave. The morphology of the V wave can reflect the severity of mitral regurgitation with stenosis, but valve areas in this setting may be better assessed by a pressure half-time method. Finally, as queried in our first patient example, V wave alternans is a reflection of left ventricular pressure alternans in a failing heart. Other signs of poor left ventricular function in Figure 1 also included an elevated <u>minimal</u> diastolic pressure and markedly elevated left ventricular end diastolic pressure.

Hemodynamic findings of poor left ventricular function will be addressed in detail in a later "Rounds."

ACKNOWLEDGMENTS

The authors wish to thank the J.G. Mudd Cardiac Catheterization Team and Donna Sander for manuscript preparation.

REFERENCES

1. Connolly DC, Kirklin JW, Wood EH. The relationship between pulmonary artery wedge pressure and left atrial pressure in man. Circ Res 2:434–440, 1954.
2. Shaffer AB, Silber EN. Factors influencing the character of the pulmonary arterial wedge pressure. Am Heart J 51:522–532, 1956.
3. Yu PN, Murphy GW, Schreiner BF Jr, James DH. Distensibility characteristics of the human pulmonary vascular bed: study of the pressure/volume response to exercise in patients with and without heart disease. Circulation 35:710–723, 1967.

4. Haskell RJ, French WJ. Accuracy of left atrial and pulmonary artery wedge pressure in pure mitral regurgitation in predicting left ventricular end-diastolic pressure. Am J Cardiol 61:136–141, 1988.

5. Walston A, Kendall ME. Comparison of pulmonary wedge and left atrial pressure in man. Am Heart J 86:159–164, 1973.

6. Lappas D, Lell WA, Gabel JC, Civetta JM, Lowenstein E. Indirect measurement of left atrial pressure in surgical patients—pulmonary capillary wedge and pulmonary artery diastolic pressures compared with left atrial pressures. Anesthesiology 38:394–397, 1973.

7. Rahimtoola SH, Loeb HS, Ehwani A, Sinno M, Chuquimia R, Lal R, Rosen KM, Gummar RM. Relationship of pulmonary artery to left ventricular diastolic pressures in acute myocardial infarction. Circulation 46:283–290, 1972.

8. Pichard AD, Kay R, Smith H, Rentrop P, Holt J, Gorlin R. Large V waves in the pulmonary wedge pressure tracing in the absence of mitral regurgitation. Am J Cardiol 50:1044–1050, 1982.

9. Fuchs RM, Henser RR, Yin FCP, Brinker JA. Limitations of pulmonary wedge V waves in diagnosing mitral regurgitation. Am J Cardiol 49:849–854, 1982.

10. Braunwald E, Awe WC. The syndrome of severe mitral regurgitation with normal left atrial pressure. Circulation 27:29–35, 1963.

11. Schwinger M, Cohen M, Fuster V. Usefulness of onset of the pulmonary wedge V wave in predicting mitral regurgitation. Am J Cardiol 62:646–648, 1988.

12. Harshaw CW, Murro AB, McLaurin LP, Grossman W. Reduced systemic vascular resistance as therapy for severe mitral regurgitation of valvular origin. Ann Intern Med 83:312, 1975.

13. Libanoff AJ, Rodbard S. Evaluation of the severity of mitral stenosis and regurgitation. Circulation 33:281–320, 1966.

14. Fredman C, Pearson AC, Labovitz AJ, Kern MJ. Comparison of hemodynamic pressure half-time method and Gorlin formula to Doppler and echocardiographic determinations of mitral valve area in patients with combined mitral stenosis and regurgitation. Am Heart J 119:121–129, 1990.

15. Lange RA, Moore DM Jr, Cigarroa RG, Hillis LD. Use of pulmonary capillary wedge pressure to assess severity of mitral stenosis: Is true left atrial pressure needed in this condition? J Am Coll Cardiol 13:825–829, 1989.

Chapter 15

The Tricuspid Valve

Morton J. Kern, MD, and Ubeydullah Deligonul, MD

INTRODUCTION

One of the most commonly observed hemodynamic waveforms is the pressure in the right atrium, reflecting function of and flow across the tricuspid valve. This hemodynamic rounds will examine different right atrial pressure waveforms as one of the main indicators of tricuspid valve function. The physiology of constrictive pericardial disease and atrial filling patterns will be addressed in detail at a later hemodynamic rounds. When assessing the small but clinically important gradients across the tricuspid valve, 2 simultaneous, matched pressures from 2 equisensitive transducers will provide the most precise hemodynamics. Before presenting case material, we will review the normal right atrial waveform.

NORMAL RIGHT ATRIAL WAVEFORM

Simultaneous right ventricular and right atrial pressure waves using fluid-filled transducer systems were measured in a 40-year-old woman with a history of dyspnea and Chronic Obstructive Pulmonary Disease (COPD) (Fig. 1). Identical matching of the right atrial and right ventricular diastolic pressures is the norm. The "A" wave (atrial contraction) of the right atrial pressure corresponds to the "A" wave of the right ventricle. The "V" wave corresponds to the opening of the tricuspid valve on the downslope of the right ventricular pressure tracing. Note that pressure immediately after the "A" wave, the X descent, falls and does not begin to increase until late in systole. As right ventricular pressure falls below right atrial pressure, the tricuspid valve opens, releasing atrial pressure (the Y descent of the "V" wave). Not shown on this tracing is a "c" wave of ventricular contraction apparent on some beats as a

"notch" immediately after an "A" wave or the initial upstroke of ventricular pressure.

The higher ejection velocity and faster development of the right ventricular pressure causes more oscillating of the transducer system than that of the right atrial pressure, and, therefore, a high-frequency "ringing" is observed as a notch on the upstroke before the systolic peak of the right ventricle (black arrow) and a rapid dip (negative overshoot) in early diastole (open arrow). This common artifact using fluid-filled systems is important to recognize when assessing tricuspid and pulmonary gradients.

X AND Y TROUGHS

Compare the typical hemodynamic normal example (Fig. 1) of tricuspid valve function to right and left atrial pressure waveforms in a 62-year-old man with aortic stenosis (Fig. 2). These pressures were measured continuously on pullback of a fluid-filled transseptal Brockenbrough catheter. The mean left atrial pressure is elevated approximately 22 mm Hg with striking "A" and "V" waves. There are 2 principal negative or downward motions of the right (and left) atrial pressure waves. The X trough results from movement of the tricuspid (or mitral) valve away from the atrium when intrapericardial pressure is decreasing immediately after ventricular contraction begins and left ventricular volume falls. The Y trough occurs with opening of the tricuspid valve [1]. There is a reciprocal relationship between pressure and right atrial or venous flow. Flow is virtually absent at times of peak positive "A" and "V" waves [2,3]. The left atrial "V" wave is giant (i.e., twice the mean pressure) and occurs, in this particular patient, in the absence

101

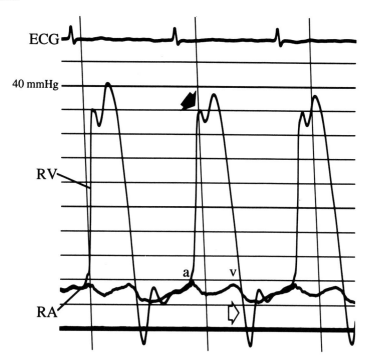

Fig. 1.   Simultaneous right ventricular (RV) and right atrial (RA) pressures measured through two fluid-filled catheters (0–40 mm Hg scale). See text for details.

of mitral regurgitation. The "V" wave reflects the pressure-volume relationship of the atrium and will be discussed in detail in a subsequent "rounds". A non-compliant or stiff ventricle often is associated with large "A" and "V" waves. The differences between left and right atrial pressures are easily appreciated. The left atrial "V" waves are generally greater than "V" waves on the right atrial pressure where the "A" wave predominates. The "c" waves, again, are not evident. Also note that atrial arrhythmias may significantly alter the waveforms (first right atrial beat after *, a¹).

CARDIAC RHYTHM AND RIGHT ATRIAL PRESSURE

Right atrial pressure waves may be distorted during cardiac arrhythmias. Consider the right atrial pressure wave obtained in a 66-year-old man following myocardial infarction (Fig. 3). Cardiac rhythm disturbances were noted on the resting electrocardiogram on day 3. The right atrial pressure wave was recorded using a fluid-filled catheter. Examine the pressure waves and consider the following: What is the etiology of the large, spiked waves ("C"). Is the tricuspid valve normal? What accounts for the "C" spike variation from 16 to 24 mm Hg? What is responsible for the change in waveform on beats 6 and 7?

These large, spiked waves represent "C" waves or (giant) cannon waves. This occurs when atrial contraction falls out of sequence with normal ventricular systole and the atria contract against a tricuspid valve closed by the increased right ventricular pressure during ejection. The size of the "C" wave is dependent on the timing of atrial contraction relative to ventricular filling (and the position of the tricuspid valve). When the atrial contraction precedes ventricular contraction in its normal synchronous mode, normal "A" waves are generated (beats 6 and 7). When atrial synchrony is lost, the cannon waves return. These cannon waves can be observed on bedside physical examination in the jugular venous pulse and should be differentiated from systolic tricuspid regurgitant waves (to be identified below). Iatrogenic induced (pacemaker) or spontaneous abnormalities of conduction also can produce similar types of cannon waves of atrial activity out of synchrony with ventricular contraction.

Large spiked pressure waves appeared in the right atrial tracing of a 78-year-old woman with a ventricular pacemaker (Fig. 4). Examine the rhythm first. The pressure tracing demonstrates brief, sharp peaked waves, less prominent than the atrial contraction waves of the previous tracing. The dysynchronous ventricular pacemaker timing relative to atrial dissociated contraction appears responsible. Note the wider "c" type wave of beat 3 with the "P" wave falling on the QRS. The high pres-

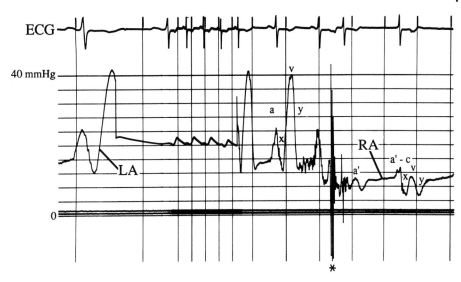

Aortic Stenosis

Fig. 2. Continuous pressure recording from left atrium (LA) to right atrium (RA) on pullback (*) across the intra-atrial septum demonstrating phasic waveforms "A" and "V" and X and Y descents, respectively, for the two atria. See text for details.

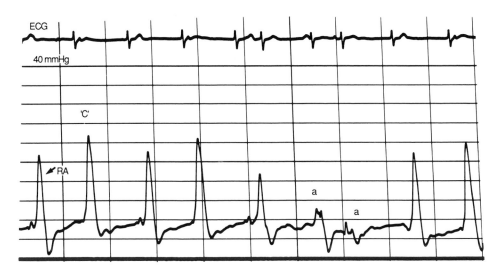

Fig. 3. Right atrial (RA) pressure (0–40 mm Hg scale) in a patient after myocardial infarction. See text for details.

Cannon A-waves in pt. c̄ AV Dyssynchrony.

sure spike with very narrow width also suggested artifact from catheter impaction, but the timing sequence also is highly consistent with "cannon" type waves.

SYSTOLIC REGURGITANT WAVES

In contrast to large cannon ("c") type waves, positive systolic pressure waves on the right atrial tracing may also be due to an incompetent or occasionally a stenotic tricuspid valve. A 50-year-old woman with atrial fibrillation and history of rheumatic fever has increasing pedal edema and dyspnea. Simultaneous right ventricular and right atrial pressures were measured with two fluid-filled catheters (Fig. 5). The right atrial pressure, matching right ventricular pressure in diastole, rose across the systolic period of right ventricular ejection, the most common pressure wave pattern of tricuspid regurgitation [4]. As anticipated in atrial fibrillation, the right atrial and ventricular "A" waves are absent. A prominent Y descent occurs after the point of the maximal right atrial pressure ("V" wave) and falls sharply with the drop in right ventricular pressure. Although the slope of the atrial pressure during right ventricular ejection is generally proportional to the severity of tricuspid regurgitation [4], the compliance or pressure-volume relationship of the atrium will determine the size and character of the

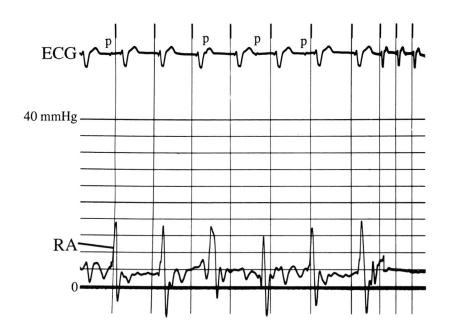

Fig. 4. Right atrial (RA) pressure (0–40 mm Hg scale) in a patient with compensated heart failure. See text for details.

Pt. c̄ AV ~~Dyssync~~ Dissynchrony 2° V-Pacing

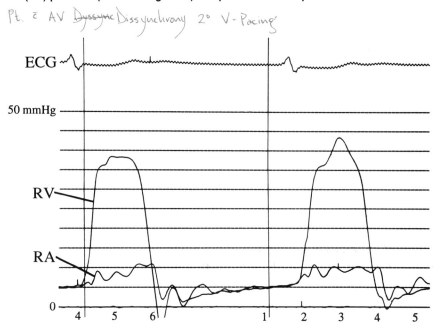

Fig. 5. Right atrial (RA) pressure (0–40 mm Hg scale) with a varying murmur along the right sternal border. See text for details.

Tricuspid Regurgitation in pt. c̄ AFib. Note gradual rise of systolic RA pressure — with inspiration

pressure wave. Note that the diastolic pressure of the right atrial and right ventricular tracings are nearly identical throughout the majority of diastole. If the catheters are zeroed, calibrated properly, and the resonant features and sensitivity of the two fluid-filled systems are matched, small diastolic gradients of tricuspid stenosis can be reliably determined.

PULSATILE VENOUS WAVES

A 39-year-old woman with severe ascites and dyspnea at rest has large "V" waves during jugular vein examination and a pulsatile liver. The simultaneous right ventricular and right atrial pressures (Fig. 6) show the marked and more striking upslope of right atrial pressure

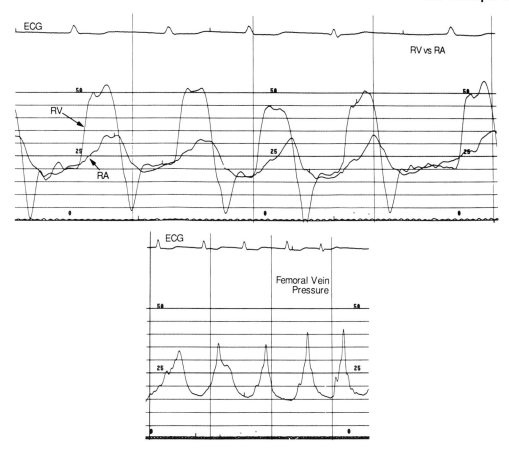

Fig. 6. Simultaneous right ventricular (RV) and right atrial (RA) pressures (0–50 mm Hg scale) through two fluid-filled channels in a patient with pulsatile neck veins. See text for details.

during right ventricular ejection with a "V" or "S" (systolic) wave to 32 mm Hg. The more rapid rise of right atrial pressure indicates severe tricuspid regurgitation (compared to Fig. 5). Early diastolic right ventricular pressure drop is associated with an early right atrial-right ventricular pressure gradient which equilibrates before the first one-third of diastole following a rapid decline, reflecting mostly high flow and not necessarily significant tricuspid valvular stenosis. The faster heart rate (than the previous patient, Fig. 5) may also contribute to the early right atrial-right ventricular diastolic gradient. The regurgitant "S" wave, occurring slightly earlier than a "V" wave, is very prominent on physical examination and can be seen in the neck and even transmitted down to the femoral vein (lower panel, Fig. 6). The marked regurgitant waves seen on the lower panel are measured in the femoral vein. Femoral vein pressure may be as high as 35 mm Hg. Thus, on puncture of the femoral vein, a "venous" pressure pulse may be observed. The timing of the "V" wave is coincident with the electrocardiographic "T" wave, but may be easily confused as an arterial pulse of low amplitude.

RIGHT ATRIAL-RIGHT VENTRICULAR GRADIENTS

Right atrial and right ventricular pressures were measured in a 49-year-old woman with increasing abdominal girth, dyspnea at rest and exercise, and systolic and diastolic murmurs that vary markedly with respiration (Fig. 7). The right atrial pressure (upper panel) demonstrated prominent regurgitant wave with fusion of "A" and "V" waves with an absent X trough and a marked Y descent. Is there truely an "A" wave? No, the rhythm is atrial fibrillation. Also observe absent "A" waves on right ventricular tracing (lower panel). The "c" wave of ventricular contraction can now be seen (arrow, lower panel). Because of the resonant qualities of some fluid-filled systems, the pressure waveform with a blunted "A" wave and X descent may occasionally be confused with the "M" configuration of constrictive or restrictive physiology [5,6] (Fig. 8) to be discussed later. The broad and wide upsloping right atrial pressure of tricuspid regurgitation is importantly associated with a persistent gradient of approximately 4 mm Hg across the tricuspid

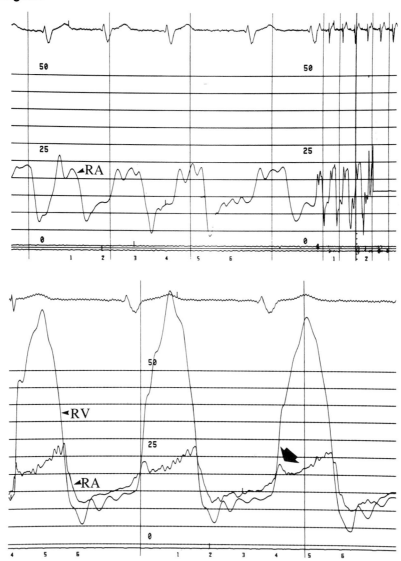

Fig. 7. Simultaneous right ventricular (RV) and right atrial (RA) pressures (0–50 mm Hg scale) through two fluid-filled channels in a patient with prominent waves in neck veins and varying murmurs. See text for details.   *Tricuspid stenosis + regurgitation + AFib. Note prominent C-waves (arrow)*

valve throughout diastole. Compare this pressure tracing to that seen on Figures 5 and 6 in which diastolic right ventricular-right atrial pressure gradients are not present. These small pressure gradients are always significant in tricuspid valve disease [5].

A 66-year-old white female had severe tricuspid regurgitation in 1985 and underwent a procedure with a symptom-free period until 5 years later. Marked increase in abdominal girth and severe lower extremity edema were the predominant complaints along with mild paraoxysmal nocturnal dyspnea and orthopnea. There was no chest pain. High flow velocities across the tricuspid valve were demonstrated by echocardiography. Moderate left ventricular dysfunction was also present. The hemodynamic tracings of the right heart pressures

were measured with fluid-prosthetic transducers through two catheters (Fig. 9). The left-hand panel of Figure 9 demonstrates the elevated and matched right atrial pressure. The rhythm was atrial bigeminy. Note the loss of distinct right atrial "A" and "V" waves. When simultaneous right ventricular and right atrial pressures are measured (right-hand panel, Fig. 9), a significant right atrial right ventricular diastolic gradient can be seen. The tricuspid valve, 5 years after bioprosthetic valve implantation, had a mean gradient of 11 mm Hg with a cardiac output of 6.4 L/min, which yielded a valve area of 1.5 cm^2. Importantly, matching of the two pressure transducers eliminated artifactual differences contributing to this gradient. As one can see, in significant tricuspid stenosis the gradient persists throughout diastole during both long

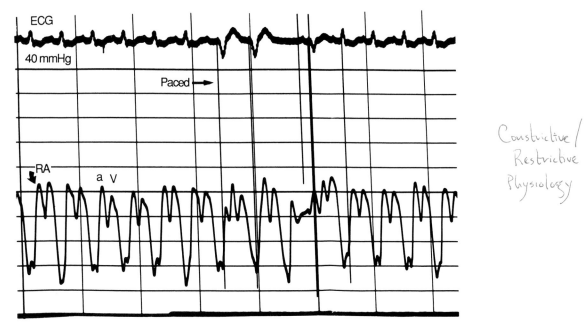

Constrictive / Restrictive Physiology

Fig. 8. Right atrial (RA) pressure in a patient with dyspnea at rest (0–40 mm Hg scale). See text for details.

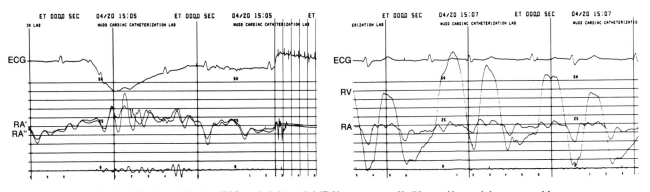

Fig. 9. Right ventricular (RV) and right atrial (RA) pressures (0–50 mm Hg scale) measured in a patient with severe ascites and peripheral edema. Left panel shows matching two fluid-filled transducers prior to crossing tricuspid valve (0–50 mm Hg scale). See text for details.

Tricuspid stenosis + AFib.

and short cycles (compared to Fig. 7). Repeat tricuspid valve replacement was subsequently performed.

RIGHT ATRIAL PRESSURE ARTIFACTS

The most common artifacts in the measurement of right atrial pressure include failure to match the zero positions or transducer gain sensitivity of the 2 fluid-filled systems. When tricuspid valve disease is suspected, precise calibration and equisensitivity of transducers are critical because small gradients may have large clinical importance.

An increase in right atrial mean pressure during inspiration is a common sign (Kussmaul's sign) of physiologic abnormalities of atrial filling, especially prevalent in patients with constrictive or restrictive physiology.

However, how does one explain the inspiratory increases in right atrial pressure in a 46-year-old woman with atypical chest pain without suspected pericardial disease (Fig. 10, top)? To the unknowing observer, this increase in right atrial mean pressure would be consistent with pathophysiology of constrictive pericarditis, but the mean right atrial pressure is only 4 mm Hg. It would be unusual for an asymptomatic, untreated person with significant constrictive physiology to have a low mean right atrial pressure. Whenever a suspected erroneous physiologic event occurs during mean pressure recording, observe the phasic waveform generating this response. As can be seen on the lower panel of Figure 10, the phasic right atrial waveform is displayed during inspiration. The initial several beats demonstrate the normal fall in right atrial pressure with an increasing Y descent and then the

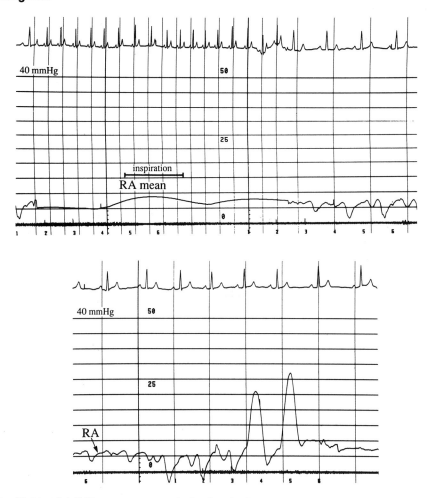

Fig. 10. Right atrial (RA) mean pressure during inspiration: Kussmaul's sign? See text for details.

catheter accidentally enters the right ventricle. The artifact of measuring right ventricular pressure during mean right atrial waveform recording is the explanation for an abnormal increase in right atrial mean pressure during inspiration in this patient in whom pericardial disease was not present.

Another common and disturbing artifact of fluid-filled pressure systems, especially in measuring right atrial and other right heart pressures, is that of excessive catheter "fling" of an underdamped pressure (catheter, tubing, transducer) system. This artifact is very common when using balloon-tipped pulmonary artery flotation catheters. The left side of Figure 11A,B shows right heart pressures recorded prior to pressure system manipulation to reduce the underdamped signal. Interpretation of waveforms and other details of these pressure tracings cannot be discerned from the rapid high-frequency "ringing" artifact of the underdamped system. To improve hemodynamic recordings while continuously measuring pressure, a 50% saline and contrast solution was instilled through the catheter. The right-hand panel

shows the distinct and strikingly elevated waveforms of a patient with congestive heart failure. The small "A" and large "V" waves with the prominent Y descent are evident [7]. In the same patient, the catheter was flushed with saline and passed to the pulmonary artery which also demonstrated marked high frequency "ringing" artifact. Contrast media was again instilled which correctly damped the pressure waveform providing accurate identification of pulmonary artery pressures (shown in the right-hand panel of Fig. 11B).

Whenever the damping characteristics of the fluid-filled systems are not satisfactory, maneuvers to improve the resonant characteristics should be made to achieve satisfactory pressure responses. Accurate determination of waveforms will aid in the determination of diseased conditions using pressure patterns.

ACKNOWLEDGMENTS

The authors wish to thank Donna Sander for manuscript preparation.

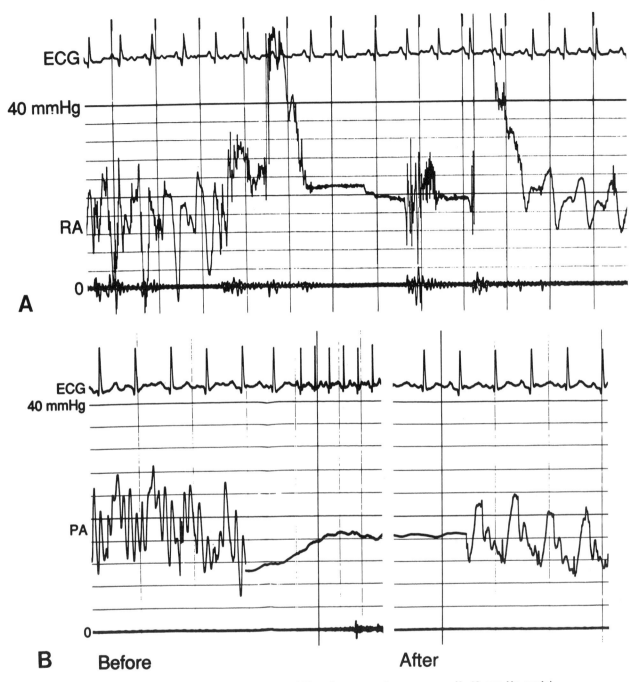

Fig. 11. A:Right atrial (RA) pressure and B) pulmonary artery pressure (0–40 mm Hg scale) with high-frequency artifact. Left panels are before and right panels after pressure system manipulation.

REFERENCES

1. Brecher GA, Hubay CA: Pulmonary blood flow and venous return during spontaneous respiration. Circ Res 3:210–214, 1955.
2. Brecher GA: Cardiac variations in venous return studied with a new bristle flow meter. Am J Physiol 176:423–430, 1954.
3. Morgan BC, Able FL, Mullins GL, et al.: Flow patterns in cavae, pulmonary artery, pulmonary vein and aorta in intact dogs. Am J Pysiol 210:903–909, 1966.
4. Lingamneni R, et al.: Tricuspid regurgitation: clinical and angiographic assessment. Cathet Cardiovasc Diagn 5:7, 1979.
5. Grossman W: Profiles in valvular heart disease. In: "Cardiac Catheterization and Angiography." Philadelphia: Lea & Febiger, 1986, p 378.
6. Tyberg JV, Taichman GC, Sith ER, Douglas NWS, Smiseth OA, Keon WJ: The relationship between pericardial pressure and right atrial pressure: an intraoperative study. Circulation 73:428–432, 1986.
7. Boltwood CM Jr, Carey JS, Feld G, Shah PM: Pericardial constraint in chronic heart failure. Am Heart J 113:847–849, 1987.

Chapter 16

The Pulmonary Valve

Morton J. Kern, MD

INTRODUCTION

Abnormalities of the pulmonary valve occur most frequently in children with rare individuals having clinically significant pulmonary valve disease in adulthood. The hemodynamics of pulmonary valve disease most often reflect that of a congenitally narrowed, domed valve of pulmonic stenosis. A minority of individuals may have a thickened or dysplastic valve. Infundibular hypertrophy may present as pulmonic stenosis with normal valve structures. Occasionally ventricular septal defects will also accompany the deformed valve. The diagnosis of pulmonary valvular (and sub- and supra-) lesions is made from echocardiography, right heart pressure recordings and right ventricular angiography [1–4]. Although uncommon, it is important to recognize the different waveforms associated with pulmonary stenosis and regurgitation and conditions which may mimic or be confused for pulmonary stenosis in the absence of true valvular abnormalities. This hemodynamic rounds will deal with right heart pressure tracings reflecting abnormalities of the pulmonary valve.

PULMONARY STENOSIS: VALVULAR OR NONVALVULAR?

A 23-yr-old young woman with a history of congenital disease developed progressive exertional shortness of breath with atypical chest pain. At 8 mo of age the patient had repair of an atrial septal defect with pulmonary artery banding. The ventricular septal defect was not repaired. At age 14 the patient had debanding of the pulmonary artery and ventricular septal patch repair. Despite a small residual ventricular septal defect, right ven-

tricular volume overload and increased right ventricular pressures were identified by echocardiography.

Because of increasing dyspnea on exertion with normal exercise tolerance, repeat echocardiography on the current examination revealed normal left ventricular systolic function, right ventricular enlargement with right ventricular overload, biatrial enlargement, and a small muscular persistent ventricular septal defect. Echocardiography suggested an increased pulmonary flow velocity and a pressure gradient across the pulmonary artery. Systemic blood pressure was 120/80 mm Hg. Pulse was 60/min. There was no jugular vein distension. Heart examination revealed normal S_1 and S_2 without gallops. A III/VI systolic murmur was heard across the precordium with radiation to the back. Lungs were clear. Electrocardiogram showed normal sinus rhythm and pseudoinferior infarction pattern.

Right and left heart catheterization was performed. The mean pulmonary capillary wedge pressure was 14 mm Hg. There was no systolic gradient across the aortic valve. There was no clinically detectable shunt by oxygen saturation measurements through the right heart. Left ventriculography revealed a left ventricular ejection fraction of 53% without mitral regurgitation. Right ventriculography revealed a trace of right to left ventricular contrast flow.

To assess the right heart pressures two catheters were placed in the pulmonary artery and pressures zeroed, matched, and recorded. Examine the pressure waveforms on Figure 1. The pressure tracings are superimposed from two fluid-filled catheters. On pullback of the first catheter into the right ventricular cavity, a pressure gradient is easily identified with right ventricular pressure equal to 95/10 mm Hg and pulmonary artery pres-

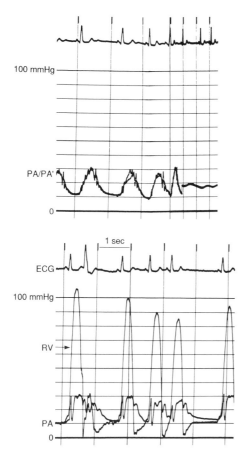

Fig. 1. Top: Two simultaneously matched pressures measuring pulmonary artery pressure beyond the pulmonary valve (0–100 mm Hg scale). The mean pressures also matched. Peak pulmonary artery pressure was 30 mm Hg. Bottom: Right ventricular pressure and simultaneous pulmonary artery pressure. Note the prominent systolic gradient. PA = pulmonary artery; RV = right ventricle. See text for details.

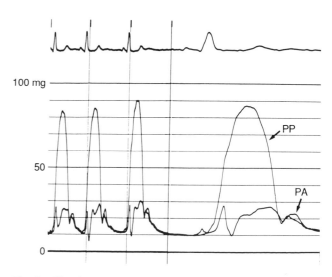

Fig. 2. Simultaneous pressures from patient example in Figure 1 measured as in Figure 1. Note the decline in peak systolic pressure. Is this pulmonic valve stenosis? PA = pulmonary artery. PP = proximal pulmonary. See text for details.

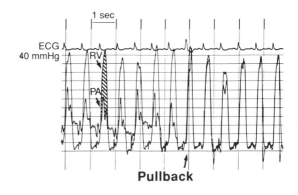

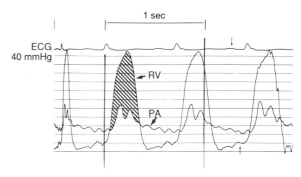

Fig. 3. Top: Hemodynamics in a patient with a systolic pulmonic murmur. Right ventricular (RV) pressure is 42 mm Hg, pulmonary artery (PA) systolic pressure is 20 mm Hg. On continuous pullback from the pulmonary artery into the right ventricle, the two pressures match. There is no subpulmonic gradient identified. Bottom: Right ventricular and pulmonary artery pressures (100 mm Hg paper speed). Note the end diastolic pressures for both pulmonary artery and right ventricular tracings are separated by 4 mm Hg. Also evident is the "a" wave on right ventricular tracing due to first degree A–V block (arrow). See text for details.

sure equal to 30/12 mm Hg. This finding is consistent with pulmonary stenosis. Does this patient have pulmonary stenosis? Examine pressure tracings on Figure 2 in the same patient. A large gradient between the higher pressure (PP) and the pulmonary artery pressure is obvious. From examining this tracing, localize where the gradient is produced. This patient does not have valvular, but supravalvular stenosis. On Figure 2, the tracing labelled PP is a proximal pulmonary artery pressure obtained above the pulmonary valve but below the area of narrowing (the site of the prior pulmonary banding) just proximal to the bifurcation of the left and right pulmonary arteries. The pressures in the distal pulmonary artery were 34/12 mm Hg, at the proximal site of the narrowing which was the previous location of the pulmonary artery band (85/12 mm Hg) and right ventricular pressure (95/10 mm Hg). Clues to the fact that this proximal pulmonary (PP) artery pressure was not the right

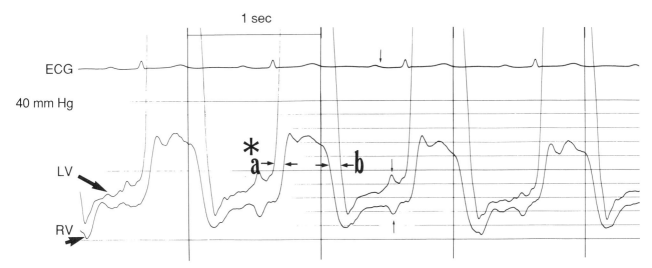

Fig. 4. Simultaneous left (LV) and right ventricular (RV) pressures in a patient with ischemic heart disease without intraventricular conduction delay on electrocardiogram. The time intervals between left and right ventricular pressures (a and b) are normal and nearly identical. Because of first degree heart block, note the prominent A wave on both left ventricular and right ventricular diastolic pressures (arrows) and unusual configuration of the right ventricular A wave.

ventricular pressure were evident by the reduction in peak systolic pressure and the matching of the diastolic to the pulmonary artery diastolic pressure. The diastolic pressures of both tracings are superimposible. The finding of valvular pulmonary artery disease is excluded by this tracing. In all patients with suspected pulmonary valvular stenosis, a careful pullback of pressures measured from the distal pulmonary artery to the left main and to the pulmonary valve, and then careful matching of the pressure to the right ventricle is essential. Compare this tracing to the next patient.

CASE 2

Examine the right heart hemodynamics (Fig. 3) of a 77-yr-old woman who had myocardial infarction in April, 1984. Because of new onset chest pain in July, 1990, the patient returned to the cardiac catheterization laboratory. This pain was similar to that of the previous myocardial infarction. Because of signs of dyspnea and a systolic murmur heard in the left parasternal area, simultaneous right and left heart catheterization was performed prior to coronary arteriography. On passage of the balloon-tipped pulmonary artery catheter, a right ventricular systolic pressure of 40 mm Hg was recognized and on passage into the pulmonary artery beyond the pulmonic valve, the pulmonary artery pressure was 20/10 mm Hg. Simultaneous pressures were then obtained using a second right heart catheter to identify the pulmonary artery-right ventricular gradient. Cardiac output was 4.9L/min and the planimetered mean pulmonary

artery gradient was 20 mm Hg. Compare the right ventricular and pulmonary artery pressures obtained on Figure 3 with the tracings of Figures 1 and 2. Note that the pulmonary artery pressure upstroke is slightly delayed and that the right ventricular pressure on pullback across the right ventricular infundibular area into the right ventricle (Fig. 3, top) shows no supra- or subpulmonic gradient. The demonstration of the matching right ventricular pressures on pullback across the pulmonary artery valve is needed to identify unsuspected infundibular narrowing as a cause of the murmur.

An aside of special interest is the effect of pulmonary stenosis with right ventricular hypertrophy and bundle branch block on the right ventricular and left ventricular pressure patterns. The normal timing of the right ventricular pressure rise relative to left ventricular pressure (shown in Fig. 4) can be delayed by abnormal impulse conduction to the right (or left) ventricle. Simultaneous right and left ventricular pressure measurements were made in patient 2 with pulmonary stenosis and myocardial ischemia (Fig. 5). Note the early onset of the right ventricular pressure relative to the left ventricular pressure and the leftward shift of right ventricular pressure beneath the left ventricular pressure curve. This timing shift may reflect the intraventricular conduction abnormality. However, with bundle branch block, a delay in right ventricular pressure would be expected. The earlier right ventricular pressure seems to indicate an earlier excitation pathway. Alternatively, one might also attribute this earlier pressure rise to a different mechanism. The widened QRS is a nonspecific conduction defect.

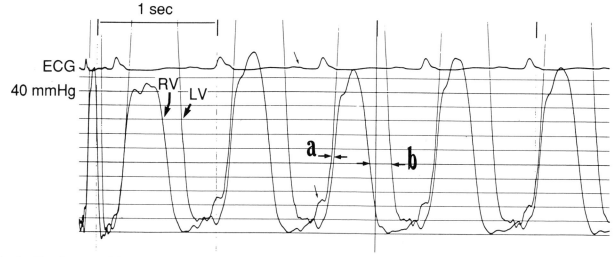

Fig. 5. Simultaneous right ventricular (RV) and left ventricular (LV) pressures in the patient in Figure 3. Note the early onset of right ventricular pressure upstroke as indicated by the distance between arrows (a) on beat 3. During ventricular relaxation, the right ventricular pressure declines earlier and more rapidly than the left ventricular pressure. The time interval between decline in right and left ventricular pressures is indicated by the distance between arrows (b) and is markedly prolonged. See text for discussion.

The possible left ventricular hypertrophy with QRS widening may cause a delay in the onset of the left ventricular upstroke, delaying the timing of left ventricular relative to right ventricular pressure. Compared to the normal simultaneous right and left ventricular pressures in Figure 4, the left ventricular pressure upstroke in Figure 5 occurs later after the R wave suggesting delay of left ventricular pressure rather than earlier activation of right ventricular pressure. The clinical significance of these findings is unknown.

COMBINED PULMONARY STENOSIS AND INSUFFICIENCY

A 36-yr-old woman had progressive shortness of breath, systolic heart murmur, and combined diastolic murmur. Echocardiography revealed high velocity jets across the pulmonary valve in systole and diastole. Simultaneous hemodynamics measuring the pulmonary artery, right ventricular, and right atrial pressures (0–50 mm Hg scale) are shown in Figure 6. These pressure waves show a modest gradient between right ventricular and pulmonary artery systolic pressures with matching of a low pulmonary artery and right ventricular end-diastolic pressures. There is a normal decline in pulmonary artery pressure across the diastolic period. Compare this tracing to Figure 3 (bottom) in which the pulmonary artery pressure declines across the diastolic period, but is maintained and elevated above right ventricular end-diastolic pressure, analogous to the hemodynamics of aortic stenosis without insufficiency in which aortic diastolic

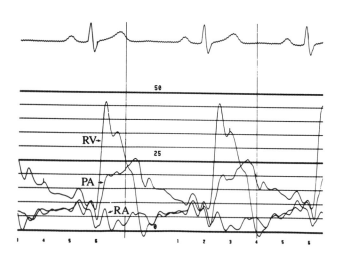

Fig. 6. Simultaneous right ventricular (RV), pulmonary artery (PA), and right atrial (RA) pressures (0–50 mm Hg scale) in a patient with systolic and diastolic murmurs. See text for details.

pressure is maintained at levels well above left ventricular end-diastolic pressure in distinction to the reduced aortic diastolic pressure seen in chronic aortic insufficiency. The wide pulmonary pulse pressure of Figure 6 was associated with echocardiographically demonstrated pulmonic insufficiency. From these tracings (Figure 6), we can also deduce that there is no tricuspid stenosis or regurgitation. The pulmonary stenosis (and less so insufficiency) can be well characterized by the combined techniques. These findings correlated angiographically with an insufficient pulmonic valve, as well as a mild doming and deformation of the pulmonary valve leaflets.

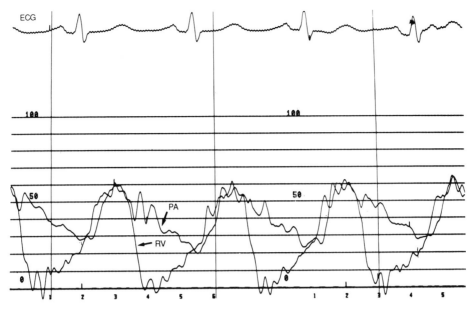

Fig. 7.   Simultaneous right ventricular (RV) and pulmonary artery (PA) pressures in a patient with continuous diastolic murmur (0–100 mm Hg scale). See text for details.

A DIASTOLIC MURMUR AND ELEVATED RIGHT VENTRICULAR END-DIASTOLIC PRESSURE

In a 45-yr-old woman, elevated and matching pulmonary artery systolic pressures (Figure 7) were observed with continuous diastolic murmur across the right upper sternal border. There was no right ventricular-pulmonary artery systolic gradient. The end-diastolic right ventricular pressure is elevated (25 mm Hg) and matches the pulmonary artery diastolic pressure at the onset of right ventricular contraction. Compare the waveforms of Figure 7 to Figures 3 and 6. The elevated pulmonary artery diastolic pressure does not normally indicate pulmonary insufficiency, but the marked distortion of the diastolic right ventricular pressure, especially at end diastole, suggests continued filling of the right ventricle or a very noncompliant chamber. Coupled with clinical and echocardiographic findings, the diagnosis is clear. Less obvious would be hemodynamic pulmonic insufficiency of Figure 6 without the striking right ventricular pressure increase during diastole. These tracings (Fig. 7) might well correspond to those seen for acute aortic insufficiency where end-diastolic left ventricular pressure increases to nearly equal that of aortic diastolic pressure.

SUMMARY

Although an uncommon lesion, when pulmonary stenosis is considered, pulmonary artery and right ventricular pressures should be assessed simultaneously on two-catheter pullback to appreciate the precise location of pulmonary-right ventricular pressure gradients. The case

examples demonstrate that the peripheral pulmonic stenosis can mimic pulmonary valve stenosis and that pulmonary artery insufficiency may be difficult to delineate on pressure alone (as is often the case with the hemodynamics of aortic insufficiency). These hemodynamic tracings are complemented by the echocardiographic and angiographic characterization of pulmonic valve lesions. Conduction defects or ventricular hypertrophy can affect the right ventricular pressure tracing and either delay or increase the timing of pressure rise and decline depending on the conduction disturbance and abnormality of myocardial contraction.

ACKNOWLEDGMENTS

The authors wish to thank the J.G. Mudd Cardiac Catheterization Laboratory team and Donna Sander for manuscript preparation.

REFERENCES

1. Grossman W: Profiles in valvular heart disease. In Grossman W (ed): "Cardiac Catheterization and Angiography," Boston: Lea & Febiger, 1986, pp 359–381.
2. Freed MD, Keane JR: Profiles in congenital heart disease. In Grossman W (ed): "Cardiac Catheterization and Angiography." Boston: Lea & Febiger, 1986, pp 446–469.
3. Hirshfeld JW: Valve function: Stenosis and insufficiency. In Pepine CJ (ed): "Diagnostic and Therapeutic Cardiac Catheterization." Baltimore: Williams & Wilkins, 1989, pp 390–410.
4. Conti CR: Cardiac catheterization and the patient with congenital heart disease. In Pepine CJ (ed): "Diagnostic and Therapeutic Cardiac Catheterization." Baltimore: Williams & Wilkins, 1989, pp 508–522.

PART II: VALVULOPLASTY

Logically following valvular hemodynamics is our discussion of valvuloplasty techniques, hemodynamic results, and clinical outcome. The use of valvuloplasty has become a standard treatment for mitral and pulmonary stenosis, and less so for aortic and tricuspid stenosis. Percutaneous balloon valvuloplasty has evolved from the single plastic balloons, to double or trifoil balloons, to the unique dumbbell-shaped Inoue balloon as the principle standard method in adults. To employ the mitral valvuloplasty technique, the approach to transseptal catheterization should be studied, an endeavor enhanced by reading several fine referenced articles on transseptal puncture. Pulmonary balloon valvuloplasty, principally used in children, is now relatively straight forward for adults, especially when employing the Inoue balloon technique.

Morton J. Kern, MD

Chapter 17

Percutaneous Balloon Valvuloplasty

Ubeydullah Deligonul, MD, and Morton J. Kern, MD

INTRODUCTION

Percutaneous balloon catheter valvuloplasty has become an important therapeutic procedure for valvular heart disease which can be safely and effectively performed in most cardiac catheterization laboratories equipped for routine hemodynamic studies. The hemodynamic changes indicating the improvement in valve function after balloon valvuloplasty are usually very prominent and are excellent examples of the effects of altered pressure and flow on the valve area. Rarely, the dramatic hemodynamic consequences of complications, such as acute valvular regurgitation, present equally interesting hemodynamic demonstrations of valve function not previously encountered outside the experimental animal laboratory.

In this hemodynamic rounds we will present and discuss several examples of pressure recordings from patients who underwent complicated and uncomplicated percutaneous balloon valvuloplasty procedures.

CASE PRESENTATIONS AND DISCUSSION

Mitral Balloon Valvuloplasty (MBV)

Introduced in 1984 by Inoue [1], MBV has now become an alternative treatment for symptomatic mitral stenosis. The immediate results of MBV are comparable to closed surgical mitral commissurotomy [2]. The published data [3–5] indicate that a typical response to MBV is a 50% or more reduction in mean mitral gradient and 100% or more increase in mitral valve area. Consider the hemodynamic tracings in a 44-yr-old woman with mitral stenosis and dyspnea (New York Heart Association class III symptoms). Before the valvuloplasty (Fig. 1, upper panel) the mean mitral valve gradient (shaded area) was 16 mm Hg and the mitral valve area was 1.0 cm^2. The technical aspects of the procedure are described in detail elsewhere [3], but in our laboratory a double balloon technique (2,18 mm $\times$ 4 cm balloons) was used. Immediately after MBV (lower panel), the mean gradient decreased to 5 mm Hg and the mitral valve area increased to 2.1 cm^2. Note the reduction of the V wave.

In some patients it is even possible to achieve completely normal appearing diastolic left atrial and left ventricular pressure tracings. Figure 2 illustrates the hemodynamic results with MBV that may be seen in occasional patients. The patient was a 75-yr-old man with increasing exertional dyspnea (New York Heart Association class III symptoms) and hemophilia B. The hemodynamics before MBV (Fig. 2, upper panel) showed a significant mean mitral gradient with prominent V waves. After MBV (Fig. 2, lower panel), there was a marked decrease in mitral gradient with normal appearance of left atrial pressure tracing. Mitral valve area increased from 1.2 cm^2 to 3.0 cm^2.

With a successful MBV the pulmonary vascular resistance decreases significantly as a result of decreased pulmonary wedge pressure and increased cardiac output. The pulmonary artery pressure may continue to decrease gradually after MBV [6–9].

Mitral Regurgitation and MBV

Mitral regurtigation is a known complication of both balloon catheter and surgical mitral commissurotomy. Although a mild increase in pre-existent mitral regurgi-

119

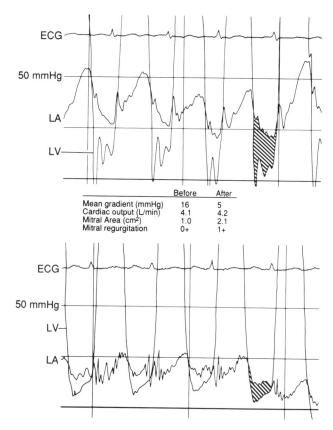

	Before	After
Mean gradient (mmHg)	16	5
Cardiac output (L/min)	4.1	4.2
Mitral Area (cm²)	1.0	2.1
Mitral regurgitation	0+	1+

Fig. 1. Hemodynamic tracings obtained before and after mitral valvuloplasty. LA = left atrium; LV = left ventricle. See text for details. Reproduced with permission from "The Cardiac Catheterization Handbook," Kern MJ. ed. Mosby Year Book, 1990.

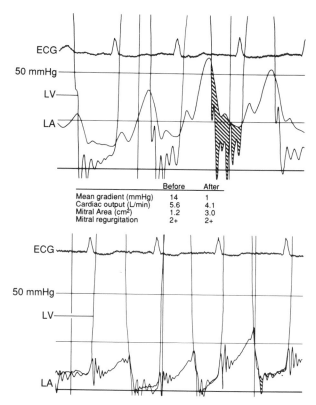

	Before	After
Mean gradient (mmHg)	14	1
Cardiac output (L/min)	5.6	4.1
Mitral Area (cm²)	1.2	3.0
Mitral regurgitation	2+	2+

Fig. 2. Hemodynamic tracings obtained before and after mitral valvuloplasty. LA = left atrium; LV = left ventricle. See text for details. Reproduced with permission from "The Cardiac Catheterization Handbook," Kern MJ. ed. Mosby Year Book, 1990.

tation or the new appearance of mild mitral regurgitation after MBV may occur in up to 55% of the patients, severe mitral regurgitation requiring valve replacement is uncommon (3–5). Examine the simultaneous left atrial and left ventricular pressure tracings before and after MBV in a patient who developed 4+ mitral regurgitation following balloon inflation (Fig. 3). Before MBV (Fig. 3, upper panel), the A wave was greater than the V wave. There was no angiographic mitral regurgitation, and the V wave morphology, likewise, did not suggest significant hemodynamic mitral regurgitation. After MBV (Fig. 3, lower panel), the V wave is somewhat larger and more peaked, but there is no "giant" V wave expected in acute severe mitral regurgitation. The enlarged and compliant left atrium (due to longstanding mitral stenosis) and left atrial decompression via the new "atrial septal defect" created to facilitate atrial septal balloon passage are potential mechanisms influencing the V wave morphology, despite severe angiographic

mitral regurgitation. The creation of a small atrial septal defect is a routine part of the MBV procedure with an incidence of 19% by oximetric method [12] increasing to 62% by dye dilution method [13]. Examination of right-sided (injection and sampling in the pulmonary artery) green dye curve (Fig. 4) in a patient with no significant "step-up" after MBV by the oximetric method reveals an early peak (arrow) indicative of left-to-right shunt. Although the left to right atrial shunting is usually small, surgery may be required rarely [14,15].

The mitral regurgitation may improve or occasionally may worsen during followup [10]. We have observed a patient with severe mitral stenosis and mild aortic regurgitation who had no mitral regurgitation after MBV, but returned 8 mo later with severe mitral regurgitation and congestive heart failure [11]. Simultaneous left atrial and left ventricular pressure tracings before, immediately after and 8 months after MBV for this patient are shown in Figure 5. On the later hemodynamic study (Fig. 5, panel

C), the development of a large V wave in the left atrial tracing and elevated left ventricular end diastolic pressure with no significant gradient at end-diastole was a striking new finding. During mitral valve surgery, no mitral leaflet tears or perforations were found. Only 1 elongated and thin chord attaching to the posterior leaflet was noted to be ruptured. In this patient, worsening aortic regurgitation after relief of mitral stenosis may also have played a role in cardiac decompensation [16,17].

Aortic Balloon Valvuloplasty (ABV)

The percutaneous balloon dilatation of calcific aortic stenosis is now limited to carefully selected patients who are not surgical candidates. Although many patients experience relief of symptoms, the high incidence of recurrence and continued high mortality in these severely ill patients have been major problems with ABV [3]. On the other hand, ABV has an important role in the treatment of congenital aortic stenosis in young age group, especially when a surgical comissurotomy is considered as the first step [18].

The typical hemodynamic response to ABV in calcific aortic stenosis is a $\geq 50\%$ decrease in the aortic mean gradient and a 25–75% increase in the aortic valve area. A 74-yr-old man with fatigue and dyspnea had aortic stenosis. Simultaneous aortic and left ventricular pressures before the ABV (Fig. 6, upper panel) show a mean aortic gradient of 76 mm Hg with aortic valve area calculated as 0.67 cm^2. After ABV (Fig. 6, lower panel), the mean aortic gradient was 35 mm Hg with a valve area of 1.0 cm^2. Note the decreased peak left ventricular systolic pressure (220 mm Hg to 180 mm Hg) and increased aortic systolic pressure (130 mm Hg to 150 mm Hg) after ABV. After the ABV, both the aortic pressure and the peripheral pulse tracing show a faster upstroke compared to the slope before ABV. A more dramatic example is shown in Figure 7. After ABV (Fig. 7, right panel), the change in aortic pressure morphology demonstrates a significantly faster systolic upstroke (130 mm Hg/sec before vs 400 mm Hg/sec after) with a higher peak systemic pressure and mild reduction in left ventricular pressure.

One of the determinants for the final result of ABV is the diameter(s) of the dilatation balloon(s). To demonstrate the influence of progressively larger balloons, examine the hemodynamic tracings in Figure 8. Simultaneous left ventricular and aortic pressures were obtained before ABV (A), after ABV using a 15 mm balloon dilatation (B) and after 18 mm balloon dilatation (C). Note the incremental improvement in aortic gradient, pulse pressure and slope with increasing balloon size. Despite reduction in aortic gradients, most patients will still have moderately severe aortic stenosis after ABV with a final valve area averaging 0.7–1.1 cm^2[3]. How-

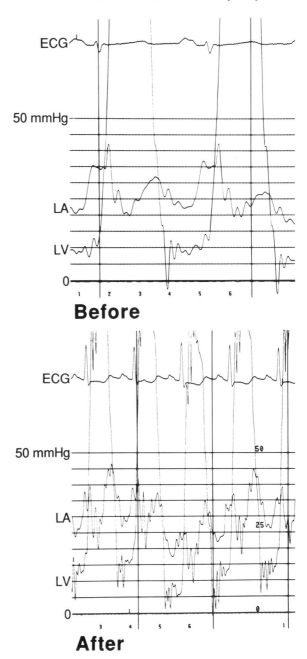

Before

After

Fig. 3. Hemodynamic tracings obtained before and after balloon valvuloplasty in a patient who developed an increased systolic murmur. See text for details.

ever, these results do not seem to preclude the symptomatic improvement [19].

Bittl et al. [20] investigated the behavior of the left ventricular pressure during balloon inflation across the aortic valve. The maximum left ventricular pressure immediately after balloon occlusion was directly-related to left ventricular function parameters and inversely related to mean circumferential end-systolic wall stress. The pa-

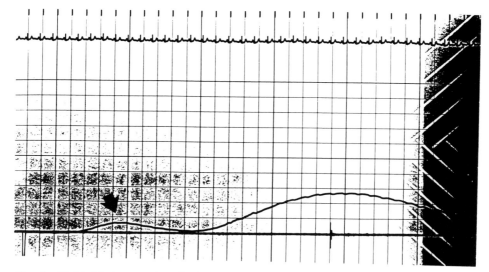

Fig. 4. Right-sided green dye dilution curve after mitral balloon valvuloplasty. The arrow shows the "bump" of early recirculation to the pulmonary artery of a small left-to-right shunt at the atrial level.

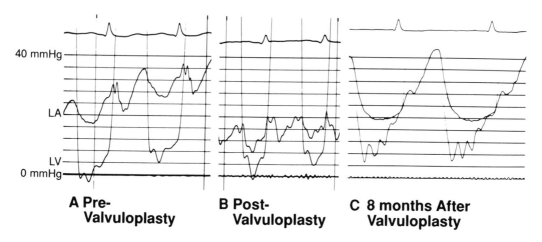

A Pre-Valvuloplasty   **B Post-Valvuloplasty**   **C 8 months After Valvuloplasty**

Fig. 5. Hemodynamic tracings in a patient before, immediately after, and 8 mo after valvuloplasty who developed progressive increase in shortness of breath. See text for details.

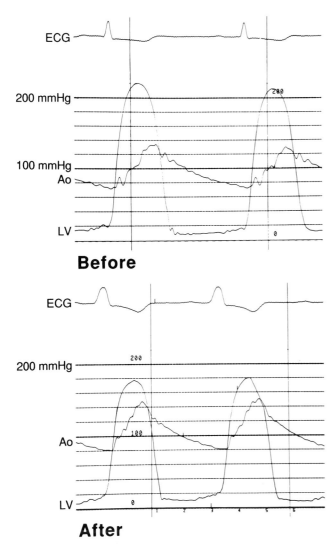

Fig. 6. Left ventricular and aortic pressure tracings in a patient undergoing aortic balloon valvuloplasty. See text for details.

tients with congestive heart failure had lower values of peak occlusion left ventricular pressures than did those without failure. An example of intraventricular pressure recording during balloon occlusion of the aortic orifice in a patient with a normal left ventricular ejection fraction is shown in Figure 9. Within a few beats after aortic out flow occlusion, the left ventricular pressure increases to a maximum level (325 mm Hg), which is followed by gradual reduction of left ventricular and aortic systolic pressures and increase in left ventricular diastolic pressure. In some patients with calcific aortic stenosis, the inflated balloon may not totally occlude the aortic orifice allowing continued ejection with an increased gradient. The degree of aortic outflow occlusion may differ among patients and even among occlusions in the same patient.

Ventricular arrhythmias, which frequently occur during balloon inflation, also make the evaluation of peak occlusion left ventricular pressure difficult to interpret.

Aortic Regurgitation After ABV

The development of severe aortic regurgitation is an occasionally observed complication. A slight increase in the degree of aortic regurgitation or new mild aortic regurgitation may occur in 1–11% of patients undergoing ABV [21,22]. Severe aortic regurgitation is less frequent, but may cause severe hemodynamic abnormalities with progressive circulatory disturbance requiring emergency aortic surgery [23]. An example of severe acute aortic regurgitation complicating ABV is shown in Figure 10. Simultaneous left ventricular and aortic pressures before ABV (Fig. 10, upper panel) show typical features of aortic stenosis. The left ventricular end diastolic pressure is 22 mm Hg and aortic diastolic pressure is 68 mm Hg. Note the several marked changes in both left ventricular and aortic pressure tracings after ABV (Fig. 10, lower panel). The left ventricular systolic pressure is decreased (228 mm Hg to 150 mm Hg) and the end diastolic pressure is markedly increased (to 40 mm Hg) indicating deteriorating left ventricular performance. In addition, the aortic diastolic pressure has fallen to 40 mm Hg so that it is now equal to the left ventricular pressure at the end of diastole. Also note the rapid increase in left ventricular diastolic pressure with the enormous amount of regurgitant blood. In some patients, early closure of the mitral valve may occur with early crossover of left atrial and left ventricular diastolic pressure tracings. The decreased aortic gradient may be due to increased aortic valve opening and/or decreased stroke volume because of left ventricular failure.

Tears involving the aortic annulus are rarely reported [24]. The aortic insufficiency may be extremely severe and may be associated with acute mitral regurgitation resulting from severe left ventricular volume overload. Hemodynamic tracings were obtained (Fig. 11) during a repeat ABV in an 86-yr-old woman with congestive heart failure. Left ventricular (220/34 mm Hg) and aortic (155/58 mm Hg) pressures yielded a peak to peak gradient of 70 mm Hg (Fig. 11, panel A) with aortic valve area of 0.47 cm^2. Immediately following the first balloon inflation, equilibration of aortic and left ventricular pressures was evident consistent with aortic insufficiency (Fig. 11, right side panel A). The stiff Amplatz guidewire across the valve was thought to be contributory. After the second balloon inflation and repositioning of the wire (Fig. 11, panel B), the left ventricular-aortic pressure gradient persists (left ventricular pressure = 170 mm Hg, aortic pressure = 90 mm Hg). There is end-diastolic equilibration of aortic and left ventricular pressures. Following the third balloon inflation (Fig. 11, right side panel B at

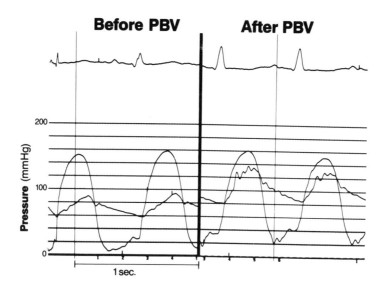

Fig. 7. Left ventricular and aortic pressure tracings in a patient undergoing aortic balloon valvuloplasty. (Left panel) The slope of the aortic upstroke is 130 mm Hg/sec before PBV. (Right panel) The aortic slope is 400 mm Hg/sec after PBV. See text for details.

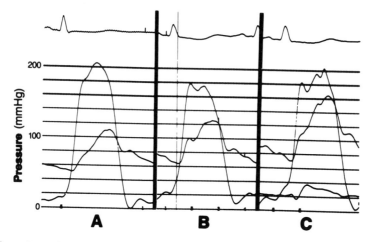

Fig. 8. Hemodynamic tracings of aortic and left ventricular pressures during balloon valvuloplasty. Panel A is the control. Panel B is after 15 mm balloon inflation. Panel C is after 18 mm balloon inflation. See text for details. Reproduced with permission from Vandormael et al., Cathet Cardiovasc Diagn 14:49–52, 1988.

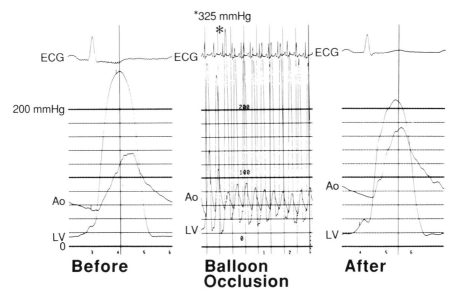

Fig. 9. Hemodynamic tracings during aortic balloon valvuloplasty. See text for details.

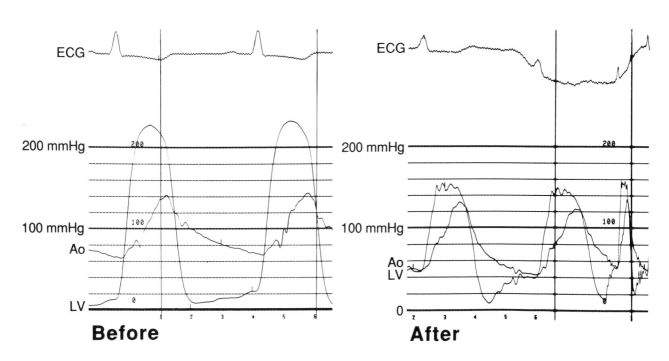

Fig. 10. Aortic (Ao) and left ventricular (LV) pressure tracings during balloon valvuloplasty. The lower panel represents hemodynamic findings at the conclusion of the procedure. A new murmur was identified.

paper speed 100 mm/sec), end-diastolic equilibration of left ventricular, aortic and pulmonary artery pressure is evident. Matching of diastolic left ventricular and pulmonary capillary wedge pressures (Fig. 11, left side panel C) is also associated with giant "V" waves. Emergency echocardiography confirmed the mitral regurgita-

tion. Complete equilibration of left ventricular (LV) and aortic (Ao) pressures demonstrates the hemodynamic severity (Fig. 11, panel D) of a torn aortic root later identified at surgery. Left ventricular and aortic pressures after administration of epinephrine prior to emergency surgery are shown in panel D.

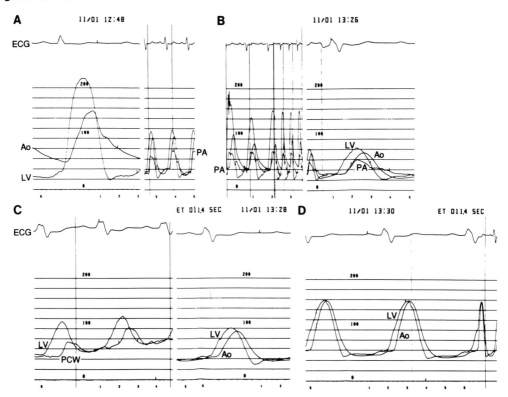

Fig. 11. Serial hemodynamic tracings during aortic balloon valvuloplasty in an 86-yr-old woman undergoing a repeat procedure. The patient required emergency surgery. See text for details. Reproduced with permission from reference 24.

Pulmonary Balloon Valvuloplasty (PBV)

PBV is now the routine treatment for significant congenital pulmonic stenosis. A significant, long-lasting decrease in the pulmonary-right ventricular gradient can be achieved with relatively low morbidity and mortality [25]. PBV is also an effective treatment for adult patients with pulmonic stenosis [26]. An ususual hemodynamic phenomenon sometimes seen after PBV is the development of a subvalvular gradient despite effective opening of the stenotic valve [27]. Review the pressure tracings obtained from an 18-yr-old man with pulmonary stenosis during PBV (Fig. 12). The baseline right ventricular systolic pressure is markedly increased (150 mm Hg) (Fig. 12, upper left hand panel) and is higher than the systemic arterial pressure (not shown). On catheter pullback from the pulmonary artery to the right ventricle before PBV, no significant subvalvular gradient was noted (Fig. 12, upper right hand panel). After PBV, catheter pullback reveals development of significant subvalvular gradient at the right ventricular outflow tract (Fig. 12, lower panel). Because of the outflow obstruction, the net right ventricular to pulmonary artery gradient did not change significantly. A similar situation may be seen after surgical valvotomy [28], probably related to hypertrophy and hyperdynamic contraction of the outflow portion of

the right ventricle. However, the subvalvular obstruction has been shown to decrease gradually after PBV. In a group of 22 patients aged 16–45 years, Fawzy et al. [29] showed that the peak pulmonary gradient decreased from an average 38 mm Hg immediately after PBV to 18 mm Hg after an average 35 mo followup. The outflow gradient was also reduced from an average 35 mm Hg to 15 mm Hg, with a significant increase in measured right ventricular outflow tract diameter.

SUMMARY

The hemodynamic findings of aortic, mitral and pulmonary balloon valvuloplasty serve to identify classical valvular lesions and their responses to graded or abrupt catheter dilation techniques. The production of mild insufficiency after valve dilation is generally well tolerated. Severe valvular insufficiency produces the expected hemodynamic alterations, but acute decompensation may be witnessed over brief periods of time. The use of extra stiff guidewires across dilated valves, especially the aortic valve, may also produce an exaggerated hemodynamic picture of insufficiency. Although gradients may be reduced, the effect of valve dilation on aortic valve area is generally small. A discussion of factors

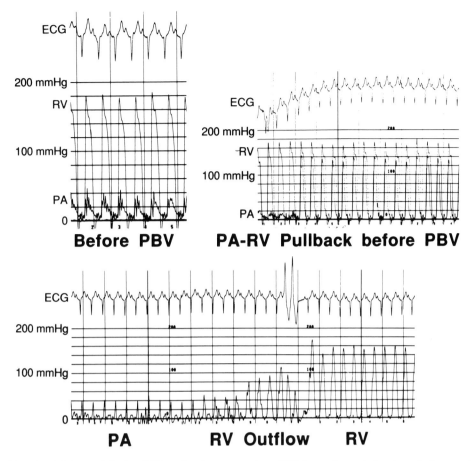

Fig. 12.   Right ventricular (RV) and pulmonary artery (PA) hemodynamic tracings before and after pulmonic balloon valvuloplasty. Note the pressure in the right ventricular outflow tract. See text for details.

influencing valve area calculations will be the subject of a future "Rounds."

ACKNOWLEDGMENTS

The authors with to thank the J.G. Mudd Cardiac Catheterization Team and Donna Sander for manuscript preparation.

REFERENCES

1. Inoue K, Owaki T, Nakamura T, Kitamura F, Miyamoto N. Clinical application of transvenous mitral commissurotomy by a new balloon-catheter. J Thorac Cardiovasc Surg 87:394, 1984.
2. Reyes VP, Raju Bs, Raju ARG, Turi ZG for the MSU-Nizam's Institute Valvuloplasty Study Group. Percutaneous balloon mitral valvuloplasty vs. surgery: results of a randomized clinical trial. Circulation 78:II–489, 1988.
3. Block PC, Palacios IF. Aortic and mitral balloon valvuloplasty: The United States experience. In Topol EJ (ed): "Textbook of Interventional Cardiology." Philadelphia: Saunders, 1990.
4. Nobuyoshi M, hamasaki N, Kimura T, Nosaka H, Yokoi H, Yasumoto H, Horiuchi H, Nakashima H, Shindo T, Mori T, Miyamoto AT, Inoue K. Indications, complications and short-term clinical outcome of percutaneous transvenous mitral commissurotomy. Circulation 80:782–792, 1989.
5. Vahanian A, Michel PL, Cormier B, Vitoux B, Michel X, Slama M, Sarano LE, Trabelsi S, Ismail MB, Acar J. Results of percutaneous mitral commissurotomy in 200 patients. Am J Cardiol 63:847–852, 1989.
6. Block PC, Palacios IF. Pulmonary vascular dynamics after percutaneous mitral valvotomy. J Thorac Cardiovasc Surg 96:39–43, 1988.
7. McKay CR, Kawanishi DT, Rahimtoola SH. Catheter balloon valvuloplasty of the mitral valve in adults using a double-balloon technique. JAMA 257:1753–1761, 1987.
8. McKay CR, Kawanishi DT, Kotlewski A, Parise K, Odom-Maryon T, Gonzalez A, Reid CL, Rahimtoola SH. Improvement in exercise capacity and exercise hemodynamics 3 months after double-balloon, catheter balloon valvuloplasty treatment of patients with symptomatic mitral stenosis. Circulation 77:1013–1021, 1988.
9. Pektas O, Isik E, Coskun M, Demirkan D, Genc C, Tore HF, Uyan C, Dokumaci B. Late hemodynamic changes in percutaneous mitral valvuloplasty. Am Heart J 119:112–120, 1990.
10. Abascal VM, Wilkins GT, Choong CY, Thomas JD, Palacios IF, Block PC, Weyman AE. Echocardiographic evaluation of mitral valve structure and function in patients followed for at least 6

months after percutaneous balloon mitral valvuloplasty. J Am Coll Cardiol 12:606–615, 1988.

11. Tatineni S, Deligonul U, Kaiser G, Kern MJ. Delayed onset of severe mitral regurgitation after successful percutaneous mitral balloon valvuloplasty. Am Heart J (1991, in press).

12. Casale P, Block PC, O'Shea JP, Palacios IF. Atrial septal defect after percutaneous mitral balloon valvuloplasty: Immediate results and follow-up. J Am Coll Cardiol 15:1300–1304, 1990.

13. Cequier A, Bonan R, Serra A, Dyrda I, Crépeau J, Dethy M, Waters D. Left-to-right atrial shunting after percutaneous mitral valvuloplasty: Incidence and long-term hemodynamic follow-up. Circulation 81:1190–1197, 1990.

14. Lefevre T, Bonan R, Serra A, Dyrda I, Crépeau J, Petitclerc R, Waters D. Atrial shunting with sub-acute right heart failure following percutaneous mitral valvuloplasty. J Invas Cardiol 1:311–318, 1989.

15. Goldberg N, Roman CF, Cha SD, Weiner R, Maranhao V, Eldredge J, Fernandez J. Right-to-left interatrial shunting following balloon mitral valvuloplasty. Cathet Cardiovasc Diagn 16:133–135, 1989.

16. Uricchio JF, Likoff W. Effect of mitral commissurotomy on co-existing aortic valve lesions. N Engl J Med 256:199–204, 1957.

17. Cohn LH, Mason DT, Ross J, Morrow AG, Braunwald E. Preoperative assessment of aortic regurgitation in patients with mitral valve disease. Am J Cardiol 19:177–182, 1967.

18. Keane JF, Perry SB, Lock JE. Balloon dilation of congenital valvular aortic stenosis. J Am Coll Cardiol 16:447–458, 1990.

19. Block PC, Palacios IF. Clinical and hemodynamic follow-up after percutaneous aortic valvuloplasty in the elderly. Am J Cardiol 62:760–763, 1988.

20. Bittl JA, Bhatia SJS, Plappert T, Ganz P, Sutton MGS, Selwyn AP. Peak left ventricular pressure during percutaneous aortic balloon valvuloplasty: Clinical and echocardiographic correlations. J Am Coll Cardiol 14:135–142, 1989.

21. Safian RD, Berman AD, Diver DJ, McKay LL, Come PC, Riley MF, Warren SE, Cunningham MJ, Wyman M, Weinstein JS, Grossman W, McKay RG. Balloon aortic valvuloplasty in 170 consecutive patients. N Engl J Med 319:125–130, 1988.

22. Letac B, Cribier A, Koning R, Bellefleur JP. Results of percutaneous transluminal valvuloplasty in 218 adults with valvular aortic stenosis. Am J Cardiol 62:598–605, 1988.

23. Dean LS, Chandler JW, Saenz CB, Baxley WA, Bulle TM. Severe aortic regurgitation complicating percutaneous aortic valve valvuloplasty. Cathet Cardiovasc Diagn 16:130–132, 1989.

24. Kern MJ, Deligonul U, Serota H, Gudipati C, Ring M, Dressler F, Aguirre F. Acute combined aortic and mitral insufficiency during balloon catheter valvuloplasty for a third recurrence of critical aortic stenosis. Am Heart J 120:1007–1011, 1990.

25. Beekman RH, Rocchini AP. Pulmonary valvuloplasty. In Topol EJ (ed): "Textbook of Interventional Cardiology." Philadelphia: Saunders, 1990, pp. 900–911.

26. Fawzy ME, Mercer EN, Dunn B. Late results of pulmonary balloon valvuloplasty in adults using double balloon technique. J Inter Cardiol 1:35–32, 1988.

27. Ben-Shachar G, Cohen MH, Sivakoff MC, Portman MA, Riemenschneider TA, Van Heeckeren DW. Development of infundibular obstruction after percutaneous pulmonary balloon valvuloplasty. J Am Coll Cardiol 5:754–756, 1985.

28. Griffith BP, Hardesty RL, Siewers RD, Lerberg DB, Ferson PF, Bahnson HT. Pulmonary valvulotomy alone for pulmonary stenosis: Results in children with and without muscular infundibular hypertrophy. J Thorac Surg 83:577–583, 1982.

29. Fawzy ME, Galal O, Dunn B, Shaikh A, Sriram R, Duran CMG. Regression of infundibular pulmonary stenosis after successful balloon pulmonary valvuloplasty in adults. Cathet Cardiovasc Diagn 21:77–81, 1990.

Chapter 18

Pulmonic Balloon Valvuloplasty

Morton J. Kern, MD, and Richard G. Bach, MD

INTRODUCTION

Although rarely seen in adults or adolescents, pulmonic stenosis represents one of the more common conditions of congenital heart disease. The traditional method for treatment of congenital pulmonic stenosis was surgical valvotomy until 1982, when Kan et al. [1] developed the technique of percutaneous balloon valvuloplasty. However, in adults and adolescents with pulmonic stenosis, the application of this technique is less well-defined. Successful reports of the procedure in adults have compiled a large experience with the technique, but the overall results have been limited. The introduction of the Inoue valvuloplasty balloon has provided a further technical advance, since the balloon diameter can be increased serially without the cumbersome exchange technique [2,3]. These hemodynamic rounds will review adult pulmonic stenosis treated with balloon valvuloplasty.

CASE REPORTS
Case 1

A 39-year-old woman complained of progressive dyspnea on exertion. She had relatively normal childhood growth and development but was noted to have had a murmur during a high school medical evaluation. No therapy was sought and the patient had been well until recently. She had had several successful deliveries without hemodynamic compromise. The patient had no risk factors for coronary artery disease and was being treated for mild systemic hypertension.

On physical examination, there was a systolic murmur over the left and right sternal borders, a single S_2, and a hyperdynamic right ventricular contraction without a diastolic murmur. There was no peripheral edema or hepatomegaly. The electrocardiogram demonstrated right ventricular hypertrophy. Two-dimensional echocardiography documented pulmonic stenosis, a large right ventricle, and minimal tricuspid regurgitation. The peak valvular gradient was estimated to be >60 mm Hg by Doppler.

At cardiac catheterization, coronary arteriography and left ventriculography were normal. There was a significant pulmonic valvular gradient (Fig. 1). The pulmonary artery pressure was 22/12 mm Hg with a right ventricular pressure of 135/12 mm Hg (Fig. 1). The aortic pressure was 195/90 mm Hg, and the left ventricular pressure was 195/12 mm Hg with a restrictive diastolic filling pattern. Cardiac output was 3.8 l/min. Oximetry was normal.

To identify infundibular or subvalvular narrowing of the right ventricular outflow tract, a second catheter was placed across the pulmonic valve. While continuously recording both pressures, the catheter was then withdrawn (Fig. 2). Right ventricular pressures beneath the pulmonic valve in the outflow tract were compared to the right ventricular pressures in the right ventricular apex (Fig. 2, top). The right ventricular pressure pullback demonstrated a small infundibular gradient of approximately 35 mm Hg (right ventricular outflow, 100/22 mm Hg; right ventricular body, 135/22 mm Hg), appreciated at both low and high recording speeds (Fig. 2, bottom).

Balloon valvuloplasty was performed with a single standard balloon catheter, as previously described [1]. A 300-cm exchange guidewire was positioned in the distal pulmonary artery, and a 20 mm × 4 cm balloon catheter (Boston Scientific Co., Boston, MA) was positioned across the valve (Fig. 3). Figure 4 demonstrates aortic and right ventricular pressures during a pulmonary balloon inflation. After two balloon inflations, hemodynamics

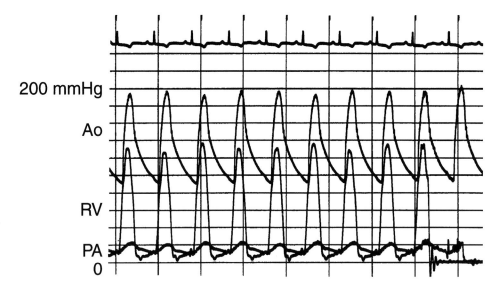

Fig. 1. Hemodynamic tracings obtained before pulmonary valvuloplasty, demonstrating aortic pressure (Ao), right ventricular pressure (RV), and pulmonary artery pressure (PA) on a 0–200 mm Hg scale. The systolic gradient across the pulmonic valve is 110 mm Hg.

demonstrated a significant decrease in pulmonary gradient.

Following removal of the balloon catheter and guidewire, hemodynamic data were again measured. The right ventricular systolic pressure decreased from 135 mm Hg to 45 mm Hg, with a corresponding reduction of the pulmonary gradient from 110 mm Hg to 25 mm Hg. The pulmonary artery pressure was minimally effected (20 mm Hg to 24 mm Hg) (Fig. 5).

The residual subvalvular obstruction was measured during pulmonary artery catheter pullback (Fig. 6). The pulmonary artery systolic pressure was 22 mm Hg (Fig. 6, left), and as the catheter entered the right ventricle two new observations were evident. First, the systolic pressure increased to 26–28 mm Hg, and also, the diastolic pressure waveform matched the right ventricular pressure. This region is the subvalvular right ventricular outflow tract, from which the residual gradient is formed.

Case 2

A 29-year-old man had tetralogy of Fallot with a large ventricular septal defect, infundibular obstruction, and valvular pulmonic stenosis detected at birth. At age 7, he underwent surgical closure of the ventricular septal defect using a Dacron patch, resection of infundibular muscle, and incision of the pulmonic valve commissures, with excellent results. He was asymptomatic until several months before admission, when he noted progressive dyspnea on mild exertion, easy fatigability, and intermittent pedal edema. His examination was notable for clear lungs, a diminished second heart sound, and a loud, harsh III/VI systolic crescendo-decrescendo murmur at the

upper left sternal border. There was no peripheral edema. The electrocardiogram demonstrated right ventricular hypertrophy.

Cardiac catheterization demonstrated normal left ventricular wall motion and normal coronary arteries. A peak systolic transvalvular pulmonic gradient of 60 mm Hg was produced by a right ventricular pressure of 85/15 mm Hg and a pulmonary artery pressure of 25/15 mm Hg (Fig. 7, top left). There was no infundibular gradient. Right ventriculography in a lateral projection showed limited motion and doming of the pulmonic valve leaflets (Fig. 8, left). Pulmonary artery angiography showed mild pulmonic insufficiency. There was poststenotic dilatation of the main pulmonary artery. Cardiac output was 4.5 l/min, and oximetry showed no evidence of intracardiac shunt.

Balloon valvuloplasty was performed. From right ventricular angiography in the left lateral projection, the pulmonic annulus was measured at 22–23 mm. After 5,000 units of intravenous heparin had been administered, a stiff 0.038″ Amplatz guidewire was placed into a distal pulmonary artery segment via a balloon-tipped wedge catheter. Multiple dilatations with a 23 mm × 4 cm balloon catheter (Boston Scientific Co.) were performed across the pulmonic valve. The balloon was noted, at times, to slip backward or forward at full inflation. These dilatations resulted in improvement but there remained a residual 30–40 mm Hg transvalvular gradient (Fig. 7, top right). Therefore, a 0.018″ guidewire was exchanged for a 0.025″ Amplatz wire and a 28-mm Inoue balloon (Toray, Inc., Tokyo, Japan) situated across the pulmonic valve. Careful torquing of the Inoue catheter through the right

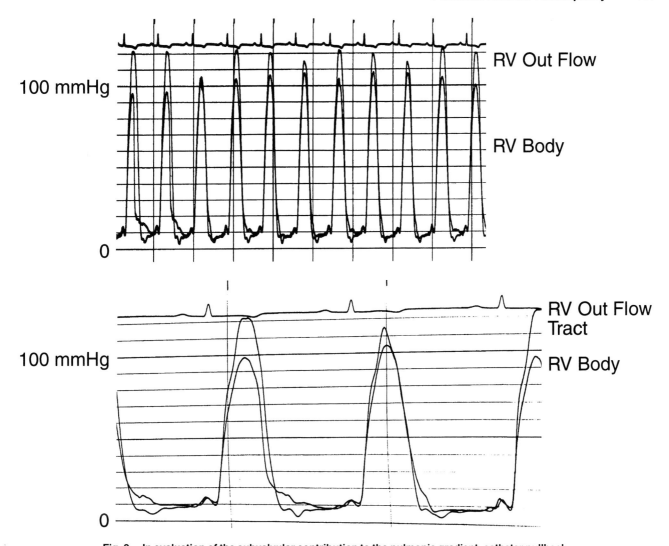

Fig. 2. In evaluation of the subvalvular contribution to the pulmonic gradient, catheter pullback from the pulmonary artery to the right ventricle was performed. The subpulmonic gradient was 20 mm Hg. The two right ventricular (RV) pressures are shown during pullback maneuver on a 0–100 mm Hg scale. The RV pullback shows the small infundibular tract outflow gradient between the RV infundibulum and outflow and the RV body. The pressures are recorded at 25-mm/sec paper speed at a 0–100 mm Hg scale (top) and at 100-mm/sec paper speed (bottom).

atrium and across the tricuspid valve was required. Taking advantage of the Inoue balloon characteristics, the tip was partially inflated in the main pulmonary artery and the balloon was pulled into the appropriate position at valve level (Fig. 8, middle and right). Sequential stepwise dilatations from 24 to 28 mm by increasing balloon volume resulted in marked reduction in the transvalvular gradient to 6–8 mm Hg, with a reduction in right ventricular systolic pressure to 45 mm Hg (Fig. 7, bottom). Pulmonary angiography showed moderate pulmonic insufficiency. Following the procedure, the patient noted resolution of his symptoms, which has been sustained for >9 months. Follow-up echocardiography at 6 months postvalvuloplasty showed no valvular resteno-

sis and mild pulmonic insufficiency. A summary of the hemodynamics is shown in Table I.

DISCUSSION

These cases illustrate typical hemodynamics of pulmonic stenosis in adults, and the typical response to catheter balloon valvuloplasty. Chen et al. [4] have described their experience in 53 adolescent or adult patients ranging in age from 13–55 years with follow-up studies at a mean of 7 ± 3 years after the procedure by Doppler echocardiography. The results indicated that after pulmonic balloon valvuloplasty, the systolic pressure gradient across the pulmonic valve decreased from

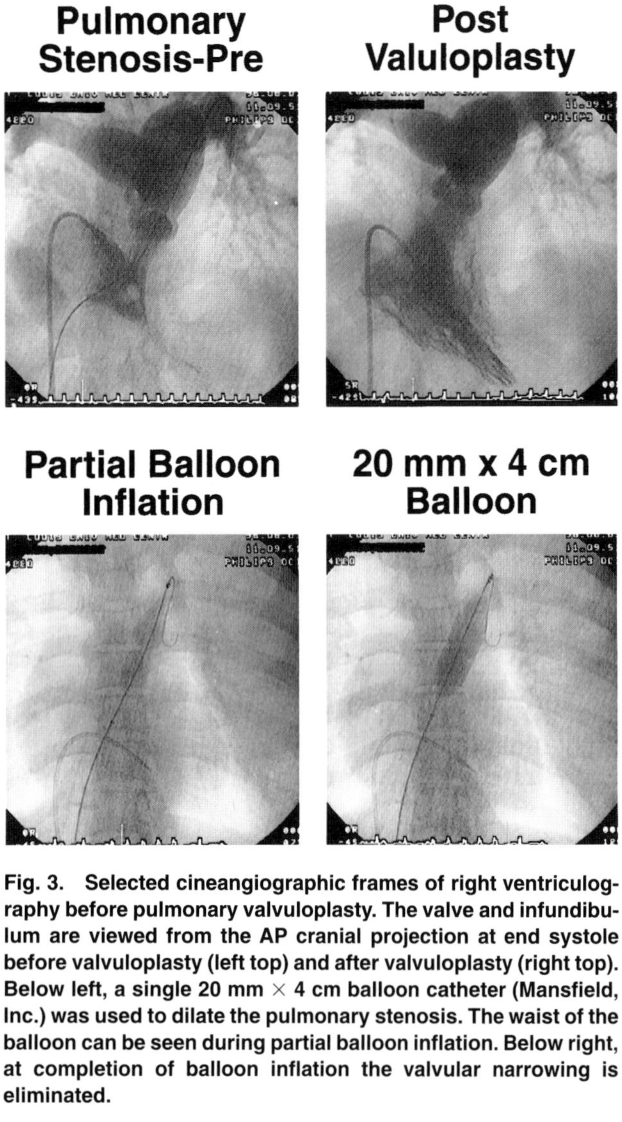

Pulmonary Stenosis-Pre

Post Valuloplasty

Partial Balloon Inflation

20 mm x 4 cm Balloon

Fig. 3. Selected cineangiographic frames of right ventriculography before pulmonary valvuloplasty. The valve and infundibulum are viewed from the AP cranial projection at end systole before valvuloplasty (left top) and after valvuloplasty (right top). Below left, a single 20 mm × 4 cm balloon catheter (Mansfield, Inc.) was used to dilate the pulmonary stenosis. The waist of the balloon can be seen during partial balloon inflation. Below right, at completion of balloon inflation the valvular narrowing is eliminated.

91 ± 46 mm Hg to 38 ± 32 mm Hg, and the diameter of the pulmonic valve orifice increased from 9 ± 4 mm to 17 ± 5 mm. At follow-up, hemodynamic data indicated that the systolic gradient continued to decrease from 107 ± 48 mm Hg before to 50 ± 29 mm Hg after valvuloplasty, and at follow-up remained at 30 ± 16 mm Hg. Pulmonic valve incompetence was noted in 7 of 53 patients (13%) after balloon valvuloplasty but was absent at follow-up examination in all patients. The investigators concluded that late adolescent or adult patients with congenital pulmonic stenosis can be treated with percutaneous balloon valvuloplasty successfully with excellent short- and long-term results, similar to those in children.

Valvuloplasty Techniques

The technique of pulmonic valvuloplasty has variably included single and double balloons as well as the use of

the recently developed Inoue two-component balloon. The method has had little modification over time since its introduction. With one (or two) vascular access sheaths, one catheter can be placed in the pulmonary artery and another catheter in the right ventricle. After assessing the transpulmonic gradient and cardiac output, the diameters of the valvular orifice and annulus are measured from the right ventricular angiogram viewed in the AP cranial or lateral projections. The ratio of the diameter of the balloon to the diameter of the valvular annulus (from 22–25 mm in diameter), in most studies, ranges between 1.1–1.2. Once the hemodynamics and angiographic data have been obtained, a long exchange guidewire guides the balloon catheter across the pulmonic valve. When using an Inoue-type balloon, the method of placement may involve a flotation approach [3]. The balloon is quickly inflated, the waist of the narrowed valve is eliminated, and the balloon is deflated and withdrawn for repeat hemodynamic measurements.

The successful results of balloon techniques have changed clinical practice so that the method of choice for pulmonic stenosis is catheter balloon valvuloplasty over the surgical valvotomy technique, except in patients with dysplastic valves [5]. The mobility of a dysplastic pulmonary valve is so impaired that surgery is most often the preferred treatment of choice. However, some patients with dysplastic valves may still do well with pulmonary catheter balloon valvuloplasty [5]. Chen et al. [4] reported on their results using the Inoue technique in adults and adolescents. The 10-year follow-up results demonstrated sustained clinical benefit.

Some investigators believe that one difference between pulmonic balloon valvuloplasty in adults and in children is the necessity to accurately select a balloon size which is not larger than the annulus of the pulmonic valve. Although this remains controversial, in children, a balloon size should be substantially larger than the annulus [6]. In addition, the results of balloon valvuloplasty are sustained for a longer period of time in adults as compared to children, where restenosis of the valve may approach 20%, which is particularly important in the youngest children [7]. The Inoue balloon provides the ability to increase balloon diameter by increasing balloon volume, which allows stepwise increases in valve expansion.

With regard to technical approaches, the Inoue balloon catheter appears to have an advantage over conventional balloon catheters. Conventional balloons with a stiff tip and long balloon material are less flexible than the shorter Inoue balloon. This difference in sizing and flexibility minimizes potential injury to the right ventricular outflow tract and the pulmonary artery. The ability of the Inoue balloon to assist in positioning itself accurately across the

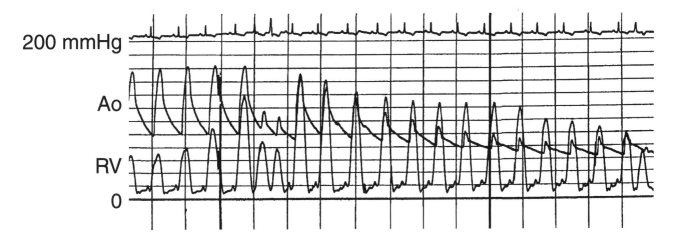

Fig. 4. Hemodynamic alterations during pulmonary valvuloplasty. The right ventricular (RV) pressure after the second balloon inflation is recorded at initiation of balloon inflation. Aortic pressure (Ao) and cardiac output fall during pulmonary artery balloon obstruction. Ventricular premature contractions can be seen. Right ventricular pressure increases to equal systemic pressure for the first three beats, and then both systemic pressure and RV pressure fall during balloon inflation and deflation. Scale is 0–200 mm Hg.

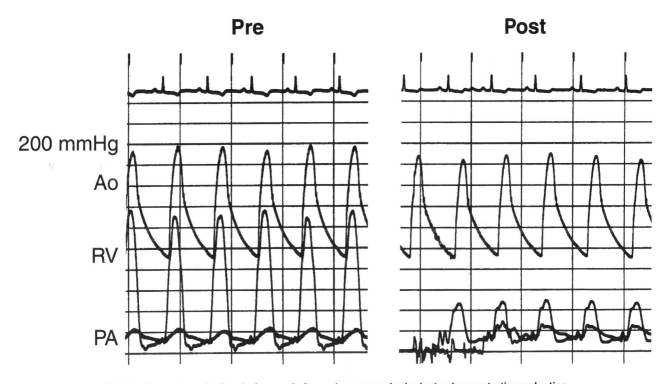

Fig. 5. Hemodynamic data before and after pulmonary valvuloplasty, demonstrating reduction in the right ventricular (RV)/pulmonary artery (PA) systolic gradient from 110 mm Hg to approximately 25 mm Hg. The residual outflow tract gradient represents that of the infundibulum, which was not affected by the balloon inflation.

most severe portion of the pulmonary valve also diminishes the abrupt forward movement which is experienced during balloon inflation with the conventional technique. The risk of overdilatation of the pulmonic valve can also be reduced using a stepwise inflation technique of the Inoue balloon method. Increments of up to 5-mm diameters can be adjusted by increasing the inflation volume. A single Inoue balloon catheter can thus replace two

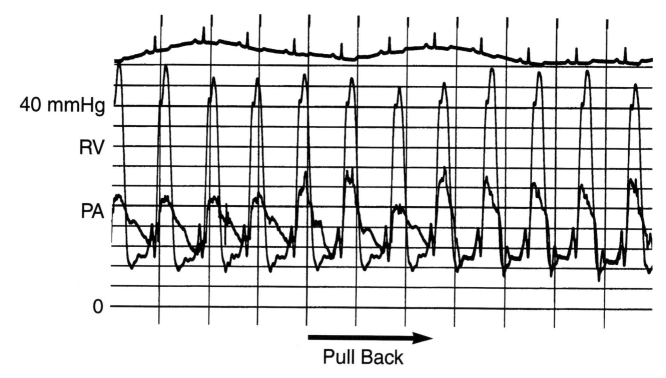

Pull Back

Fig. 6. Demonstration of right ventricular (RV) outflow tract gradient. Catheter pullback to just beneath the pulmonary valve shows an increase in systolic pressure simultaneous with RV diastolic pressure (0–40 mm Hg scale). As the catheter is pulled farther back, two RV pressures become superimposed (not shown).

traditional 15-mm-diameter balloons for valvular dilatation. Finally, the Inoue balloon catheter has larger lumens with short inflation/deflation cycle times, in most cases between 5–10 sec. The reduction of the duration of reduced cardiac output increases procedural safety and minimizes hemodynamic compromise. The profile of the Inoue balloon is also narrow enough to avoid difficulties with hemostatic control, and the balloon can be inserted without a vascular sheath. The puncture site is easily compressible, reducing blood loss and hematoma. The only major disadvantage to the Inoue balloon catheter is the cost, which has been an issue in some areas of the world.

Residual Transpulmonic Gradients

A persistent systolic gradient suggests that subvalvular stenosis of the right ventricular outflow tract may occur after successful balloon valvuloplasty. The reduction in systolic gradient at follow-up examination of the patients undergoing pulmonary valvuloplasty suggests that a delayed reduction of the gradient produces results similar to those of surgical pulmonic valvulotomy, and that the systolic gradient measured immediately after balloon valvuloplasty underestimates the long-term results of the procedure. As noted in case 1, infundibular hypertrophy caused by long-standing pulmonary stenosis may result in

residual outflow tract obstruction, which can regress over time. The regression of infundibular hypertrophy is more notable in the younger population as compared to adults [8]. The systolic gradient, measured across both the valve and the infundibulum at follow-up, although markedly reduced after valvuloplasty, suggests that there is some degree of regression of the hypertrophic infundibulum and that surgical resection for adults may not be required. This finding also supports the idea that stenosis of the infundibulum is not an absolute contraindication to percutaneous balloon pulmonic valvuloplasty.

Although the mechanism of infundibular tract systolic gradients is incompletely understood, the subvalvular muscular hypertrophy and activity of contraction in the unrestrained phase immediately on relief of valvular resistance probably produce a hyperkinetic effect. Beta-blockers have been recommended, although in most adult series these medications have not been necessary.

Complications After Pulmonic Valvuloplasty

Pulmonic insufficiency after valvuloplasty occurred in 13% of patients in the study of Chen et al. [4], none of which was of major hemodynamic consequence. Similar data have been reported by others [9,10] and appear due to the more precise sizing of the pulmonic valve by a

Pulmonary Valuloplasty

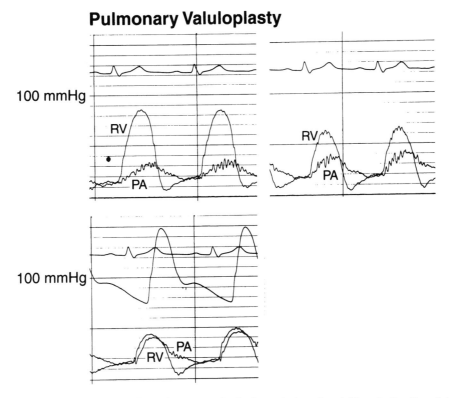

Fig. 7. Hemodynamic data for pulmonary valvuloplasty, before (top left) and after (top right) initial balloon inflations, and after (bottom) Inoue balloon inflations. RV, right ventricular pressure; PA, pulmonary artery pressure.

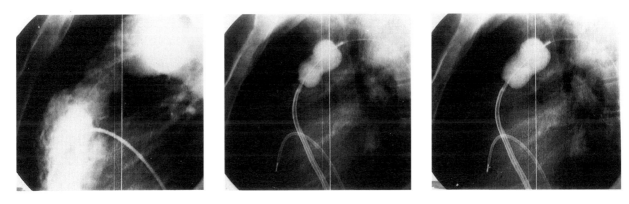

Fig. 8. Cine frames during pulmonary valvuloplasty. At left, lateral view right ventriculogram demonstrating doming stenotic pulmonary valve. At center, Inoue balloon partially inflated. At right, Inoue balloon fully inflated.

variable balloon catheter method. Unique to pulmonic stenosis is the situation of the dysplastic valve associated with complex intracardiac defects. David et al. [5] reported on the results of percutaneous balloon dilatation for pulmonic stenosis in 38 patients ranging from 9 months to 63 years in age. Thirty-four patients had typical pulmonary stenosis, with 5 having complex congenital cardiac anomalies. Thirteen patients also had a patent foramen ovale. For the group, there was significant reduction in the immediate postvalvuloplasty transpulmonic gradient from 97 mm Hg to 26 mm Hg. There was one death in the postvalvuloplasty period of a patient with class IV congestive heart failure due to right ventricular decompensation. There were no other cardiovascular complications encountered, with a mean hospital stay of 3 days. At 8-month follow-up, the transpulmonic gradient in 12 patients was 27 mm Hg, compared to the prevalvuloplasty value of 84 mm Hg. Two patients had restenosed,

TABLE I. Hemodynamic Data

	Right Ventricular Pressure (mm Hg)	Pulmonary Artery Pressure (mm Hg)	Pressure Gradient (mm Hg)	Cardiac Output (l/min)	Left Ventricular Pressure (mm Hg)	Aortic Pressure (mm Hg)
Case 1						
Before pulmonary valvuloplasty	135/12	22/12	115	3.8	195/12	195/90
After pulmonary valvuloplasty	45/12	24/12	25			190/90
Case 2						
Before pulmonary valvuloplasty	85/20	32/18	53			
After pulmonary valvuloplasty	45/18	42/15	3			

one required open-heart surgical valvotomy, and one had successful repeat balloon valvuloplasty.

CONCLUSIONS

These cases illustrate the successful treatment of severe pulmonic stenosis using balloon valvuloplasty. Pulmonic valvuloplasty should be considered an excellent alternative to surgical treatment for most, if not all, patients, regardless of age, with significant pulmonary valvular obstruction. These individuals are at risk for severely compromised hemodynamic function if the lesion is not corrected. Although only limited studies exist, the Inoue balloon may provide certain significant technical advantages for pulmonic valvuloplasty.

ACKNOWLEDGMENTS

The authors thank the J.G. Mudd Cardiac Catheterization Laboratory for technical support, and Donna Sander for manuscript preparation.

REFERENCES

1. Kan JS, White RJ Jr, Mitchell SE, Gardner TJ: Percutaneous balloon valvuloplasty: A new method for treating congenital pulmonary-valve stenosis. N Engl J Med 307:540–542, 1982.
2. Lau K, Hung J, Wu J, Chern M, Yeh K, Fu M: Pulmonary valvuloplasty in adults using the Inoue balloon catheter. Cathet Cardiovasc Diagn 29:99–104, 1993.
3. Patel JM, Dani SI, Shah SC, Shah UG, Patel TK: Inoue-balloon pulmonary valvuloplasty using a "free-float" technique. J Invas Cardiol 8:374–377, 1996.
4. Chen C, Cheng T, Huang T, Zhou Y, Chen J, Huang Y, Li H: Percutaneous balloon valvuloplasty for pulmonic stenosis in adolescents and adults. N Engl J Med 335:21–25, 1996.
5. David SW, Goussous YM, Harbi N, Doghmi F, Hiari A, Krayyem M, Ferlinz J: Management of typical and dysplastic pulmonic stenosis, uncomplicated or associated with complex intracardiac defects in juveniles and adults: Use of percutaneous balloon pulmonary valvuloplasty with eight-month hemodynamic follow-up. Cathet Cardiovasc Diagn 29:105–112, 1993.
6. Rao PS: Pulmonic stenosis. In Cheng TO (ed): "Percutaneous Balloon Valvuloplasty." New York: Igaku-Shoin Medical, 1992, pp 365–420.
7. Rao PS, Thapar MK, Kutayli F: Causes of restenosis after balloon valvuloplasty for valvular pulmonary stenosis. Am J Cardiol 62:979–982, 1988.
8. Ben-Shachar G, Cohen MH, Sivakoff MC, Portman MA, Riemenschneider TA, Van Heeckeren DW: Development of infundibular obstruction after percutaneous pulmonary balloon valvuloplasty. J Am Coll Cardiol 5:754–756, 1985.
9. Gutgesell HP: Pulmonary valve insufficiency: Malignant or benign? J Am Coll Cardiol 20:174–175, 1992.
10. O'Connor BK, Beekman RH, Lindauer A, Rocchini A: Intermediate-term outcome after pulmonary balloon valvuloplasty: Comparison with a matched surgical control group. J Am Coll Cardiol 20:169–173, 1992.

PART III: CONSTRICTIVE PHYSIOLOGY

The most important advance in hemodynamic diagnosis in the last decade has been the identification of the influence of respiratory dynamics on ventricular pressure interaction for separation of constrictive from restrictive physiology. Hurrell, Higano and colleagues from the Mayo Clinic have described this phenomenon in detail in their *Circulation* publications. This experience was derived over 10 years, collecting data from a group of patients with documented constrictive pericarditis at operation and correlating the hemodynamic findings. This landmark study has provided new dynamic criteria for the hemodynamic diagnosis of constrictive pericardial disease, increasing the sensitivity and specificity for beyond the traditional "dip and plateau" and static hemodynamic measurements. We have added three new parts to this section on the hemodynamics of constrictive physiology and believe that these descriptions and cases will enhance the reader's appreciation of this difficult but important physiology.

Morton J. Kern, MD

Chapter 19

Hemodynamics of Constrictive Physiology—Section I:
Pericardial Compressive Hemodynamics

Morton J. Kern, MD, and Frank V. Aguirre, MD

INTRODUCTION

Although pericardial effusions are common, a majority of patients are not typically symptomatic or hemodynamically compromised. Hemodynamic data obtained during pericardiocentesis provides a unique opportunity to examine the effects of right and left heart filling pressures when opposed by extrinsic pericardial pressure. Changes in pressure waveforms also provide insight into the constrictive/restrictive pathophysiologic mechanisms and the response to therapies. Pericardiocentesis often reverses the hemodynamic abnormalities, but may not normalize all pressures despite low or near zero pericardial pressure. Recent detailed hemodynamic and echocardiographic observations describe a spectrum of hemodynamic responses which have changed earlier "all or none" concepts of the severe hemodynamic compromise of cardiac tamponade [1,2]. Part I of this round will illustrate several salient features of pericardial compressive hemodynamics which may be confused with the classical findings of cardiac tamponade or the physiology of restrictive cardiomyopathy. Parts II and III will discuss further examples of pericardial constrictive physiology.

PERICARDIAL FLUID AFTER CARDIAC TRANSPLANTATION AND EARLY TAMPONADE

A 53-yr-old woman underwent orthotopic cardiac transplantation for dilated cardiomyopathy [3]. The postoperative course was uncomplicated. Medications at the time of discharge included cyclosporin, azathioprine and steroids. On the fourth hospital day, a moderate pericardial effusion without echocardiographic evidence of hemodynamic compromise was noted. Over the next week, increasing jugular venous distension, hepatomegaly and increasing abdominal girth with clear lung fields prompted a repeat echocardiogram which showed right ventricular enlargement, normal systolic left ventricular function and larger anterior and posterior pericardial effusions without echocardiographic signs of tamponade [4]. Cardiac catheterization was then performed during routine endomyocardial biopsy from the femoral approach. During the right heart catheterization, mean right atrial pressure of 20mmHg, pulmonary artery diastolic pressure of 20mmHg and mean pulmonary capillary wedge pressure of 18mmHg were recorded with equalization of left and right ventricular diastolic pressures (Figs. 1,2). Note the prominent Y descent on the right atrial tracing and the dip-and-plateau configuration of the right ventricular pressure (Fig. 1). Left ventricular and pulmonary capillary wedge pressures were also mildly elevated and equilibrated (Fig. 2). No biopsy evidence of transplant rejection was found. Because pericardial effusion and abnormal hemodynamics of this type have been described early after cardiac transplant [5,6], diuretics, nitrates and isoproterenol were prescribed, but without effect on jugular venous distension or dyspnea on minimal exertion. One week later, the patient was dyspneic with a systolic blood pressure of 85mmHg and a pulsus paradoxus (> 10mmHg) not previously observed (Fig. 3). Equilibration of right atrial and pulmonary artery pressure was present. Urgent periocardiocentesis was performed. Before assessing the results of the pericardiocentesis, consider the following issues: based on the

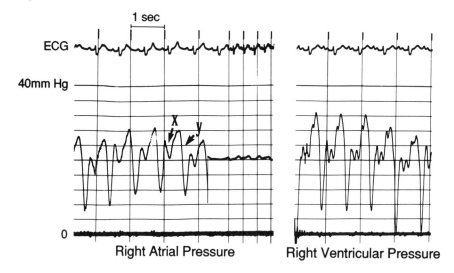

Fig. 1. Right atrial and right ventricular pressure waves showing exaggerated Y descents and early diastolic dip-and-plateau on right ventricular tracing. ECG = electrocardiogram (0–40mmHg pressure scale). See text for details.

right atrial waveforms, does this patient more likely have pericardial constriction, early tamponade or both? Does equilibration of right and left ventricular pressures favor constriction or tamponade? Finally, based on hypotension with newly observed pulsus paradoxus, does one delay pericardiocentesis until after confirmation by echocardiography?

Pericardiocentesis was performed from the subxyphoid approach with hemodynamic monitoring [7]. Pericardial pressure was initially measured through the long 18 gauge pericardial needle. After passing the J-tipped guidewire and an 8 French dilator, a multiple sidehole catheter was advanced into the pericardial space for fluid drainage and pressure measurement. A balloon-tipped catheter measured pressures in the right heart. A 5 French sheath was placed in the femoral artery.

Hemodynamic data at the time of pericardiocentesis (Fig. 4) again showed equalization of diastolic pressures with a mean right atrial pressure of 26mmHg and a dip-and-plateau configuration of the right ventricular tracing as in Figure 2. Arterial pressure was 85/58mmHg. A 2-dimensional echocardiogram, performed at bedside, confirmed the larger pericardial effusion and moderate depression of both right and left ventricular systolic function. Right atrial and right ventricular diastolic collapse, although present, were not striking.

Surprisingly, intrapericardial pressure was elevated to only 10mmHg (Fig. 4). After removal of 250cc of serosanguinous pericardial fluid, the pericardial pressure fell to zero with no change in right atrial or systemic pressure, or cardiac output. Note the absence of waveform alteration of right atrial pressure and persistence of hypotension with pulsus paradoxus after pericardiocentesis.

A presumptive diagnosis of cardiac allograft rejection was confirmed by biopsy. Treatment of allograft rejection permitted the patient to be discharged with resolution of the symptoms and hemodynamic abnormalities. Repeat right heart catheterization two months later showed only mild elevation of right heart pressures without diastolic pressure equalization.

This patient initially demonstrated hemodynamics of constrictive physiology in association with a pericardial effusion. Later development of hypotension and pulsus paradoxus suggested early cardiac tamponade. Most surprising was the fact that pericardial pressure was significantly lower than right atrial pressure and hence, pericardiocentesis did not alter the systemic hemodynamic response. With treatment of allograft rejection, the hemodynamics reverted toward normal. Restrictive physiology was the true pathophysiologic explanation of the hemodynamics [8].

THE THREE PHASES OF CARDIAC TAMPONADE

Cardiac tamponade was initially thought to be an *all or none* phenomena with hypotension and decreased cardiac output as a result of fluid accumulation reaching a critical level impairing ventricular filling [1]. The all or none hypothesis stated that increased pericardial pressure produced equilibration with right ventricular pressure and thus limited ventricular filling and cardiac output. Early in the course of effusion, cardiac pressures remain unchanged. With increasing fluid, both the pericardial and right ventricular filling pressures increase together, eventually equilibrating with left ventricular pressure. At this point, elevated right ventricular pressure without de-

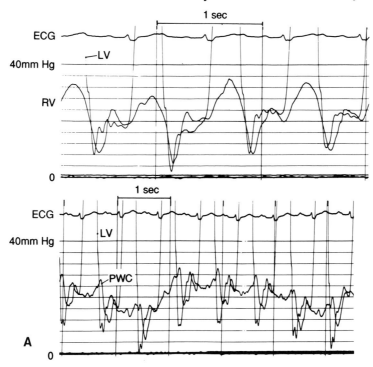

Fig. 2. A: (Top) Left (LV) and right ventricular (RV) pressure waves (0–40mmHg full scale). (Bottom) LV and pulmonary capillary wedge pressure (PCW) demonstrating diastolic equalization in a patient with pericardial effusion after cardiac tamponade. See text for details. With permission from reference #3.

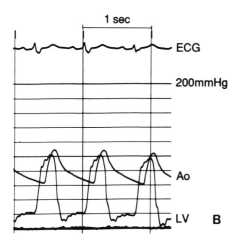

Fig. 2. B: Aortic and left ventricular pressures prior to hemodynamic compromise in a patient with pericardial effusion. Note the pattern of left ventricular filling with early but moderate diastolic dip with a plateau phase over the second two-thirds of the diastolic filling period. Arterial pressure is satisfactory despite symptoms of dyspnea at this time. Ao=aortic pressure; LV=left ventricular pressure.

pression of cardiac output or pulsus paradoxus may be evident. Reddy et al. [1] described this intermediate presentation as right heart tamponade. With continued fluid accumulation, pericardial, right ventricular and left ventricular filling pressures increase and equilibrate, de-

creasing cardiac output and producing pulsus paradoxus. Thus, 3 phases of cardiac tamponade can be readily appreciated.

Reddy et al. [2] have subsequently modified their earlier observations (Fig. 5). Phase I cardiac tamponade occurs when intrapericardial pressure is less than right ventricular and pulmonary capillary wedge (left ventricular filling) pressures. A characteristic hemodynamic response on pericardiocentesis in phase I patients decreases pericardial and right atrial pressures with minimal change in the inspiratory decrease in arterial systolic pressure and no change in cardiac output. Phase II cardiac tamponade occurs when intrapericardial pressure equilibrates with right ventricular, but not pulmonary capillary wedge pressure. Pericardiocentesis in phase II decreases pericardial, right atrial and, to some extent, pulmonary capillary wedge pressures with a larger change in the inspiratory decrease in arterial pressure (paradox) with a modest increase in cardiac output. Classical phase III cardiac tamponade is observed when intrapericardial pressure equilibrates with right ventricular and pulmonary capillary wedge (left ventricular filling) pressures. Pericardiocentesis in phase III decreases pericardial, right atrial and pulmonary capillary wedge pressures with normalization of the exaggerated inspiratory decrease in arterial systolic pressure and a pronounced increase in cardiac output. The changes after pericardi-

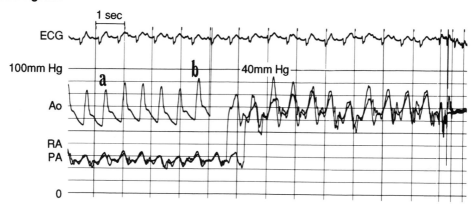

Fig. 3. Hemodynamics after an episode of hypotension with echocardiographic signs of hemodynamic compromise. Arterial pressure (Ao), right atrial (RA) and pulmonary artery (PA) pressures are shown on 0–100mmHg scale (left side) and 0–40mmHg (right side). Note the change in inspiratory systolic pressure (a to b) during a respiratory phase without alteration of the right atrial or pulmonary artery pressures. Equilibration of right atrial and pulmonary artery pressures are striking as shown on the right side of panel.

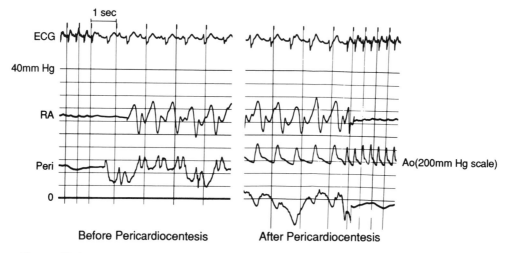

Before Pericardiocentesis   After Pericardiocentesis

Fig. 4. Right atrial (RA) and intrapericardial pressure (peri) before (left) and after (right) pericardiocentesis (0–40mmHg scale). Note: absence of change in RA waveform and low arterial pressure after pericardial fluid removed. See text for details. With permission from reference #3.

ocentesis indicate that pericardial effusion and tamponade physiology exhibits the greatest abnormalities in phase 3, and is associated with significant abnormalities of pressure and flow in phase 2 and with only pressure alterations in phase 1. As Reddy et al. [2] conclude, cardiac tamponade is not an all-or-none phenomena. The severity of hemodynamic derangement rather than its mere presence should be assessed in patients with pericardial effusion. Echocardiography has significantly improved out ability to assess the hemodynamic phases of cardiac tamponade.

ROLE OF ECHOCARDIOGRAPHY IN CARDIAC TAMPONADE

Levine et al. [9] emphasize that two-dimensional echocardiography not only has improved the detection of pericardial effusion, but also indicates with high degree of sensitivity probable tamponade (although not which phase) as defined by right heart chamber collapse during diastole in the presence of pericardial effusion. As described in the hemodynamic spectrum above [2], many patients with moderate pericardial effusion may have only minimal hemodynamic compromise with systolic pressures > 100mmHg with at least half having cardiac index of > 2.3L/min/m^2 (9). Pericardiocentesis in these patients resulted in hemodynamic improvement, but did not alleviate symptoms of dyspnea or modify tachycardia. Subtle or early evidence of hemodynamic compromise was obtained in distinction to the classic reports of cardiac tamponade in decades past where only phase III patients with severe hemodynamic compromise were recognized. Correlation between echocardiographic evi-

Pathophysiology of Cardiac Tamponade

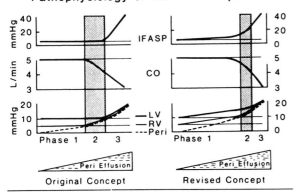

Fig. 5. Diagram of concepts of the 3 phases of cardiac tamponade. Previous concept on left has been modified by including data and theories of ventricular compliance on right side. Hemodynamic changes of pericardial pressure (peri), right ventricular (RV), left ventricular (LV) pressure and inspiratory increase in arterial systolic pressure (IFASP) and cardiac output (CO) are demonstrated with increasing pericardial effusion for a given patient. The height of the triangle from left to right is the amount of pericardial effusion accumulating. Phase 2 is represented by the stipled bar. See text for details. With permission from reference #2.

dence of tamponade and hemodynamic findings indicate a fair, but wide, range of results suggesting a qualitative difference exists with regard to unmeasured variables in such studies. Echocardiography should not delay pericardiocentesis when clinical features and hemodynamics indicate phase II or III tamponade is present.

PULSUS PARADOXUS

A 68-year-old man with chronic renal failure on dialysis presents with increasing shortness of breath and dyspnea over 2 months. His cardiac silhouette on chest X-ray was reported to be enlarged compared to previous film. A marked inspiratory decline in arterial pressure was noted by the referring physician. The patient was being treated for persistent hypertension and had recently had cardiac catheterization for a chest pain syndrome which showed normal coronary arteries and moderately diminished left ventricular function. Echocardiography revealed a large pericardial effusion with right heart chamber collapse in diastole. Pericardiocentesis was performed with technique used in patient #1. Arterial pressure (Fig. 6) varied from 180/120mmHg to 145/95mmHg over a single respiratory cycle. The inspiratory decline in arterial pressure was 40mmHg. Corresponding with the labored inspiration was the marked increase and decrease in the matching right atrial and pericardial pressures. Of note is the abbreviated Y descent on the right atrial tracing. The inspiratory increase in right atrial and intrapericardial pressures was also abnormal. Compare

the right atrial pressure wave to that obtained in patient #1 prior to pericardiocentesis. Several differences can be seen. The inspiratory increase in right atrial (and pericardial) pressures is not as prominent. The striking Y descent is absent in patient #2. The severity of pulsus paradoxus is also greater in patient #2. Pericardial catheter drainage removed 450cc of serosanguinous fluid, reducing the pericardial pressure to 2–3mmHg and the right atrial pressure from a mean of 18mmHg to a mean of 10mmHg (Fig. 6, lower right panel). Release of pericardial pressure changed the right atrial pressure waveform toward normal with restoration of the X and Y filling patterns, especially prominent during inspiration. The A and V waves with the corresponding X and Y descents are altered to various degrees depending on the type of pericardial physiology present (Table I).

This patient example demonstrates the remarkable feature of extreme pulsus paradoxus that can occur in the absence of classical tamponade (hypotension, narrow pulse pressure, low cardiac output and tachycardia). The resolution of pulsus paradoxus, evident after pericardiocentesis, corresponded to improvement in dyspnea with slowing of the heart rate. Incidentally, the pulmonary artery oxygen saturation, obtained with an oximetric catheter before pericardiocentesis, had risen from 48% to 72%, demonstrating a marked increase in cardiac ouput. This patient in phase II cardiac tamponade had a clear symptomatic and hemodynamic indication for a therapeutic pericardial drainage due to uremic pericarditis. Note that the right atrial pressure did not normalize (< 8mmHg). The failure to normalize right atrial pressure suggests a continuing restrictive or occult effusive constrictive physiology [10,11] to be discussed in future rounds.

Pulsus paradoxus is the exaggeration of the normal inspiratory decrease in arterial systolic pressure and is defined as an inspiratory decline of > 12mmHg during regular rhythm or as a > 9% inspiratory decline of arterial sytemic pressure [12]. Pulsus paradoxus occurs to variable degree depending on the equilibration of pericardial and ventricular filling pressures as determined by venous return. In phase I, a compensatory increase in venous pressure usually maintains ventricular volume close to basal levels. Right and left ventricular pressures are generally higher than pericardial pressure and thus the inspiratory decrease in arterial pressure may be exaggerated but rarely reaches the diagnostic level. In phase 2, pericardial pressure increases more than ventricular filling pressures, equilibrating first with the right then with the left ventricular pressure. Venous pressures may compensate by increasing venous return but with inadequate ventricular filling to maintain baseline cardiac output. The inspiratory decrease in arterial systemic pressure is further exaggerated beyond that observed in

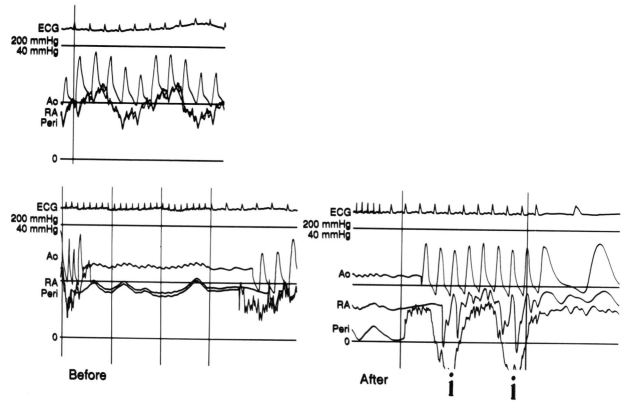

Fig. 6. Hemodynamics in a patient with large pericardial effusion and dyspnea. Ao = aortic pressure; RA = right atrial pressure; Peri = pericardial pressure. Top panel shows initial hemodynamics with inspiratory alterations in arterial pressure and right atrial and pericardial pressures. Mean right atrial and pericardial pressures shown on the lower panel before pericardiocentesis demonstrate marked inspiratory increase in these waveforms. After pericardiocentesis (right side, lower panel), pericardial and right atrial pressures are reduced. (i) shows influence of normal inspiration on right atrial and pericardial pressure waveforms. See text for details.

TABLE I. Clinical and Hemodynamic Findings in Compressive Pericardial Disease

	Tamponade	Subacute constriction	Chronic constriction
Etiology	Idiopathic Neoplasm Trauma	Idiopathic Uremic Radiation malignancy Collagen vascular disease Infectious (e.g. tuberculosis)	Idiopathic Infectious (e.g. tuberculosis)
Pulsus paradoxus (> 10mmHg)	Marked	Moderately prominent	Usually slight
Right atrial pressure waveforms[a]	X, Xy	Xy, XY	XY, xY
LV-RV equilibration	¶	±	+
RA = PCW	¶	±	+
CXR pericardial calcification	—	±	+
Cardiomegaly	¶	±	+

[a]X = large or prominent, x = diminished or absent, ± = occasionally present, + = present, — = absent.
¶ = depending on which phase of cardiac tamponade.

phase 1 and reaches diagnostic level for pulsus paradoxus in some but not all patients, depending on ventricular compliance. In phase 3, increased pericardial pressure equilibrates with right and left ventricular pressures and initiates severe hemodynamic compromise. Cardiac output declines markedly and pulsus paradoxus may often exceed a > 20mmHg inspiratory decline in pressure.

CONCLUSION

The hemodynamic findings typically associated with cardiac tamponade, subacute (elastic) pericardial constriction or chronic (rigid) pericardial constriction are compared on Table I. As noted in patient #1, the prominent Y descent favors a more constrictive pericarditis, whereas in patient #2 with cardiac tamponade, the X is prominent with a blunted Y descent. The elevation and equilibration of the ventricular diastolic pressures may be seen in all 3 conditions and does not distinguish one from the other. Restriction to diastolic filling, the dip and plateau is more prominent with the constrictive physiology than tamponade, but may be seen with either depending on the hemodynamic phase in the spectrum of cardiac tamponade.

Cardiac tamponade is a clinical syndrome characterized by a spectrum of hemodynamic abnormalities, but usually associated with an elevated venous pressure, exaggerated inspiratory fall in arterial pressure (pulsus paradoxus) and as a late (phase III) event, arterial hypotension. Echocardiographic evidence of right atrial and right ventricular collapse are useful signs differentiating hemodynamically insignificant pericardial effusion from tamponade. The change in pressure waveforms after pericardial pressure reduction will reflect the atrial and ventricular filling related to myocardial compliance and occult pericardial disease. Examples of low pressure cardiac tamponade, tamponade in the setting of left ventricular dysfunction and abnormal pericardial pressures during cardiac pacing will be the subject of future rounds.

ACKNOWLEDGMENTS

The authors thank the J.G. Mudd Cardiac Catheterization Laboratory and Donna Sander for manuscript preparation.

REFERENCES

1. Reddy PS, Curtiss EI, O'Toole JD, Shaver JA: Cardiac tamponade: Hemodynamic observations in man. Circulation 58: 265–272, 1978.
2. Reddy PS, Curtiss EI, Uretsky BF. Spectrum of hemodynamic changes in cardiac tamponade. Am J Cardiol 66:1487–1491, 1990.
3. Seacord LM, Miller LW, Pennington DG, McBride LR, Kern MJ: Reversal of constrictive/restrictive physiology with treatment of allograft rejection. Am Heart J 120:455–459, 1990.
4. Singh S, Wann LS, Schuchard GH, et al.: Right ventricular and right atrial collapse in patients with cardiac tamponade. Am J Cardiol 50:1018–1021, 1982.
5. Tamburino C, Vaissier E, Gandjbakhch I, Pavie A, Cabrol A, Cabrol C: Hemodynamic parameters one and four weeks after cardiac tansplantation. Am J Cardiol 63:635–637, 1989.
6. Corcos T, Tamburino C. Leger P, Vaissier E. Rossant P, Mattie MF, Daudon P, Gandjbakhch I, Pavie A, Cabrol A, Cabrol C: Early and late hemodynamic evaluation after cardiac transplantation: A study of 28 cases. J Am Coll Cardiol 11:264–269, 1988.
7. Serota H: "Special Techniques" in: "Cardiac Catheterization Handbook." Deligonul U, Ring M, Kern MJ (eds). St. Louis, Mosby Year-Book, 1991, pp 360–364.
8. Young JB, Leon CA, Short HD III, Noon GP, Lawrence EC, Whisennand HH, Pratt CM, Goodman DA, Weilbaecher D, Quinones MA: Evolution of hemodynamics after orthotopic heart and heart-lung transplantation: Early restrictive patterns persisting in occult fashion. J Heart Transplant 6:34–43, 1987.
9. Levine MJ, Lorell BH, Diver DJ, Come PC: Implications of echocardiographically assisted diagnosis of pericardial tamponade in contemporary medical patients: Detection before hemodynamic embarrassment. J Am Coll Cardiol 17:59–65, 1991.
10. Bush CA et al.: Occult constrictive pericardial disease. Circulation 56:924, 1977.
11. Hancock EW: Subacute effusive constrictive pericarditis. Circulation 43:183, 1971.
12. Curtiss EI, Reddy PS, Uretsky BF, Cecchetti AA: Pulsus paradoxus: Definition and relation to the severity of cardiac tamponade. Am Heart J 115:391–398, 1988.

Chapter 20

Hemodynamics of Constrictive Physiology—Section II:
Pericardial Compressive Hemodynamics

Morton J. Kern, MD, and Frank V. Aguirre, MD

INTRODUCTION

Compressive pericardial hemodynamics result from pericarditis with or without the accumulation of pericardial fluid. The effects of increasing pericardial pressure, producing the hemodynamic spectrum of cardiac tamponade, were discussed in the earlier rounds (part I).

A common feature in compressive pericardial hemodynamics is the impaired atrial and ventricular filling patterns indicating diastolic dysfunction. The extrinsic cardiac compression, with or without various degrees of an intrinsic myopathic component, prevents adequate diastolic filling of both atria and ventricles in the stepwise fashion [1–3]. An inadequate preload, relative to the impairment in diastolic filling, reduces stroke volume despite the elevated diastolic pressures. The diastolic filling pressures and systemic venous return vary abnormally over the respiratory cycle, producing the characteristic findings of pulsus paradoxus and Kussmaul's sign [4–6]. This hemodynamic rounds will illustrate several distinctive features of different types of constrictive hemodynamic waveforms.

PERICARDIAL CONSTRAINT

A 49 yr old woman with mild renal failure secondary to systemic lupus erythematosus presented with progressive dyspnea and easy fatigue. Jugular venous distension with moderate cardiac enlargement on chest x-ray was recently reported. Echocardiography revealed a small pericardial effusion and mildly diminished ventricular function. Echocardiographic signs of tamponade [7,8] were not appreciated. Right heart cardiac catheterization was performed with an 8F balloon-tipped flotation cath-

eter using fluid-filled transducers from the right femoral vein. The hemodynamic tracings are shown in Figure 1. What characteristics of the pressure tracings indicate pericardial constraint is present? Is pericardial tamponade (phase I or II) also a possibility?

The right atrial pressure was elevated (15 mm Hg) with an exaggerated and prominent Y descent and attenuated X descent. There was no decrease in the mean right atrial pressure with inspiration. The right ventricular pressure demonstrated prominent early diastolic dip preceding atrial contraction, but without a plateau phase. The pulmonary capillary wedge pressure also demonstrated striking V waves, prominent Y descents, and equilibration to the mean right atrial pressure of approximately 15 mm Hg. This patient demonstrated classic features of constrictive pericarditis with the exception of a prolonged diastolic pressure plateau of the right ventricle. Left ventricular pressure is not shown in this individual, but matched right ventricular diastolic pressure as shown in Figure 2. The corresponding right and left ventricular pressures are equilibrated and elevated with early impaired diastolic filling. As a hemodynamic detective, examine the ventricular tracings of the Figures 1 and 2. What is the major difference? Figure 2 was obtained in a patient who was in atrial fibrillation, a rhythm which is very common for pericarditis. The abnormal hemodynamics of the "dip and plateau" may be obscured during short RR intervals and depend on the duration of diastole.

Pericardial constriction usually impairs diastolic filling of all chambers of the heart. Right and left ventricular diastolic pressures are equilibrated and elevated, usually equal or within 5 mm Hg [9]. Atrial pressures, that is, pulmonary capillary wedge (left) and right atrial pres-

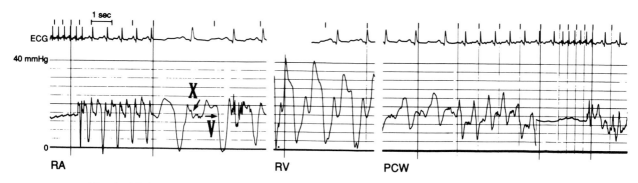

Fig. 1. Right atrial (RA), right ventricular (RV), and pulmonary capillary wedge (PCW) pressures in a patient with renal failure and lupus erythematosus presenting with fatigue. Right atrial pressure is elevated along with right ventricular diastolic and pulmonary capillary wedge pressure mean. See text for details.

sure, may not be equal since the associated A or V waves may differ between atrium. In the first patient (Fig. 1), the pulmonary capillary wedge pressure and right atrial pressure means were equivalent. Larger V waves were noted in the pulmonary capillary wedge tracing than in the right atrial pressure. Note that right ventricular pressure (36/20 mm Hg) was mildly elevated. In general in pericardial compression, pulmonary artery and right ventricular systolic pressures are usually mildly elevated between 35 and 45 mm Hg, reflecting the elevated end-diastolic and increased pulmonary venous pressures [9].

As with all clinical determinations based on hemodynamics, the data must be reliable and precise. The transducers should be calibrated simultaneously to a mercury manometer at bedside and checked immediately prior to recordings for accurate zero starting points.

THE DIASTOLIC PLATEAU

Pericardial constriction alters the rate and amount of ventricular filling. Moderate pericardial constriction usually is observed with right atrial pressures between 12 and 15 mm Hg. Consider the hemodynamic data obtained in a 56 yr old man with minimal dyspnea 3 yr after bypass surgery (Fig. 3). Right atrial and right ventricular pressures were recorded through a balloon-tipped fluid-filled catheter. Note the prominent "dip and plateau" in the right ventricular pressure and end-diastolic equilibration with right atrial pressure. Does this patient have constrictive pericarditis or low pressure tamponade? The characteristic waveform of right ventricular "dip and plateau" is certainly present, although the right ventricular pressure is only 24/6 mm Hg with a normal right atrial pressure (4–5 mm Hg) and normal configurations for the X and Y descents. Bradycardia produced long diastolic filling periods. The beta blocker for angina caused bradycardia. The minimal elevation of the right ventricular pressure speaks against clinically important

constrictive physiology. Bradycardia is one of the conditions which may produce a striking "dip and plateau" configuration of both left and right ventricular pressures which may be confused for constrictive physiology. The left ventriculogram and echocardiogram were normal. This patient did not have clinically apparent pericardial disease.

LOW PRESSURE TAMPONADE

Occult pericardial constriction or low pressure tamponade has been described in conditions of hypovolemia, especially prevalent in patients who have received diuretics prior to cardiac catheterization [10,11]. Occult pericardial constriction can be revealed by the administration of rapid infusion of normal saline which produces an elevation and equilibration of diastolic pressures consistent with pericardial constrictive physiology. However, the sensitivity and specificity of the volume challenge are still poorly defined and congestive heart failure may be a side effect of massive volume infusion.

Reddy et al. [2] indicate that the compensatory increase in venous pressure may be attenuated because of hypovolemia and thus cardiac output may be compromised in the presence of low ventricular filling pressures equilibrated with intrapericardial pressure defining the syndrome of low pressure tamponade [2,11]. A subgroup of patients with equilibration of pericardial and ventricular pressures of < 10 mm Hg may experience significant increase in cardiac output after pericardiocentesis [2].

Intrapericardial pressure closely follows changes in right atrial pressure and volume during the cardiac cycle [1–3]. Pressure changes within the pericardium reflect the volume of fluid as influenced by myocardial chamber size during filling and emptying. The pericardial pressure waves generally parallel right atrial pressure when early tamponade is present, but distinctly different wave-

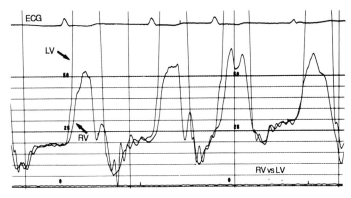

Fig. 2. Simultaneous right (RV) and left ventricular (LV) pressures on a 0–50 mm Hg scale in a patient with shortness of breath. See text for details.

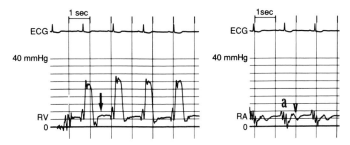

Fig. 3. Right ventricular (RV) and right atrial (RA) pressures (0–40 mm Hg scale) in a 56 yr old man with dyspnea 3 yr after coronary artery bypass surgery. See text for details.

forms are seen in patients without cardiac tamponade. Examine the hemodynamic tracings of a 64 yr old woman admitted for elective pericardiocentesis because of increasing fatigue with moderate pericardial effusion and early tamponade physiology [12] (Fig. 4). The patient had a DDD pacemaker which had intermittent failure to sense and capture the atrium with periods of atrial ventricular dissociation. Pericardiocentesis was performed with hemodynamic monitoring and measurement of right atrial pressure with a 7F balloon-tipped flotation catheter. Arterial pressure was measured with a 5F sheath with fluid-filled catheter. As can be observed in Figure 4A, there was minimal pulsus paradoxus. The right atrial mean and pericardial mean pressures were both 9 mm Hg. The mean pulmonary capillary wedge pressure was 14 mm Hg. Of interest are the large negative pericardial pressure waves occurring during atrial ventricular dissociation. The decline in pericardial pressure is especially evident on beats #2 and #6. These negative waves occur during atrial systole against a closed tricuspid valve. Large atrial cannon waves are coupled with a negative mirror image pericardial wave of a proportional size. The effect was most evident on the longest and largest cannon waves (compare beat #6 vs.

#7). After pericardiocentesis (Fig. 4B), the mean right atrial pressure was 6 mm Hg with mean intrapericardial pressure of 0 mm Hg. Echocardiography revealed absence of pericardial fluid and no signs of tamponade physiology. Pericardial pressure continued to demonstrate large negative waves associated with right atrial cannon waves. Normally right atrial pressure and volume decrease after atrial systole and before ventricular systole, producing an X descent. As ventricular volume decreases during ejection, pericardial pressure decreases, increasing transmural (that is, right atrial-pericardial pressure gradient) pressure, resulting in venous influx into the right atrium during late ventricular systole (beginning the V wave). In A-V dissociation, atrial systole may occur during ventricular systole resulting in a large venous cannon wave. The decrease in atrial volume produces a proportional decrease in intrapericardial pressure (a negative cannon wave) exaggerated by atrial and ventricular contraction and volume reduction at the same time. This unusual observation demonstrates the interesting pressure changes that occur normally within the pericardium. The clinical syndrome of this patient was attributed to loss of the atrial contribution to cardiac output rather than to pericardial fluid.

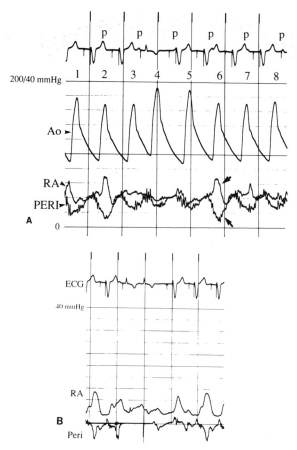

Fig. 4. A: Hemodynamic data during DDD pacing before pericardiocentesis. Ao=femoral artery pressure; RA=right atrial
pressure; Peri=pericardial pressure; P=p waves. Scale is 0–
200 mm Hg for arterial pressure and 0–40 mm Hg for right atrial
and pericardial pressures. With permission from reference #12.
B: Hemodynamic data after pericardiocentesis. See text for details. With permission from reference #12.

ATRIAL WAVEFORMS AND PERICARDIAL CONSTRAINT

A rapid Y descent indicates an exaggerated and
abruptly terminating right atrial emptying after tricuspid
(or mitral) valve opening. The Y descent is followed by
a moderate but often sharp A wave with its X descent of
atrial diastole. When atrial relaxation is impaired, the X
descent is attenuated. Pericardial constraint produces a
characteristic M or W configuration which can be readily
appreciated with moderately fast pressure recording
speeds. These M and W configurations are not exclusive
nor diagnostic for pericardial disease.

A 73 yr old man with congestive heart failure and
coronary artery disease was admitted for evaluation of
shortness of breath and easy fatigability. Jugular venous
distension and mild pedal edema were present. The electrocardiogram showed irregular rhythm with intermittent
paced and sinus beats. Arterial pressure was 100/60 mm

Hg without pulsus paradoxus. The right atrial pressure,
shown in Figure 5, is increased with a mean of 14 mm
Hg (not shown). The M pattern is distinct. Based on this
waveform, consider the following: Can a restrictive
myocardial process be differentiated from a constrictive
pericardial process from this tracing? Are the waves
"A" and "V" true filling waves or artifact? What hap-
pens to alter the waveform on beats #7, #8, and #9?

MECHANISM OF THE "M" CONFIGURATION

The "M" configuration of right atrial pressure is composed of abbreviated "A" and "V" waves with a brief
and attenuated X descent between the "A" and "V"
waves. The Y descent following the "V" wave is prominent, demonstrating rapid atrial emptying with restraint
of ventricular filling by the end of the first one-third of
diastole. This prominent "Y" is immediately followed
by the sequential "A" and "V" waves, producing the
"M" pattern. This waveform may be exaggerated in
tachycardia, as shown in this patient, or may be inverted,
having a slightly wider X descent, and appear as a "W"
configuration in patients with slower heart rates. This
configuration is commonly seen in patients with restrictive or constrictive physiology from any cause including
chronic congestive heart failure, as well as other restrictive myocardial fibrotic processes [13]. There are no differentiating features between constriction and restriction
on the basis of right atrial pressure alone. The tricuspid
valve is generally normal and contributes little to this
pathologic waveform. The M pattern is the result of the
effect of attenuation of diastolic filling on atrial pressure
and flow. It should be noted that an underdamped pressure transducer system showing ringing of the atrial pressure wave may also produce this M or W configuration
through artifact.

What accounts for the altered M pattern on beat #9?
On the first two paced beats (#7, #8) indicated by the
vertical lines, the "A" and "V" pattern is disturbed. On
beat #9, one can observe a pause and continued increase
in right atrial pressure prior to a fusion beat with an A
wave after the atrial pacing spike preceding the ventricular pacing spike. Compare this right atrial waveform to
that in Figure 3 and 6 with the X descent slightly greater
than the Y descent for a normal right atrial pressure.

KUSSMAUL'S SIGN

Constrictive pericardial compression prevents negative intrathoracic inspiratory pressure from being normally transmitted to the intrapericardial space and right
heart chambers. Normally venous return and right atrial
pressure decline during inspiration with an increase in
the Y descent and slight increase in the X descent (both

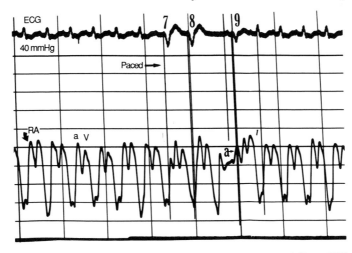

Fig. 5. Right atrial (RA) pressure in a patient with congestive heart failure. "M" or "W" configuration? See text for details.

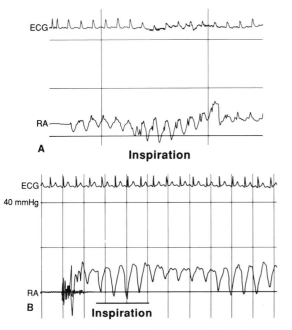

Fig. 6. A: Phasic right atrial (RA) pressure during inspiration. See text for details. B: Right atrial (RA) pressure in a patient with shortness of breath during inspiration. See text for details.

A and V waves decline) and then return to normal (Fig. 6A). In patients with constrictive physiology inspiration produces an increase in the right atrial pressure mean augmenting the Y descent (Fig. 6B). The pericardial pressure offsets the negative inspiratory pressure and venous return continues unchanged or increases during normal inspiration. This paradoxical increase in right atrial pressure during inspiration is known as Kussmaul's sign [3,4]. The lack of phasic augmentation of right heart filling during inspiration occurs during cardiac tamponade. In cardiac tamponade, pulsus paradoxus, the exag-

gerated inspiratory fall in arterial pressure, is due to right heart filling during inspiration at the expense of left ventricular filling. Kussmaul's sign is, however, non-specific and may be seen in any condition producing constrictive physiology, such as restrictive cardiomyopathy, right ventricular infarction, tricuspid stenosis, or pulmonary embolism.

CONSTRICTIVE OR RESTRICTIVE PHYSIOLOGY?

Differentiating the underlying causative process of constrictive physiology may not be possible by hemodynamic data alone. The equilibration of left and right ventricular pressures of < 5 mm Hg with impaired diastolic filling pattern is one hallmark of constrictive physiology. Consider the right and left heart hemodynamics (Fig. 7) recorded in a patient with congestive heart failure 1 yr following cardiac surgery. Mean right atrial pressure was elevated (12 mm Hg) with a Kussmaul's sign during inspiration (Fig. 7, upward arrow). The right atrial Y descent was more prominent than the X descent. Simultaneous right atrial and right ventricular pressures also demonstrated diastolic equilibration with early diastolic dip and matching of diastolic pressures. Because of the rapid heart rate, the plateau phase was not appreciated until a pause from an atrial premature beat was observed (Fig. 7A, second beat from right, downward arrow). The left and right ventricular diastolic pressures appear equilibrated on the 0–100 mm Hg scale (Fig. 7B, left side), but the left ventricular pressure is 4–5 mm Hg higher than the right ventricular pressure on the higher 0–40 mm Hg scale (Fig. 7B, right side). The pressures track equally but are not superimposed. Because of the rapid heart rate, the diastolic period shows continued filling (i.e., increasing pressure). This patient had constrictive

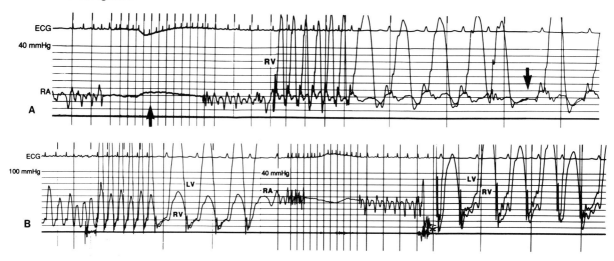

Fig. 7. **(A)** Simultaneous right atrial (RA), right ventricular (RV) (0–40 mm Hg scale), and **(B)** left ventricular (LV) pressures (0–100 mm Hg scale) in a patient with shortness of breath 1 yr following coronary artery bypass surgery. See text for details.

physiology, but a degree of restrictive cardiomyopathy (due to earlier myocardial infarctions and fibrosis) could not be excluded from either the non-invasive or hemodynamic data.

Of interest, a right ventricular systolic pulsus paradoxus is seen (Fig. 7B, left side). The > 10% inspiratory decrease in systolic pressure is generally reflected in systemic pressure occurring when diastolic pressures are equilibrated with an elevated pericardial pressure [1]. Right ventricular filling in this patient was occurring against the stiffness of the pericardium, causing both ventricles to be filled to the same degree with equal back pressure. Respiratory changes in intrathoracic pressure alternately favor left and right ventricular filling leading to a pulsus paradoxus. During inspiration, pulmonary venous pressure decreases below systemic venous pressure, whereas the reverse occurs during expiration [1–3]. Pulsus paradoxus is most commonly observed to occur in patients whose right ventricular filling pressures are equilibrated with pericardial, but not left ventricular, filling pressures [1,2]. Ventricular septal interaction has been called upon to explain the complex mechanism of pulsus paradoxus in patients in whom only right ventricular pericardial equilibration occurs. In these patients, the right-left ventricular interaction appears to be exaggerated as the ventricles are increasingly stiffened by pericardial effusion.

SUMMARY

Constrictive physiology characteristically alters atrial and ventricular waveforms. Normal pressure and flow responses to inspiration are blocked or reversed. The impairment of early diastolic filling is the common fea-

ture of restrictive myocardial, as well as diseased pericardial, processes. Low pressure tamponade can limit cardiac output, but may be difficult to detect by clinical signs alone. Examination of the pressure waveforms may provide clues to the diagnosis of constrictive physiology in these patients.

ACKNOWLEDGMENTS

The authors wish to thank the J.G. Mudd Cardiac Catheterization Laboratory and Donna Sander for manuscript preparation.

REFERENCES

1. Reddy PS, Curtiss EI, O'Toole JD, Shaver JA: Cardiac tamponade: hemodynamic observations in man. Circulation 58:265–272, 1978.
2. Reddy PS, Curtiss EI, Uretsky BF: Spectrum of hemodynamic changes in cardiac tamponade. Am J Cardiol 66:1487–1491, 1990.
3. Shabetai R, Fowler NO, Guntheroth WG: The hemodynamics of cardiac tamponade and constrictive pericarditis. Am J Cardiol 26:480–489, 1970.
4. Hancock EW: Constrictive pericarditis: clinical clues to diagnosis. JAMA 232:176, 1975.
5. Gabe IT, Mason DT, Gault JH, Ross J, Jr., Zelis R, Mills CJ, Braunwald E, Schillingford JP: Effect of respiration on venous return and stroke volume in cardiac tamponade. Br Heart J 32: 592–596, 1970.
6. Shabetai R, Fowler NO, Fenton JC, Masangkay M: Pulsus paradoxus. J Clin Invest 44:1882–1898, 1965.
7. Leimgruber PP, Klopfenstein HS, Wann LS, Brooks HL: The hemodynamic derangement associated with right ventricular diastolic collapse in cardiac tamponade: an experimental echocardiographic study. Circulation 68:612–620, 1983.
8. Singh S, Wann LS, Schuchard GH, Klopfenstein HS, Leimgruber

PP, Keelan MH, Jr., Brooks HL: Right ventricular and right atrial collapse in patients with cardiac tamponade—a combined echocardiographic and hemodynamic study. Circulation 70:966–971, 1984.

9. Grossman W (ed): "Cardiac Catheterization and Angiography, 4th Edition." Philadelphia: Lea & Febiger, 1990, p 634.

10. Bush CA, Stang JM, Wooley CF, Kilman JW: Occult constrictive pericardial disease: diagnosis by rapid volume expansion and correction by pericardiectomy. Circulation 56:924–930, 1977.

11. Antman EM, Cargill V, Grossman W: Low-pressure cardiac tamponade. Ann Intern Med 91:403–406, 1979.

12. Gudipati CV, Deligonul U, Janosik D, Vandormael M, Kern MJ: Intrapericardial "negative" cannon waves during atrioventricular dissociation in large pericardial effusion. Am Heart J 119:964–965, 1990.

13. Shabeti R, Fowler NO, Fenton JC: Restrictive cardiac disease: pericarditis and the myocardiopathies. Am Heart J 69:271, 1965.

Chapter 21

Hemodynamics of Constrictive Physiology—Section III:
Pericardial Compressive Hemodynamics

Morton J. Kern, MD, and Frank V. Aguirre, MD

INTRODUCTION

The differentiation between constrictive and restrictive hemodynamics has been the subject of numerous papers and studies attempting to identify precise and characteristic abnormalities which might give a clue to the underlying pathophysiologic process [1–6]. The clinical features of restrictive cardiomyopathy such as that caused by hypertension, infiltrative diseases (i.e., amyloidoses or hemochromatosis), or metabolic storage diseases are often similar to the hemodynamics produced from compressive and constrictive pericarditis [4–6]. The common hemodynamic finding is impairment of diastolic filling with elevated ventricular filling pressures and a fixed stroke volume, often with normal systolic function. In some patients with an elastic or effusive pericardial constrictive process, a typical series of hemodynamic waveforms has been reported with an intermediate presentation between encasing or non-elastic constrictive pericarditis and restrictive cardiomyopathy [5,6]. As in parts I and II, this rounds will examine common and uncommon hemodynamic examples after pericardial fluid withdrawal to illustrate several distinctions between restrictive cardiomyopathy, effusive-constrictive pericarditis, and compressive hemodynamics of cardiac tamponade.

THE EMPTY PERICARDIUM

A 32-yr-old woman with an acute viral syndrome is admitted to the intensive care unit with progressive dyspnea, tachycardia, and hypotension. The viral prodrome was associated with mild cough. There were no associ-

ated illnesses nor other prior significant medical conditions. There was jugular venous distention and mild pedal edema. Chest x-ray demonstrated an enlarged cardiac silhouette. Echocardiography showed a large pericardial effusion with right ventricular diastolic collapse (Fig. 1). Because of the signs of cardiac tamponade, the patient was brought to the cardiac catheterization laboratory for pericardiocentesis. A 6F sheath was positioned in the right femoral artery and an 8F sheath in the femoral vein was used for right heart pressure measurements with a balloon-tipped catheter. Right and left heart hemodynamics (with 5F pigtail catheter) were obtained using fluid-filled transducers before and after pericardiocentesis. Prior to pericardiocentesis, arterial pressure was 105/80 mm Hg with a 12 mm Hg pulsus paradoxus. Pericardiocentesis was performed with simultaneous hemodynamic and electrocardiographic monitoring. Immediately after entering the pericardium, clear yellow fluid was aspirated and pericardial, right atrial, and arterial pressures were recorded (Fig. 2A). The right atrial pressure and pericardial pressure were both elevated and equilibrated at 15 mm Hg. The Y descent was markedly attenuated and X descent nearly obliterated. There was no change in right atrial pressure during inspiration prior to pericardiocentesis.

The differences in pressure after the removal of 450 cc of clear yellow fluid are shown in Figure 2A–D. Note the marked decline in right atrial pressure after pericardiocentesis (Fig. 2B). Mean right atrial pressure fell from 12 to 2 mm Hg with restoration of A and V waves of nearly equal magnitude. An inspiratory decline in right atrial pressure was now present. The right ventricular diastolic pressure (Fig. 2C) showed equilibration with right atrial

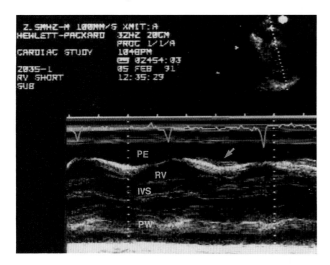

Fig. 1. M mode echocardiogram demonstrating right ventricular (RV) diastolic collapse (arrow). Diastole is delineated by the timing of the electrocardiogram. PE = pericardial effusion; IVS = intraventricular septum; PW = posterior wall.

pressure with a sharp initial diastolic dip before pericardiocentesis. A diastolic pressure plateau was absent because of the tachycardia. Following pericardiocentesis, right ventricular systolic pressure is nearly the same, but the diastolic pressure is now reduced with a normal diastolic pattern during the slower heart rate. The left ventricular diastolic and pulmonary wedge pressures were also elevated and equilibrated (Fig. 2D, before pericardiocentesis). The prominent V waves and significant Y descent seen are ameliorated following pericardiocentesis with reduction of both left ventricular end-diastolic and pulmonary capillary wedge pressure to approximately 6–8 mm Hg. Note the change in the V wave and Y descent after pericardiocentesis. A comparison of right and left atrial (PCW) pressures also demonstrates the unequal influences of intrinsic chamber and pericardial pressure activity on the two atria. Differences in atrial compliances can be appreciated by the pressure pattern responses.

TECHNICAL NOTES FOR PERICARDIOCENTESIS

In our laboratory, hemodynamic monitoring during pericardiocentesis has proven to be extremely informative and effective in identifying intrapericardial positioning of the aspirating needle. Although not routinely used, a two-ended alligator clamp connecting the needle to the V_1 lead of the electrocardiogram also provides a safety indicator to avoid contact with surface of the myocardium. This procedure has been used most often when satisfactory hemodynamic measurements cannot be obtained. Figure 3 illustrates the effect of the pericardiocentesis needle contacting the myocardium during peri-

cardiocentesis using the electrode clip. The right atrial pressure is elevated with an attenuated Y descent consistent with the hemodynamics of tamponade described earlier. The amplitude of the electrocardiogram (lead V_1) is small. Note the marked ST elevation and injury pattern on the electrocardiogram when the pericardial needle touches the myocardium. The needle was withdrawn slightly and intrapericardial hemodynamics were confirmed. The insertion of a J-tipped guidewire with subsequent placement of a multiple side-holed catheter for pericardial drainage was completed without incident.

A successful pericardiocentesis can be documented by improvement in the hemodynamics with four specific indicators: 1) reduction of intrapericardial pressures to levels of 0 ± 3 mm Hg; 2) return of right atrial pressure to near normal levels with separation between right and left ventricular diastolic filling pressures; 3) increase in cardiac output; and 4) restoration of normal inspiratory response of the right atrial and arterial pressures with disappearance of the pulsus paradoxus. The presence of persistent elevation and (near) equilibration of right and left ventricular diastolic pressures, as we will see, suggests a continued constricting pericardial process (e.g., effusive-constrictive pericarditis) [6].

In many instances, the post-pericardiocentesis management includes suturing of the pericardial catheter to the skin and attaching the catheter to a closed drainage system. Diluted heparin may prevent catheter clotting. The installation of carbon dioxide or air into the pericardial space to outline the pericardium at the end of the procedure is not advocated. The catheter should be removed within 48 h to reduce the risk of infection into the pericardial space. Assessment of pericardial fluid drainage and serial echocardiography at 24 h intervals will identify whether pericardial fluid reaccumulation is rapid and may require a more definitive drainage by a surgical pericardial window.

THE EMPTY PERICARDIUM WITH ELEVATED RIGHT ATRIAL PRESSURE

The first patient example demonstrated a remarkable decline in right atrial pressure on removal of pericardial fluid with all hemodynamics returning to normal (Fig. 2A–D). There was no reaccumulation of the pericardial fluid caused by a viral pericarditis. However, not all patients have such dramatic hemodynamic responses to pericardial evacuation. An effusive or exudative fibrin layer organizing around the heart may not permit normalization of hemodynamics. These patients may have effusive-constrictive pericarditis often due to uremia, infection, or neoplastic pericardial or myocardial infiltration [6].

An examination was made of the hemodynamics dur-

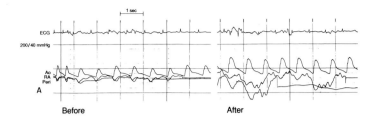

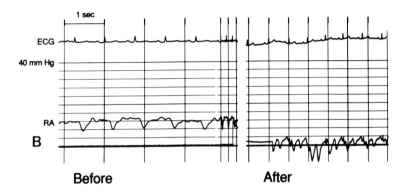

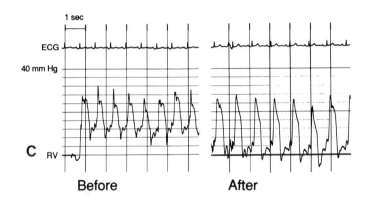

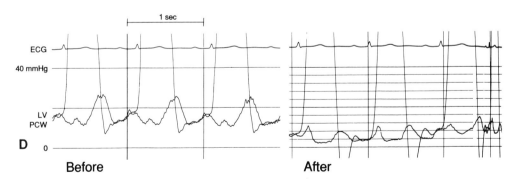

Fig. 2. A: Hemodynamic tracings of aortic (Ao), right atrial (RA), and pericardial (peri) pressures before and after pericardiocentesis in a 32-yr-old woman with increasing dyspnea. B: Right atrial (RA) pressure before and after pericardiocentesis. C: Right ventricular (RV) pressure before and after pericardiocentesis. D: Left ventricular (LV) and pulmonary capillary wedge (PCW) pressures before and after pericardiocentesis. See text for details.

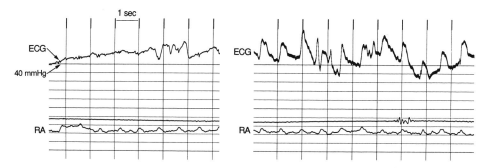

Fig. 3. Hemodynamic and electrocardiographic simultaneous measurements during pericardiocentesis. Left panel shows small electrocardiogram obtained from the pericardiocentesis needle connected to the V₁ lead by a double-ended alligator clamp. Right atrial pressure is elevated at a mean of approximately 10 mm Hg with blunted X and Y descents. On insertion of the needle (right panel), the electrocardiogram shows ST elevation and injury pattern consistent with contact of the needle to the myocardial surface. The needle was withdrawn, hemodynamic data obtained, and successful pericardiocentesis conducted. See text for details.

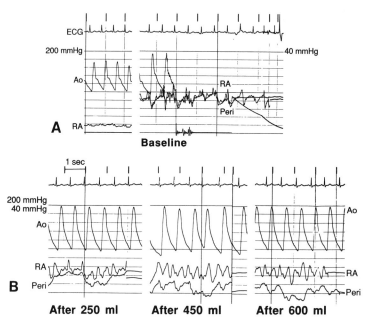

Fig. 4. A: Right atrial (RA) and aortic (Ao) pressures before pericardiocentesis. Middle panel shows simultaneous right atrial and pericardial (peri) pressures after removal of approximately 10 cc of pericardial fluid. Note the increase in arterial pressure with withdrawal of the small amount of pericardial fluid. B: Serial hemodynamics obtained after 250, 450, and 600 ml of fluid are removed from the pericardial space. At the conclusion of the procedure, right atrial (RA) pressure mean was 10 mm Hg and pericardial (peri) pressure mean was 2 mm Hg. Ao = aortic pressure. See text for details.

ing pericardiocentesis in a 39-yr-old woman with metastatic breast carcinoma with increasing dyspnea and pericardial effusion. Because of the increasing symptoms with echocardiographic and clinical signs of cardiac tamponade, pericardiocentesis was performed with hemodynamic monitoring (Fig. 4). The arterial pressure was approximately 150/88 mm Hg with a 14 mm Hg pulsus paradoxus. Right atrial and pericardial pressures were elevated and equilibrated at approximately 18 mm Hg. On removal of the first 10 cc of serosanguinous fluid, there was a marked increase in arterial pressure (Fig. 4A,

middle panel) suggesting relief of pericardial constraint. Serial hemodynamic measurements were obtained again after removal of 250, 450, and 650 ml of serosanguinous pericardial fluid (Fig. 4B). Note the arterial pressure has now risen to nearly 200/100 mm Hg, consistent with a prior history of hypertension. A decline in both right atrial and pericardial pressures was observed. However, right atrial pressure fell to a mean of 10 mm Hg with pericardial pressure falling to near 0 mm Hg. The restoration of the right atrial wave forms is evident on removal of <200 ml of fluid. Pericardial waveforms remained

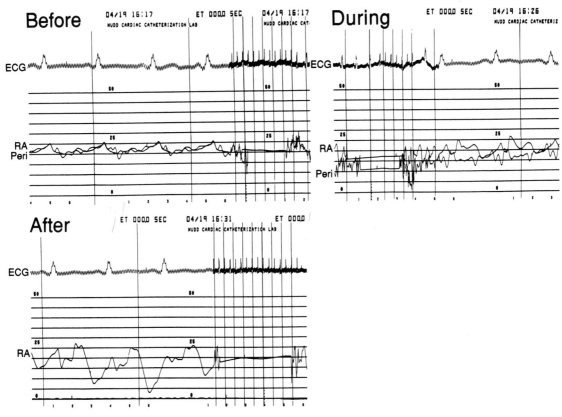

Fig. 5. Right atrial (RA) and pericardial (peri) pressures before and after pericardiocentesis. Note persistence of Y descent on right atrial pressure with elevated mean right atrial pressure after pericardiocentesis in this patient. See text for details.

poorly defined even after 650 ml was removed. The higher right atrial pressure probably reflects a degree of restrictive (effusive-constrictive) physiology, but may also be due to continued cardiac dysfunction from an underlying myopathic process.

A more striking example of the continued elevation of right atrial pressure with features of constrictive physiology is shown in Figure 5. The hemodynamic tracings were obtained in 42 yr old man with a history of alcohol abuse and renal failure. The clinical examination revealed intermittent fevers, dyspnea, and an enlarging cardiac silhouette. Renal dialysis was to be performed in 2 days. Coagulopathy and GI bleeding were present. An intermittent pericardial friction rub, hepatomegaly, and pedal edema were also observed. Sinus tachycardia with non-specific ST-T wave changes was noted. Echocardiography showed a large pericardial effusion. The blood pressure was 116/70 mm Hg with a pulsus paradoxus of 12 mm Hg. Heart rate was 120 beats/min with labored respirations. In the cardiac catheterization lab, pericardiocentesis was again performed measuring right heart pressures; 500 cc of bloody pericardial fluid was removed. The hemodynamic tracings (Fig. 5) demon-

strated equilibration and elevation of the pericardial and right atrial pressures to approximately 20 mm Hg. After removal of the pericardial fluid, pericardial pressure declined to approximately 6 mm Hg. No further fluid could be removed at this time. The echocardiogram showed a nearly empty pericardial space. Despite a low pericardial pressure, the right atrial pressure was persistently elevated to approximately 20 mm Hg with the appearance of a marked Y descent. Right atrial pressure waveforms after emptying of the pericardial space indicated a persistent constrictive/restrictive physiology in the setting of cardiomyopathy.

Although not illustrated here, cardiac tamponade may present with different hemodynamics in patients who have coexistent severe left ventricular systolic dysfunction. In experimental animal models, Hoit et al. [9] indicated that pulsus paradoxus (> 10 mm Hg inspiratory decline) was present in all animals with cardiac tamponade before left ventricular dysfunction, but in only one animal after left ventricular dysfunction was induced. Left ventricular dysfunction caused a leftward and upward shift of pericardial pressure-volume relationship. This shift in the pericardial pressure volume relationship

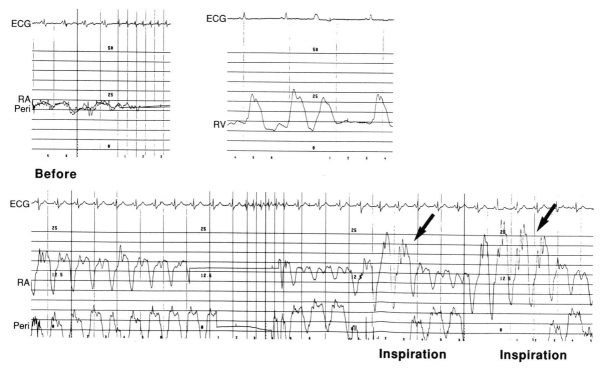

Fig. 6. Pericardial (peri) and right atrial (RA) pressures in a patient with cardiac tamponade. Right ventricular (RV) pressure was elevated and equilibrated with right atrial pressure (upper right panel). After pericardiocentesis (lower panel), inspiration produced a marked increase in right atrial pressure with augmentation of a systolic murmur. See text for details.

produced findings of right atrial and ventricular collapse with significantly smaller pericardial fluid volumes. Pulsus paradoxus may thus be absent in cardiac tamponade with coexisting left ventricular dysfunction and unequal filling pressures. Echocardiographic signs of cardiac tamponade may occur even with small effusions in the presence of left ventricular dysfunction.

INSPIRATORY AUGMENTATION OF A RIGHT HEART MURMUR

Consider the findings in a 67-yr-old woman with increasing dyspnea on exertion. The blood pressure was 100/60 mm Hg with a pulse of 70 beats/min; a large pericardial effusion was seen with right atrial and right ventricular diastolic collapse. Only minimal pulsus paradoxus (< 10 mm Hg) was noted. The heart sounds were quiet with no significant murmurs. The electrocardiogram showed a normal sinus rhythm with diffusely low voltage and non-specific ST-T wave abnormalities. Pericardiocentesis was performed, withdrawing 1,000 cc of clear yellow fluid. The hemodynamic tracings (Fig. 6) showed elevated (22 mm Hg) and equilibrated right atrial, pericardial, and right ventricular diastolic pressures. After removal of pericardial fluid, an exaggerated Y descent and an elevated right atrial pressure (mean 17

mm Hg) with an "M" configuration were consistent with persistent constrictive physiology. In addition, after pericardiocentesis, a varying intensity of a systolic murmur and right atrial pressure were observed during inspiration (Fig. 6, lower panel). What physiologic mechanism might explain this phenomenon? Echocardiography after pericardiocentesis demonstrated significant tricuspid regurgitation. The hemodynamics of effusive constrictive physiology are responsible for the persistently elevated right atrial pressure. The inspiratory increase in right atrial pressure occurs despite the low pericardial pressure (1–2 mm Hg). Recall the waveform of tricuspid regurgitation with a primary large systolic wave and increased Y descent [7]. In tricuspid regurgitation, the intensity of the systolic murmur varies and increases with inspiration (Carvallos's sign [8]), but often fails to correlate with the hemodynamic severity of the regurgitant pressure wave. Murmurs of other valvular disease may obscure the subtleties of Carvallo's observation. With dilatation of the right ventricle, the point of maximal intensity of the tricuspid murmur may be shifted toward the left, resulting in an erroneous interpretation of mitral regurgitation. Accentuation of the murmur of tricuspid regurgitation with inspiration is a well known feature that has been documented phonocardiographically, but rarely seen hemodynamically. The accentuation of V waves and the marked rise in right atrial pressure during inspiration parallel the change of the classic venous pulse tracings. Carvallo's sign is not invariably present in tricuspid regurgitation and can be abolished by right ventricular failure preventing the inspiratory augmentation of right ventricular filling.

SUMMARY

Failure of right atrial pressure to normalize after pericardial pressure is relieved suggests persistent effusive-constrictive physiology, myocardial failure, or cardiomyopathy which may have indistinguishable hemodynamic pressure waveforms. Clinical characteristics, ancillary testing, and endomyocardial biopsy may be required to obtain a definite diagnosis in such cases. The hemodynamic waveforms obtained during pericardiocentesis provide insight into the pathophysiologic processes, producing symptoms of dyspnea in this interesting patient group.

ACKNOWLEDGMENTS

The authors wish to thank the J.G. Mudd Cardiac Catheterization Laboratory Team and Donna Sander for manuscript preparation.

REFERENCES

1. Benotti JR, Grossman W, Cohn PF: Clinical profile of restrictive cardiomyopathy. Circulation 61:1206, 1980.
2. Ramsey HW, Sbar S, Elliott LP, Eliot RS: The differential diagnosis of restrictive myocardiopathy and chronic constrictive pericarditis with calcification: value of coronary arteriography. Am J Cardiol 25:635–638, 1970.
3. Little WC, Primm RK, Karp RB, Hood WP, Jr.: Clotted hemopericardium with the hemodynamic characteristics of constrictive pericarditis. Am J Cardiol 45:386–388, 1980.
4. Shabetai R, Fowler NO, Guntheroth WG: The hemodynamics of cardiac tamponade and constrictive pericarditis. Am J Cardiol 26:480–489, 1970.
5. Meaney E, Shabetai R, Bhargava V, Shearer M, Weidner C, Mangiardi LM, Smalling R, Peterson K: Cardiac amyloidosis, constrictive pericarditis and restrictive cardiomyopathy. Am J Cardiol 38:547–556, 1976.
6. Hancock EW: Subacute effusive-constrictive pericarditis. Circulation 43:183–192, 1971.
7. Kern MJ, Deligonul U: Hemodynamic rounds: interpretation of cardiac pathophysiology from pressure waveform analysis. II. The tricuspid valve. Cathet Cardiovasc Diagn 21:278–286, 1990.
8. Rivero-Carvallo JM: Signo para el diagnostico de las insuficiencias tricuspidias. Arch Inst Cardiol Mex 16:531, 1946.
9. Hoit BD, Gabel M, Fowler NO: Cardiac tamponade in left ventricular dysfunction. Circulation 82:1370–1376, 1990.

Chapter 22

Hemodynamics of Constrictive Physiology—Section IV:
Influence of Respiratory Dynamics on Ventricular Pressures

Stuart T. Higano, MD, Elie Azrak, MD, Naeem K. Tahirkheli, MD, and Morton J. Kern, MD

INTRODUCTION

Traditional hemodynamic criteria for the diagnosis of constrictive pericardial disease have been based on diastolic equalization of intraventricular pressures with a characteristic abrupt cessation of ventricular filling early in diastole. Such hemodynamic criteria have limitations, especially in patients who may have coexisting myopathic abnormalities associated with impaired diastolic ventricular function. Although noninvasive imaging modalities have been helpful to identify patients with a high likelihood of constrictive pericarditis [1–5], some patients remain in a class of diagnostic uncertainty with regard to the contribution of myocardial or pericardial disease responsible for their symptom complex despite a complete noninvasive hemodynamic evaluation. Echocardiographic imaging can eliminate alternative etiologies of diastolic dysfunction, such as systolic dysfunction, significant valvular dysfunction, pulmonary hypertension, and pericardial effusion with early tamponade physiology [1]. Symptomatic constrictive pericarditis with severe elevation of right heart pressures requires a definitive diagnosis because of the poor outcome with medical therapy and the excellent outcome with surgical pericardiectomy [6,7]. Several traditional hemodynamic criteria for increasing the confidence in the diagnosis of constrictive pericarditis in the cardiac catheterization laboratory have been proposed, but they have only moderate diagnostic sensitivity and specificity. The value of dynamic respiratory changes in right and left ventricular pressures in patients with constrictive pericarditis, as proposed by Hurrell et al. [8], appears to advance our understanding of the physiology of constrictive pericardial disease. We present several patients with suspected constrictive pericarditis who illustrate the value of dynamic respiratory changes in right and left ventricular pressures for the diagnosis of constrictive pericarditis.

CASE REPORT
Case 1

A 65-year-old male presented with progressive dyspnea on exertion, edema, and ascites. He had a history of coronary artery disease and had undergone four-vessel coronary artery bypass surgery 1 year earlier for class 3–4 angina. Two weeks postoperatively, he developed sharp chest pains and shortness of breath. An echocardiogram showed normal left ventricular function but small pericardial and pleural effusions. He was treated with indomethacin and improved. Over the next year, he developed progressive dyspnea on exertion, but no angina. He gained 50 pounds of weight with edema and ascites. He was treated with diuretics and intermittent paracentesis, with removal of up to 4 liters at various times. He also had hepatic enzyme abnormalities with negative hepatitis serologies, findings consistent with passive hepatic congestion.

On referral to Mayo Clinic, he was noted to have significantly elevated jugular venous pressure with rapid Y-descent, severe bilateral lower extremity edema and ascites. An ultrafast CT scan of the heart showed mild to moderate pericardial thickening and inferior vena cava dilation. At catheterization, there were features consistent with constrictive pericarditis. The bypass grafts were patent. Pericardiectomy was then performed. The procedure was long and complex. Intraoperatively, there were dense pericardial adhesions and a very thickened pericardium. It took in excess of 5 hr of continuous dissection to free up the right atrium, right ventricle, and the apical portion of the left ventricle. However, the anterior and lateral areas of the left ventricle were not completely dissected due to the fear of damaging the left internal mammary artery bypass graft and the phrenic nerve, as these structures could not be identified in the dense adhesions.

The postoperative course was quite complicated with a low cardiac output state, increasing liver dysfunction, and bacterial peritonitis. Echocardiograms could not confirm residual constriction; however, they were limited, given mechanical ventilation with positive pressure ventilation and postoperative atrial fibrillation. Clinical examination was suggestive of residual constriction. Repeat catheterization was performed 4 weeks after the initial operation. Many of the traditional hemodynamic criteria for constrictive pericarditis were seen, including elevation and equalization (<5 mm Hg difference) of the end-diastolic pressures, rapid X- and Y-descent in right atrial pressure, and dip and plateau configuration (Figs. 1–3). The right ventricular end diastolic pressure (RVEDP) was also $>\frac{1}{3}$ of right ventricular systolic pressure (RVSP). With respiration, dynamic changes in the right and left heart pressures were also seen that were consistent with persistent constrictive pericarditis. With inspiration, there was a decrease in the early transmitral gradient, suggesting dissociation of the intrathoracic and intracardiac pressures. The right and left ventricular systolic pressures were also discordant, suggesting ventricular interdependence. With inspiration, the left ventricular systolic pressure decreased and the right ventricular systolic pressure increased. This case demonstrates the classic dynamic respiratory changes seen in constrictive pericarditis.

Repeat pericardiectomy was undertaken and again very severe pericardial thickening and constriction were noted, which were removed with great difficulty. The patient did not recover postoperatively and support was withdrawn at family's request. A postmortem examination confirmed the diagnosis of cardiac cirrhosis from constrictive pericarditis.

Case 2

A 58-year-old male was referred for evaluation of significant dyspnea on exertion with symptoms and signs of right-sided heart failure. He had a Björk Shiley aortic valve replacement 12 years earlier for severe symptomatic aortic stenosis. Two years ago, he developed atrial fibrillation followed by increasing dyspnea and lower extremity swelling. Recent evaluation had revealed normal prosthetic and left ventricular systolic function on

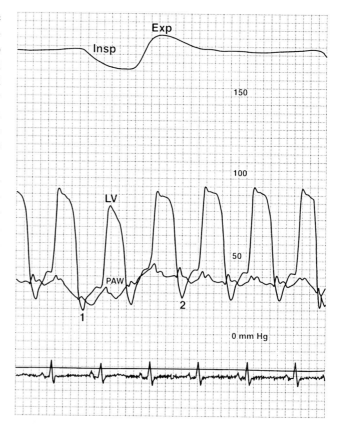

Fig. 1.   Case 1: Simultaneous recordings of left ventricular and pulmonary capillary wedge pressures demonstrating dissociation of intrathoracic and intracardiac pressures. Note the fall in early diastolic gradient with inspiration (beat 1) and the rise with expiration (beat 2). The nasal respirometer tracing is also shown. Insp, inspiration; Exp, expiration.

echocardiography; diastolic function was not evaluated. Cardiac catheterization raised the possibility of constrictive pericarditis, but a definitive diagnosis could not be made. He was referred for further evaluation. On examination, the jugular venous pressure was elevated with a rapid Y-descent, and a V-wave. Also noted was a right-sided diastolic filling sound on the (pericardial knock vs. right-sided third heart sound). Echocardiography failed to show classic mitral inflow changes on Doppler examination; however, the patient was in atrial fibrillation. An ultrafast CT scan showed moderate thickening of pericardium and indentation of the LV, consistent with constrictive pericarditis.

In the catheterization laboratory, several of the traditional hemodynamic criteria for constrictive pericarditis were present (Figs. 4–6), including elevated and equalized end-diastolic pressures with dip and plateau configuration, and an absence of decrease in mean right atrial pressure with inspiration. Also, the right ventricular systolic pressure was less than ≤55 mm Hg and right ventricular end-diastolic pressure was elevated ($>\frac{1}{3}$ of

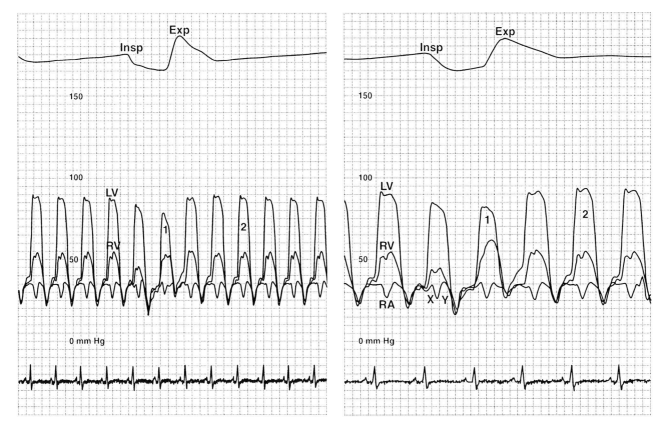

Fig. 2. Case 1: Simultaneous recordings of left ventricular, right ventricular, and right atrial pressures demonstrating ventricular interdependence. Note the discordance in left and right ventricular systolic pressures with respiration (beats 1 and 2). There is a marked "W" or "M" pattern in the right atrial pressure tracing with absent fall with inspiration (Kussmaul's sign). The nasal respirometer tracing is also shown. Insp, inspiration; Exp, expiration; LV, left ventricle; RV, right ventricle.

Fig. 3. Case 1: Simultaneous recordings of left ventricular, right ventricular, and right atrial pressures again demonstrating ventricular interdependence. Note the discordance in left and right ventricular systolic pressures with respiration. There is a marked rise in right ventricular pressure during inspiration (beat 1), during which time the left ventricular pressure is falling. Note the rapid X- and Y-descents in the right atrial tracing. The nasal respirometer tracing is also shown. Insp, inspiration; Exp, expiration; LV, left ventricle; RV, right ventricle; RA, right atrium.

RVSP). With respiration, dynamic changes in the right and left heart pressures were also seen that were consistent with persistent constrictive pericarditis. The right and left ventricular systolic pressures were also discordant, suggesting ventricular interdependence. With inspiration, the left ventricular systolic pressure decreased and the right ventricular systolic pressure increased. The early diastolic transmitral gradient did not vary with respiration, indicating normal transmission of intrathoracic pressures to intracardiac pressure (or lack of dissociation of the intrathoracic and intracardiac pressures). This finding is less sensitive than ventricular interdependence for diagnosing constrictive pericarditis [8,9]. This case demonstrates one of the classic dynamic respiratory changes seen in constrictive pericarditis. Note that temporary right ventricular pacing was used to "regularize" the rhythm and facilitate pressure analysis. The patient subsequently underwent radical pericardiectomy with improvement in his dyspnea, exercise capacity, and right-sided failure.

Case 3

A 73-year-old physician from Iowa was referred for evaluation of dyspnea on exertion, edema, and weight gain. He had previously been healthy except for non–insulin-dependent diabetes mellitus. In the preceding year, he had developed progressive dyspnea on exertion, lower extremity swelling, abdominal bloating, and weight gain. On examination, he was tachycardic with an irregular rhythm. The jugular venous pressure was elevated. There was evidence of bilateral pleural effusions, ascites, and extensive lower extremity edema (graded 3/4). The chest X-ray showed bilateral pleural effusions and cardiomegaly.

Comprehensive echocardiography (with respirometer assessment) revealed normal left ventricular systolic function with an ejection fraction of 55%, a posterior pericardial effusion measuring 2.8 cm, severe tricuspid regurgitation, and pulmonary hypertension (estimated

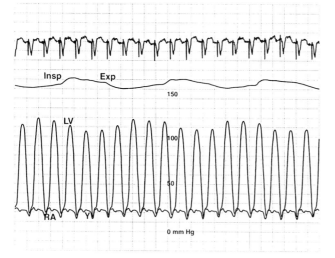

Fig. 4. Case 2: Simultaneous recordings of left ventricular and right atrial pressures. Note the rapid Y-descent in the right atrial pressures. The nasal respirometer tracing is also shown. Insp, inspiration; Exp, expiration; LV, left ventricle; RA, right atrium.

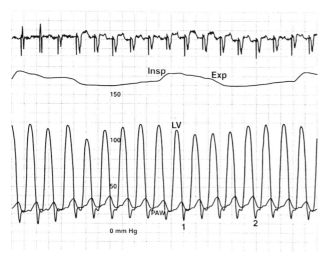

Fig. 5. Case 2: Simultaneous recordings of left ventricular and pulmonary capillary wedge pressures demonstrating lack of dissociation of intrathoracic and intracardiac pressures. This finding is less sensitive than ventricular interdependence for diagnosing constrictive pericarditis. Note the nearly constant early diastolic gradient with respiration (beats 1 vs. 2). The nasal respirometer tracing is also shown. Insp, inspiration; Exp, expiration; LV, left ventricle; PAW, pulmonary artery wedge.

pulmonary artery systolic pressure of 70 mm Hg). No significant respiratory changes in mitral inflow (E-wave) were noted. Systolic flow reversals were noted in the hepatic veins, consistent with severe tricuspid regurgitation. Interestingly, the reversals became exaggerated with expiration. A definitive diagnosis of constrictive pericarditis could not be made due to atrial fibrillation and tricuspid regurgitation.

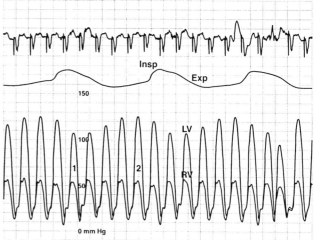

Fig. 6. Case 2: Simultaneous recordings of left and right ventricular pressure demonstrating ventricular interdependence. Note the discordance in left and right ventricular systolic pressures with respiration (beat 1 at peak inspiration vs. beat 2 at peak expiration). The nasal respirometer tracing is also shown. Insp, inspiration; Exp, expiration; LV, left ventricle; RV, right ventricle.

An ultrafast CT scan showed pleural and pericardial effusions; however, the actual pericardial thickness was difficult to measure due to the difficulty in separating the pericardium from the fluid. The impression was that the pericardial thickness was normal. Additionally, the ventricular morphology appeared normal and did not suggest tamponade or constriction.

In the catheterization laboratory, several of the traditional hemodynamic criteria for constrictive pericarditis were absent (Figs. 7–9). The pulmonary artery systolic pressure (PASP) was >55 mm Hg and the right ventricular end-diastolic pressure was less than $\frac{1}{3}$ of the right ventricular systolic pressure. However, there was end-diastolic equalization of pressures (<5 mm Hg difference). The mean right atrial pressure did not decrease with inspiration (Kussmaul's sign) and there was dip and plateau configuration of ventricular diastolic pressures, consistent with a traditional diagnosis of constrictive pericarditis. Note the absence of the X-descent and the V-wave from tricuspid regurgitation. The diagnosis remains indeterminate using the traditional hemodynamic criteria.

Using the dynamic respiratory criteria, however, it was quite clear that this patient had restrictive cardiomyopathy. The early diastolic transmitral gradient did not vary with respiration, indicating normal transmission of intrathoracic pressures to intracardiac pressure (or lack of dissociation of the intrathoracic and intracardiac pressures). This finding is less sensitive than ventricular interdependence for diagnosing constrictive pericarditis [1,2]. However, ventricular concordance is noted in the

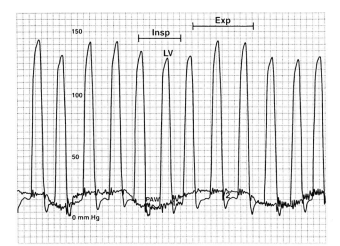

Fig. 7.   Case 3: Simultaneous recordings of left ventricular and pulmonary capillary wedge pressures demonstrating what appears to be dissociation of intrathoracic and intracardiac pressures (beat 1 vs. 2). A fluid-filled catheter was used for obtaining the pulmonary capillary wedge pressure. Note the excessive oscillations from underdamping typical of fluid-filled catheter systems. The poor fidelity of these tracings makes interpretation problematic. Insp, inspiration; Exp, expiration; LV, left ventricle; PAW, pulmonary artery wedge.

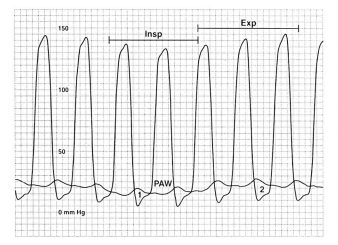

Fig. 8.   Case 3: Simultaneous recordings of left ventricular and pulmonary capillary wedge pressures demonstrating lack of dissociation of intrathoracic and intracardiac pressures. Both tracings are from high-fidelity micromanometer catheters. Note the nearly constant early diastolic gradient with respiration (beat 1 vs. 2). The high-fidelity tracings more clearly demonstrate the lack of dissociation of intrathoracic and intracardiac pressures than the fluid-filled tracings. Insp, inspiration; Exp, expiration; PAW, pulmonary artery wedge.

right and left ventricular systolic pressures. With inspiration, the left ventricular systolic pressure decreased along with the right ventricular systolic pressure. A right ventricular endomyocardial biopsy revealed only nonspecific changes and did not identify any specific disease entity.

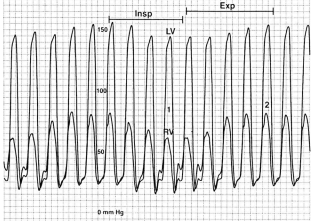

Fig. 9.   Case 3: Simultaneous recordings of left and right ventricular pressures demonstrating absent ventricular interdependence. Note the concordance in left and right ventricular systolic pressures with respiration. With inspiration, the left ventricular systolic pressure decreased along with the right ventricular systolic pressure (beat 1 vs. 2). Insp, inspiration; Exp, expiration; LV, left ventricle; RV, right ventricle.

The patient's idiopathic restrictive cardiomyopathy was treated with aggressive diuresis and afterload reduction. During the subsequent 3 years on medical therapy, he has done well without recurrent edema or ascites.

Case 4

A previously healthy 59-year-old male was referred for a 1-year history of 25- to 30-pound weight loss, dysphagia, muscle weakness, dyspnea on exertion, and lower extremity edema. Extensive prior evaluation had shown significant biventricular hypertrophy and bilateral pleural effusions. A complete gastroenterologic evaluation was negative.

At Mayo Clinic, the physical examination was consistent with biventricular failure and bilateral pleural effusions. Skin fragility was also noted. An echocardiogram showed normal left ventricular size with borderline low function and an ejection fraction of 50%. The wall thickness was increased and the myocardial texture appeared typical of amyloid infiltration. There was a small- to moderate-sized circumferential pericardial effusion measuring between 10 and 17 mm. The Doppler-derived pulmonary artery systolic pressure was 55 mm Hg. The mitral inflow showed restrictive pattern, with an E/A ratio >2 and a deceleration time of 150 milliseconds. Doppler of the pulmonary vein revealed predominant diastolic flow consistent with restrictive filling.

At catheterization, the coronary angiogram revealed mild atherosclerosis. Several of the traditional hemodynamic criteria for constrictive pericarditis were present (Figs. 10–12). There was severe elevation and near

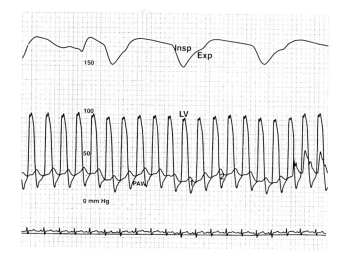

Fig. 10. Case 4: Simultaneous recordings of left ventricular and pulmonary capillary wedge pressures demonstrating lack of dissociation of intrathoracic and intracardiac pressures. Note the constant early diastolic gradient with respiration (beat 1 vs. 2). Both tracings are from high-fidelity micromanometer catheters. The nasal respirometer tracing is also shown. Insp, inspiration; Exp, expiration; LV, left ventricle; PAW, pulmonary artery wedge.

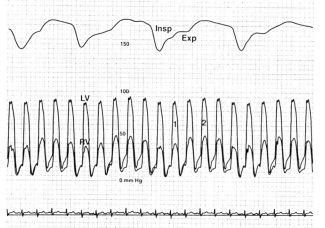

Fig. 11. Case 4: Simultaneous recordings of left and right ventricular pressures demonstrating absent ventricular interdependence. Note the concordance in left and right ventricular systolic pressures with respiration. With inspiration, the left ventricular systolic pressure decreased along with the right ventricular systolic pressure (beat 1 vs. beat 2). The nasal respirometer tracing is also shown. Insp, inspiration; Exp, expiration; LV, left ventricle; RV, right ventricle.

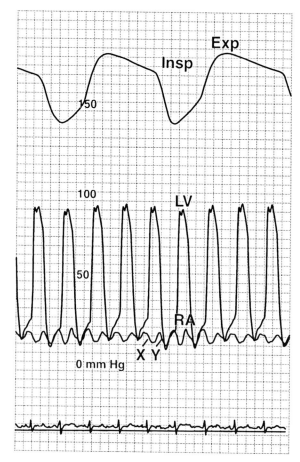

Fig. 12. Case 4: Simultaneous recordings of left ventricular and right atrial pressures. Note the marked "W" or "M" pattern in the right atrial pressure tracing with prominent X- and Y-descents and with no fall with inspiration (Kussmaul's sign). The nasal respirometer tracing is also shown. Insp, inspiration; Exp, expiration; LV, left ventricle; RA, right atrium.

equalization of diastolic pressures. There was a dip and plateau configuration of ventricular diastolic pressures. The right atrial pressure had the typical "W" or "M" configuration and the mean right atrial pressure did not decrease with inspiration (Kussmaul's sign). The pulmonary artery systolic pressure was <50 mm Hg and the right ventricular end-diastolic pressure was >⅓ of the right ventricular systolic pressure. These criteria would suggest constrictive pericarditis. Using the dynamic respiratory criteria, however, a diagnosis of restrictive cardiomyopathy was made. There was ventricular concordance and no evidence of dissociation of the intrathoracic and intracardiac pressures. There was no change in early transmitral gradient with respiration. Additionally, a cardiac biopsy was positive amyloidosis on Congo red staining. Serum immunoelectrophoresis also revealed a monoclonal protein consistent with systemic amyloidosis. The patient was given chemotherapy and did respond to the regimen initially. However, he finally expired of intractable heart failure 26 months after the diagnosis.

DISCUSSION

These case examples illustrated difficulty in using traditional hemodynamic criteria in the cardiac catheter-

TABLE I. Traditional Hemodynamic Criteria for Diagnosing Constrictive Pericarditis[a]

	Constrictive pericarditis	Restrictive cardiomyopathy
End-diastolic pressure equalization	LVEDP − RVEDP ≤5 mm Hg	LVEDP − RVEDP >5 mm Hg
Pulmonary artery pressure	PASP <55 mm Hg	PASP >55 mm Hg
High RVEDP	RVEDP/RVSP >⅓	RVEDP/RVSP ≤⅓
Dip plateau morphology	LV rapid filling wave >7 mm Hg	LV rapid filling wave ≤7 mm Hg
Kussmaul's sign	Lack of respiratory variation in mean RAP	Normal respiratory variation in mean RAP

[a]LVEDP − RVEDP = left and right ventricular end-diastolic pressure difference; PASP = pulmonary artery systolic pressure; RVSP = right ventricular systolic pressure; RVEDP = right ventricular end-diastolic pressure; LV = left ventricle; RAP = right atrial pressure.

TABLE II. Comparison of Traditional Hemodynamic Criteria With Dynamic Respiratory Criteria for Diagnosing Constrictive Pericarditis[a]

Criteria	Sensitivity (%)	Specificity (%)	PPV (%)	NPV (%)
Traditional				
LVEDP − RVEDP ≤5 mm Hg	60	38	4	57
RVEDP/RVSP >⅓	93	38	52	89
PASP <55 mm Hg	93	24	47	25
LV RFW ≥7 mm Hg	93	57	61	92
Respiratory change in RAP <3 mm Hg	93	48	58	92
Dynamic respiratory				
PCWP/LV respiratory gradient ≥5 mm Hg	93	81	78	94
LV/RV interdependence	100	95	94	100

[a]LVEDP − RVEDP = left and right ventricular end-diastolic pressure; RVSP = right ventricular systolic pressure; PASP = pulmonary artery systolic pressure; PPV = positive predictive value; NPV = negative predictive value; RFW = rapid filling wave; RAP = right atrial pressure; PCWP = pulmonary capillary wedge pressure; LV = left ventricle; RV = right ventricular. (Reproduced with permission from Hurrell DG, Nishimura RA, Higano ST, Appleton CP, Danielson GK, Holmes Jr DR, Tajik AJ. Value of dynamic respiratory changes in left and right ventricular pressures for the diagnosis of constrictive pericarditis. Circulation 1996;93: 2007–2013. Copyright 1996 William and Wilkins, Baltimore, MD.)

ization lab for the diagnosis of constrictive pericarditis. Elevation and equalization of right and left ventricular diastolic pressures with cessation of early ventricular filling can occur in restrictive diseases as well as constrictive pericarditis [10,11]. Restrictive diseases include other disorders with restrictive diastolic filling, such as restrictive cardiomyopathy, cardiac amyloidosis, or other infiltrative myocardial diseases. Traditional hemodynamic criteria used in the cardiac catheterization laboratory for the diagnosis of constrictive pericarditis include end-diastolic pressure equalization (left ventricular end-diastolic pressure minus right ventricular end-diastolic pressure less than or equal to 5 mm Hg), pulmonary artery pressure less than 55 mm Hg, right ventricular end-diastolic pressure divided by right ventricular systolic pressure greater than ⅓, dip and plateau diastolic pressure morphology as reflected by the height of the left ventricular rapid filling wave (greater than 7 mm Hg), and Kussmaul's sign (lack of an inspiratory fall in mean right atrial pressure) [12–19]. The traditional hemodynamic criteria are shown in Table I. Unfortunately, these traditional criteria have been shown to be neither specific nor sensitive in diagnosing constrictive pericarditis as demonstrated by Hurrell et al. [8], who compared patients with surgically proven constrictive pericarditis (group 1) with other causes of heart failure (group 2) (see Fig. 8 and Table II). Other restrictive diseases have altered diastolic filling properties and also have many of these traditional hemodynamic criteria (Fig. 13). It is critically important to distinguish constrictive pericarditis from the other restrictive diseases because of the excellent results of pericardiectomy.

Normal and Abnormal Ventricular Filling Physiology

Both restrictive diseases and constrictive pericarditis have impaired diastolic filling with elevated diastolic

pressures that results in dyspnea, edema, fatigue, ascites, and other signs and symptoms of right heart failure. However, restrictive diseases have a decrease in ventricular chamber compliance (due to increased myocardial stiffness), which results in an abnormal increase in impedance throughout diastole and reduced atrial filling component at end diastole. The result is a shortened deceleration time in the mitral and tricuspid valve inflows [21,22]. In contrast, the ventricular chamber compliance is normal in early diastole in constrictive pericarditis. In middiastole, ventricular filling is abruptly decelerated as the intracardiac volume approaches the relatively fixed volume of the rigid constricting pericardium. The relatively fixed intracardiac volume results in an increase in ventricular interdependence, or ventricular coupling [23]. The ventricles can not fill independent of each other. The filling of one ventricle impairs the filling of the opposite ventricle. The constricting pericardium also produces a dissociation of the intrathoracic and intracardiac pressures. In other words, changes in intrathoracic pressure do not fully transmit through the diseased pericardium to the intracardiac structures. These differences in the physiology between restrictive diseases and constrictive pericarditis should, in theory, allow for accurate discrimination of constrictive pericarditis from other restrictive diseases.

The hemodynamics of cardiac tamponade, as described by Sharp et al. [24] in 1960, can be used to further our understanding of constrictive pericarditis. While cardiac

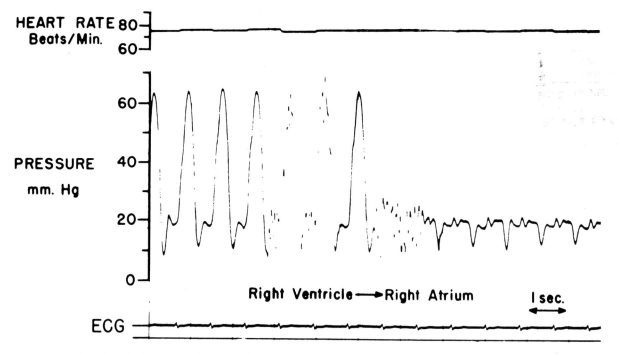

Fig. 13. Photokymographic recording from a patient with amyloid disease demonstrating the dip and plateau morphology in the right atrial and ventricular pressures previously felt to be pathognomonic for constrictive pericarditis. (Reproduced with permission from Hetzel PS, Wood EH, Burchell HB. Pressure pulses in the right side of the heart in a case of amyloid disease and in a case of idiopathic heart failure simulating constrictive pericarditis. Proc Staff Mayo Clinic 1953;28:107–112. Copyright 1953 Mayo Clinic.)

tamponade and constrictive pericarditis have important pathophysiologic differences, they share many of the same characteristics in terms of ventricular interdependence and dissociation of intrathoracic and intracardiac pressures. In the normal state, respiratory muscle contraction produces inspiration by reducing intrathoracic pressure, which in turn leads to a fall in pulmonary capillary wedge pressure (Fig. 14, top). The lowered intrathoracic pressure is transmitted through the normal pericardium and there is a nearly equivalent fall in intrapericardial and intracardiac pressure. The pressure gradient driving blood flow into the left heart (i.e., the pulmonary capillary wedge pressure minus the intracardiac pressure, or effective filling gradient) is maintained at a nearly constant level throughout the respiratory cycle. In contrast, the tense pericardial effusion in cardiac tamponade raises the intrapericardial and intracardiac pressures, resulting in an elevated pulmonary capillary wedge pressure (Fig. 14, bottom). The inspiratory fall in intrathoracic pressure is unchanged and produces a similar fall in pulmonary capillary wedge pressure. The drop in pressure is not transmitted to the intrapericardial space or intracardiac chambers and the effective filling gradient is significantly reduced. These early theoretical observations have since been confirmed using Doppler methods in experimental models and in patients with cardiac tamponade [25,26]. During inspiration, there is a reduction in transmitral

filling velocities and an elevation in velocities during expiration. These respiratory variations are not present in normals and resolve after pericardiocentesis. Dissociation of intrathoracic and intracardiac pressures also occurs in constrictive pericarditis, although the mechanism is from a rigid, thickened pericardium rather than a tense pericardial effusion.

In constrictive pericarditis, the respiratory changes in ventricular filling along with the relatively fixed intrapericardial volume results in enhanced ventricular interdependence, or coupling [23,26]. Inspiration results in a fall in left ventricular filling and a reduced left ventricular volume allowing for increased right ventricular filling within the relatively fixed intrapericardial volume.

Doppler Criteria

In 1989, Hatle et al. [9] recognized the pathophysiologic changes of constrictive pericarditis and further characterized the changes in the Doppler echocardiographic laboratory. In a landmark study, these authors described the characteristic Doppler cardiographic findings in constrictive pericarditis and demonstrated the ability of Doppler echocardiography to distinguish constrictive pericarditis from other restrictive diseases. They demonstrated that patients with constrictive pericarditis had marked changes in the mitral flow velocities with respiration that were not present in either normals or

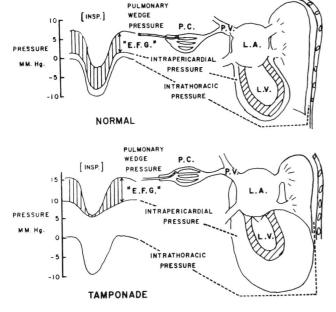

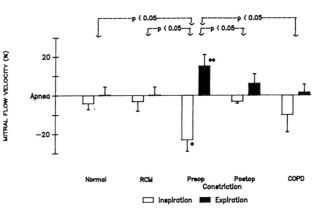

Fig. 15.   Bar graphs demonstrating the amplitude and direction of the mean percent change from apnea in inspiratory and expiratory values for peak early mitral flow velocity. There are significant respiratory changes in the mitral flow velocity in constrictive pericarditis, while normals and restrictive cardiomyopathy (RCM) have minimal changes. The respiratory variations seen in constrictive pericarditis were reduced after pericardiectomy. Patients with chronic obstructive pulmonary disease (COPD) also demonstrated respiratory variations. (Reproduced with permission from Hatle LK, Appleton CP, and Popp RL. Differentiation of constrictive pericarditis and restrictive cardiomyopathy by Doppler echocardiography. Circulation 1989;79: 357–370. Copyright 1989 William and Wilkins, Baltimore, MD.)

Fig. 14.   The top half of the figure represents the normal situation where changes in intrathoracic pressure are transmitted to both the pericardial sac and the pulmonary veins. The effective filling gradient (EFG) changes only slightly during respiration. The bottom half of the figure represents cardiac tamponade where changes in intrathoracic pressure are transmitted to the pulmonary veins but not to the pericardial sac. The EFG falls during inspiration. Abbreviations, Insp, inspiration; PC, pulmonary capillaries; PV, pulmonary veins; LA, left atrium; LV, left ventricle. (Reproduced with permission from Sharp JT, Bunnell IL, Holand JF, Griffith GT, Greene DG. Hemodynamics during induced cardiac tamponade in man. Am J Med 1960;25: 640–646. Copyright 1960 Elsevier Science.)

patients with restrictive cardiomyopathy (Fig. 15). There were opposite changes noted in the tricuspid inflow velocities. Furthermore, they demonstrated that these changes in transvalvular flow velocities normalized following pericardiectomy. The dissociation of intrathoracic and intracardiac pressures was clearly demonstrated to be present in constrictive pericarditis using Doppler techniques. The tricuspid regurgitant velocities have also been shown to be useful for diagnosing constrictive pericarditis. Klodas et al. [27] demonstrated that respiratory changes in Doppler-derived tricuspid regurgitation peak velocity and velocity duration are increased in patients with surgically confirmed constrictive pericarditis compared with heart failure due to other causes.

Another finding in the echocardiographic laboratory highly suggestive of constrictive pericarditis is the ventricular septal shift that occurs with respiration due to ventricular interdependence, as described above [28]. During inspiration, the left ventricle filling is reduced and right ventricular filling is augmented, causing the ventricular septum to shift leftward.

Respiratory Hemodynamic Criteria

The landmark Doppler study by Hatle et al. [9] also contained a wealth of invasive hemodynamic information regarding constrictive pericarditis and restrictive diseases. All patients underwent right and left heart catheterization in addition to comprehensive echocardiographic examination. The invasive pressure measurements demonstrated dissociation of intrathoracic and intracardiac pressures and enhanced ventricular interdependence. There was respiratory variation in the pressure gradient from the pulmonary capillary wedge position to the left ventricle in early diastole in constrictive pericarditis but not in restrictive disease (Figs. 16 and 17). This was direct confirmation of dissociation of intrathoracic and intracardiac pressures, the hypothesis initially presented by Sharp et al. [24], and likely accounted for the variability in mitral flow velocities seen in constrictive pericarditis.

However, the most marked differences between constrictive pericarditis and restrictive diseases were seen in the right and left ventricular systolic pressures. In constrictive pericarditis, the left ventricular pressure falls during inspiration while the right ventricular pressure rises, presumably due to the reduced and augmented stroke volumes in the respective ventricles (see Fig. 17). The ventricular pressures have been termed *discordant* and are due in part to ventricular interdependence. In restrictive diseases, as well as normals, the right and left ventricular systolic pressures change in a similar direction throughout the respiratory cycle and have been

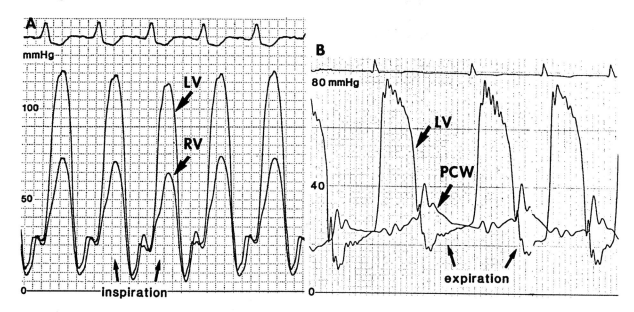

Fig. 16. Tracings of left ventricular (LV), right ventricular (RV), and pulmonary capillary wedge (PCW) pressures obtained from a patient with restrictive cardiomyopathy. Note the concordant changes in LV and RV pressures, despite end-diastolic pressure equalization and dip plateau morphology. There is also a lack of variability in the early diastolic PCW-LV gradient with respira- tion. (Reproduced with permission from Hatle LK, Appleton CP, and Popp RL. Differentiation of constrictive pericarditis and restrictive cardiomyopathy by Doppler echocardiography. Circu- lation 1989;79:357–370. Copyright 1989 William and Wilkins, Baltimore, MD.)

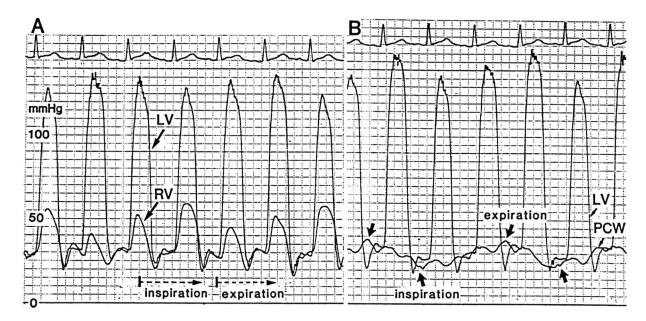

Fig. 17. Tracings of left ventricular (LV), right ventricular (RV), and pulmonary capillary wedge (PCW) pressures obtained from a patient with constrictive pericarditis. Note the discordant changes in LV and RV pressures and the variability in the early diastolic PCW-LV gradient with respiration. (Reproduced with permission from Hatle LK, Appleton CP, and Popp RL. Differentia- tion of constrictive pericarditis and restrictive cardiomyopathy by Doppler echocardiography. Circulation 1989;79:357–370. Copyright 1989 William and Wilkins, Baltimore, MD.)

termed *concordant* (see Fig. 16). The parameter that was the most significantly different between constrictive peri- carditis and other restrictive diseases was the change in right and left ventricular systolic pressures with respira-

tion (Fig. 18). From this information, two new dynamic respiratory hemodynamic criteria were developed for diagnosing constrictive pericarditis based on the prin- ciples of dissociation of intrathoracic and intracardiac

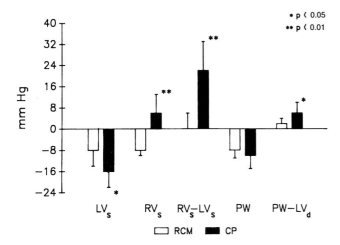

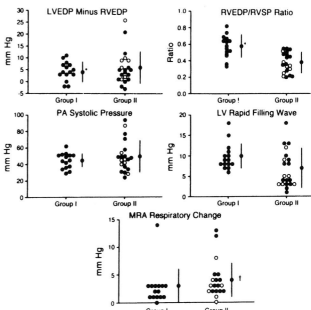

Fig. 18. Bar graph of the magnitude and directional change in the left (LV$_S$) and right (RV$_S$) ventricular systolic, pulmonary wedge (PW), and early diastolic difference in wedge to left ventricular (PW-LV$_d$) pressures from expiration to inspiration in patients with restrictive cardiomyopathy (RCM) and constrictive pericarditis (CP). The most significant differences between RCM and CP are in the inspiratory change in RV$_S$ minus inspiratory change in LV$_S$ (RV$_S$ − LV$_S$). (Reproduced with permission from Hatle LK, Appleton CP, and Popp RL. Differentiation of constrictive pericarditis and restrictive cardiomyopathy by Doppler echocardiography. Circulation 1989;79:357–370. Copyright 1989 William and Wilkins, Baltimore, MD.)

Fig. 19. Traditional hemodynamic criteria used to differentiate constrictive pericarditis (group 1) from other restrictive diseases (group 2, other causes of heart failure). Open circles indicate patients with restrictive cardiomyopathy. There is a large overlap between individuals in each group. MRA = mean right atrial pressure. *$P < 0.05$, +n = 19 patients. Value of dynamic respiratory changes in left and right ventricular pressures for the diagnosis of constrictive pericarditis. (Reproduced with permission from Hurrell DG, Nishimura RA, Higano ST, Appleton CP, Danielson GK, Holmes Jr DR, Tajik AJ. Value of dynamic respiratory changes in left and right ventricular pressures for the diagnosis of constrictive pericarditis. Circulation 1996;93:2007–2013. Copyright 1996 William and Wilkins, Baltimore, MD.)

pressures and ventricular interdependence: the early diastolic pulmonary capillary wedge to left ventricular pressure gradient and the left and right ventricular concordance, respectively.

In 1996, Hurrell et al. [8] further demonstrated the value of these dynamic respiratory changes for diagnosing constrictive pericarditis (Fig. 19). These authors examined dynamic respiratory changes in left and right ventricular pressures in 36 patients; 15 with surgically proven constrictive pericarditis and 21 with congestive heart failure. The dissociation of the intrathoracic and intracardiac pressures were assessed at end inspiration and end expiration by comparing the pulmonary capillary wedge pressure minus the minimum left ventricular early diastolic pressure gradient. Ventricular interdependence was assessed by examining simultaneously obtained right and left ventricular pressures during respiration for concordance or discordance. The degree of concordance or discordance in these systolic pressures was quantified by calculation of the "RV index." The minimum and maximum ventricular systolic pressures throughout the respiratory cycle were assigned values of 0% and 100%, respectively. The RV index was defined as the right ventricular percentage at peak inspiration.

The dissociation of intrathoracic and intracardiac pressures was significantly greater in those with constrictive pericarditis than restrictive diseases; however, there was some overlap between the groups (Fig. 20). However, the patients with constrictive pericarditis frequently demon-

strated ventricular interdependence with an RV index of 100%. During peak inspiration, there was an increase in right ventricular systolic pressure and decrease in left ventricular systolic pressure. In contrast, patients with congestive heart failure usually demonstrated concordant changes right and left ventricular systolic pressures during peak respiration. Right ventricular systolic pressure was at its maximum during peak inspiration in all patients with constrictive pericarditis, where as all but one patient in the group with congestive heart failure had right ventricular systolic pressures concordant with left ventricular systolic pressures (Fig. 21). This finding was 100% sensitive and 95% specific for the diagnosis of constrictive pericarditis. The sensitivity, specificity, predictive positive and negative values are summarized in Table II.

Catheterization Technique

Catheter evaluation of patients with suspected constrictive pericarditis involves the basic techniques of simultaneous right and left heart catheterization with several caveats. It is of utmost importance to obtain accurate pressures simultaneously in the right and left heart

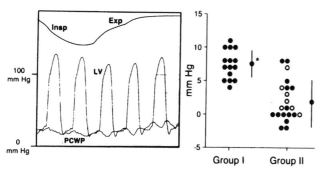

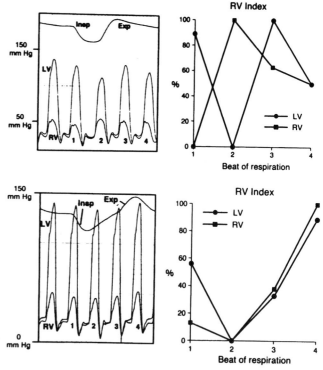

Fig. 20. Respiratory changes in early diastolic transmitral pressure gradient as estimated by the pulmonary capillary wedge pressure (PCWP) and the left ventricular (LV) minimum pressure. Left: Pressure waveforms of PCWP and LV with respirometer from a patient with constrictive pericarditis. Right: Individual data from patients with constrictive pericarditis (group 1) and other causes of heart failure (group 2) demonstrating the difference between the PCWP-LV early diastolic pressure gradient during expiration (Exp) minus inspiration (Insp). Open circles are patients with restrictive cardiomyopathy. Although there is a significant difference between the two groups (*$P < 0.05$), there is significant overlap between individuals in each group. Value of dynamic respiratory changes in left and right ventricular pressures for the diagnosis of constrictive pericarditis. (Reproduced with permission from Hurrell DG, Nishimura RA, Higano ST, Appleton CP, Danielson GK, Holmes Jr DR, Tajik AJ. Value of dynamic respiratory changes in left and right ventricular pressures for the diagnosis of constrictive pericarditis. Circulation 1996;93:2007–2013. Copyright 1996 William and Wilkins, Baltimore, MD.)

Fig. 21. Respiratory changes in left (LV) and right (RV) ventricular systolic pressures in patients with constrictive pericarditis (group 1) (top left) and other causes of heart failure (group 2) (bottom left). The RV indexes for these specific examples are also shown (right panels), which demonstrate discordance in patient with constrictive pericarditis and concordance in the patient with heart failure. Value of dynamic respiratory changes in left and right ventricular pressures for the diagnosis of constrictive pericarditis. (Reproduced with permission from Hurrell DG, Nishimura RA, Higano ST, Appleton CP, Danielson GK, Holmes Jr DR, Tajik AJ. Value of dynamic respiratory changes in left and right ventricular pressures for the diagnosis of constrictive pericarditis. Circulation 1996;93:2007–2013. Copyright 1996 William and Wilkins, Baltimore, MD.)

chambers during the respiratory cycle. Fluid-filled catheters generally do not provide high-fidelity pressure recordings required for assessing the subtle changes in pressure with respiration, especially in the wedge to left ventricle pressure gradient. Therefore, in most cases, we would recommend that high-fidelity micromanometers be used.

The procedure begins with placement of 7 French arterial and venous sheaths, usually in the femoral region. Two venous sheaths may be required if a temporary pacemaker is to be used. Right heart pressures are obtained through a large lumen 7 French Lehman catheter starting in the wedge position. High-fidelity pressures are obtained by positioning a 2 French micromanometer-tipped wire near the distal end of the Lehman catheter. Left ventricular pressures are obtained with a 7 French pigtail catheter placed retrogradely across the aortic valve into the left ventricle. High-fidelity pressures are obtained in one of two ways. Either a small 2 French micromanometer-tipped wire is positioned at the tip of the pigtail or a specially designed micromanometer-tipped pigtail catheter is used. In all systems, the fluid-filled pressure waveforms are also available for zeroing the high-fidelity pressure waveform. The micromanometers need to be zeroed and balanced using the fluid-filled waveforms as a reference whenever the catheters are moved to account

for the hydrostatic effects of varying heights within the chest. A nasal thermistor is used as a respirometer and is recorded on the tracings. Temporary pacing is used in patients with atrial fibrillation, or other irregular rhythms, to eliminate the effect of varying RR intervals on pressure. The patients were then coached to breathe deeply and smoothly during the dynamic respiratory measurements.

Case Discussion

Both the traditional and the new dynamic respiratory criteria for diagnosing constrictive pericarditis are shown in Table III. The two cases of constrictive pericarditis met all the traditional criteria for the diagnosis. As indicated in the work of Hurrell et al. [8], these traditional findings are sensitive for diagnosing constrictive pericarditis, but are not very specific. The two cases of restriction also had many of these findings and may have been mistaken for

TABLE III. Hemodynamic Criteria of Constrictive Pericarditis[a]

Criteria	Case 1 constriction	Case 2 constriction	Case 3 restriction	Case 4 restriction
Traditional				
LVEDP − RVEDP ≤5				
mm Hg	+	+	+	+
RVEDP/RVSP >⅓	+	+	−	+
PASP <55 mm Hg	+	+	−	+
LV RFW ≥7 mm Hg	+	+	+	+
Respiratory change in				
RAP <3 mm Hg	+	+	+	+
Dynamic respiratory				
PCWP/LV respiratory				
gradient ≥5 mm Hg	+	−	−	−
LV/RV interdependence	+	+	−	−

[a]LVEDP − RVEDP = left and right ventricular end-diastolic pressure; RVSP = right ventricular systolic pressure; PASP = pulmonary artery systolic pressure; PPV = positive predictive value; NPV = negative predictive value; RFW = rapid filling wave; RAP = right atrial pressure; PCWP = pulmonary capillary wedge pressure; LV = left ventricle; RV = right ventricular.

constrictive pericarditis. The new dynamic respiratory criteria helped make the correct diagnosis, although the reduced accuracy of the dissociated intrathoracic and intracardiac pressures was illustrated in case 2. However, the clear ventricular interdependence confirms the diagnosis of constrictive pericarditis.

Miscellaneous Features

Other conditions may result in similar Doppler findings to those of constrictive pericarditis. For example, severe lung disease with marked respiratory changes and intrathoracic pressures can cause changes in mitral flow velocity mimicking those reported in constrictive pericarditis [1]. Other entities, such as obesity, right ventricular infarction, or severe tricuspid regurgitation may also be problematic. Low filling pressures have been reported to cause "occult" constrictive pericarditis, which can only be unmasked with fluid challenge [29]. If the LVEDP is less than 15 mm Hg, then a 500–1,000 ml of saline challenge should be administered. One needs to be cautious when administering the fluid challenge, as excessive increases in preload can result in marked changes in diastolic function and even normal hearts may appear restrictive or possibly constrictive [30,31]. Conversely, severely elevated filling pressures may mask the more subtle respiratory variations in pressure. Frequently, upright tilting can bring out these characteristic findings of constrictive pericarditis in the Doppler echocardiographic laboratory [32].

Furthermore, irregular heart rhythms, including atrial fibrillation, may obscure the significance of the mitral flow velocity variations. Varying RR intervals cause fluctuations in the mitral inflow velocities that can mask or mimic the findings of constrictive pericarditis. Similarly, pressure measurements in the catheterization labora-

tory fluctuate with varying RR intervals. A large percentage of patients with constrictive pericarditis have atrial fibrillation on presentation. In the cardiac catheterization laboratory, the varying RR intervals of atrial fibrillation can be regularized with temporary ventricular pacing at rates just above the ventricular response. This maneuver is critical for assessing patients with constrictive pericarditis and can only be performed in the catheterization laboratory.

Radiation is a fairly common cause of constrictive pericarditis, which can often present a confusing mixed picture. In addition to thickening or scarring the pericardium, radiation can cause late myocardial scarring with restrictive filling physiology. These patients present with mixed disease, including both constrictive and restrictive physiology. The results of pericardiectomy are less satisfactory, as they frequently have residual diastolic filling abnormalities from the restrictive myocardial disease [33,34].

The traditional hemodynamic criteria used in the cardiac catheterization laboratory appear to be insensitive and nonspecific for diagnosing constrictive pericarditis. Using the principles of enhanced ventricular interdependence and dissociation of intrathoracic and intracardiac pressures, new dynamic respiratory changes can be identified in constrictive pericarditis. The dynamic respiratory changes in left and right ventricular pressures appear to augment the sensitivity and specificity of the diagnosis and should be incorporated into hemodynamic assessment of all patients with suspected constrictive pericarditis.

REFERENCES

1. Oh JK, Hatle LK, Seward JB, Danielson GK, Schaff HV, Reeder GS, Tajik AJ. Diagnostic role of Doppler echocardiography in constrictive pericarditis. J Am Coll Cardiol 1994;23:154–162.
2. Vaitkus PT, Kussmaul WG. Constrictive pericarditis versus restrictive cardiomyopathy: a reappraisal and update of diagnostic criteria. Am Heart J 1991;122:1431–1441.
3. Moncada R, Baker M, Salinas M, Demos TC, Churchill R, Love L, Reynes C, Hale D, Cardoso M, Pifarre R, Gunnar RM. Diagnostic role of computed tomography in constrictive pericardial disease. Am Heart J 1982;103:263–282.
4. Isner JM, Carter BL, Bankoff MS, Pastore JO, Ramaswamy K, McAdam KP, Salem DM. Differentiation of constrictive pericarditis from restrictive cardiomyopathy by computed tomographic imaging. Am Heart J 1983;105:1019–1025.
5. Soulen RL, Stark DD, Higins CB. Magnetic resonance imaging of constrictive pericardial disease. Am J Cardiol 1985;55:480–484.
6. McCaughan BC, Schaff HV, Piehler JM, Danielson GK, Orszulak TA, Puga FJ, Pluth J, Connolly DC, McGoon DC. Early and late results of pericardiectomy for constrictive pericarditis. J Thorac Cardiovasc Surg 1985;89:340–350.
7. Tuna IC, Danielson GK. Surgical management of pericardial diseases. Cardiol Clin 1990;8:683–696.
8. Hurrell DG, Nishimura RA, Higano ST, Appleton CP, Danielson GK, Holmes DR Jr, Tajik AJ. Value of dynamic respiratory changes in left and right ventricular pressures for the diagnosis of constrictive pericarditis. Circulation 1996;93:2007–2013.

9. Hatle LK, Appleton CP, Popp RL. Differentiation of constrictive pericarditis and restrictive cardiomyopathy by Doppler echocardiography. Circulation 1989;79:357–370.

10. Lorell BH, Grossman W. Profiles in constrictive pericarditis, restrictive cardiomyopathy, and cardiac-tamponade. In: Grossman W, editor. Cardiac catheterization and angiography, 3rd ed. Philadelphia: Lea & Febiger; 1986. p 427–445.

11. Shabetai R. Pathophysiology and differential diagnosis of restrictive cardiomyopathy. Cardiovasc Clin 1988;19:123–132.

12. Bloomfield RA, Lauson HD, Cournand A, Breed ES, Richards DW. Recording of right heart pressures in normal subjects and in patients with chronic pulmonary disease and various types of cardio-circulatory disease. J Clin Invest 1946;25:639–664.

13. Yu PNG, Lovejoy FW Jr, Joos HA, Nye RE Jr, Mahoney EB. Right auricular and ventricular pressure patterns in constrictive pericarditis. Circulation 1953;7:102–107.

14. Shabetai R, Fowler NO, Guntheroth WG. The hemodynamics of cardiac tamponade and constrictive pericarditis. Am J Cardiol 1970;26:480–489.

15. Kesteloot H, Denef B. Value of reference tracings in diagnosis and assessment of constrictive epi- and pericarditis. Br Heart J 1970;32:675–682.

16. Hirschmann JV. Pericardial constriction. Am Heart J 1978;97:110–122.

17. Fowler NO. Constrictive pericarditis: new aspects. Am J Cardiol 1982;50:1014–1017.

18. Janos GG, Arjunan K, Meyer RA, Engel P, Kaplan S. Differentiation of constrictive pericarditis and restrictive cardiomyopathy using digitized echocardiography. J Am Coll Cardiol 1983;1:541–549.

19. Appleton CP, Hatle LK, Popp RL. Central venous flow velocity patterns can differentiate constrictive pericarditis from restrictive cardiomyopathy. J Am Coll Cardiol 1987;9:119A.

20. Hetzel PS, Wood EH, Burchell HB. Pressure pulses in the right side of the heart in a case of amyloid disease and in a case of idiopathic heart failure simulating constrictive pericarditis. Proc Staff Mayo Clinic 1953;28:107–112.

21. Appleton CP, Hatle LK, Popp RL. Demonstration of restrictive ventricular physiology by Doppler echocardiography. J Am Coll Cardiol 1988;11:757.

22. Benotti JR, Grossman W, Cohn PF. Clinical profile of restrictive cardiomyopathy. Circulation 1980;61:1206–1212.

23. Santamore WP, Bartlet R, Van Buren SJ, Dowd MK, Kutcher MA. Ventricular coupling in constrictive pericarditis. Circulation 1986;74:597.

24. Sharp JT, Bunnell IL, Holand JF, Griffith GT, Greene DG. Hemodynamics during induced crdiac tamponade in man. Am J Med 1960;25:640–646.

25. Burstow DJ, Oh JK, Bailey KR, Seward JB, Tajik AJ. Cardiac tamponade: characteristic Doppler observations. Mayo Clin Proc 1989;64:312–324.

26. Gonzalez MS, Basnight MA, Appleton CP. Experimental cardiac tamponade: a hemodynamic and Doppler echocardiographic reexamination of the relation of right and left heart ejection dynamics to the phase of respiration. J Am Coll Cardiol 1991;18:242–252.

27. Klodas E, Nishimura RA, Appleton CP, Redfield MM, Oh JK. Doppler evaluation of patients with constrictive pericarditis: use of tricuspid regurgitation velocity curves to determine enhanced ventricular interaction. J Am Coll Cardiol 1996;28:652–657.

28. Gibson TC, Grossman W, McLaurin LP, Moos S, Craige E. An echocardiographic study of the interventricular septum in constrictive pericarditis. Br Heart J 1978;38:738.

29. Bush CA, Stang JM, Wooley CF, Kilman JW. Occult constrictive pericardial disease; diagnosis by rapid volume expansion and correction by pericardiectomy. Circulation 1977;56:924–930.

30. Hurrell DG, Nishimura RA, Ilstrup DM, Appleton CP. Utility of preload alteration in assessment of left ventricular filling pressure by Doppler echocardiography: a simultaneous catheterization and Doppler echocardiographic study. J Am Coll Cardiol 1997;30:459–467.

31. Nishimura RA, Abel MD, Housmans PR, Warnes CA, Tajik AJ. Mitral flow velocity curves as a function of different loading conditions: evaluation by intraoperative transesophageal Doppler echocardiography. J Am Soc Echocardiol 1989;2:79–87.

32. Oh JK, Tajik AJ, Appleton CP, Hatle LK, Nishimura RA, Seward JB. Preload reduction to unmask the characteristic Doppler features of constrictive pericarditis; a new observation. Circulation 1997;95:796–799.

33. Ling LH, Oh JK, Danielson GK, Schaff HV, Mahoney DW, Seward JB, Tajik AJ. Outcome following pericardiectomy for constrictive pericarditis: influence of an evolving disease. Circulation 1997;96(suppl):129.

34. Senni M, Redfield MM, Ling LH, Iwase M, Oh JK. Left ventricular systolic and diastolic function after pericardiectomy in patients with constrictive pericarditis: postoperative and serial Doppler echocardiographic findings. Circulation 1997;96(suppl):I30.

Chapter 23

Hemodynamics of Constrictive Physiology—Section V:
Respiratory Dynamics

Elie Azrak, MD, and Morton J. Kern, MD

INTRODUCTION

The definitive diagnosis of symptomatic constrictive pericarditis with severe elevation of right heart pressures is difficult to establish by traditional static hemodynamic criteria [1–5]. Using the traditional hemodynamic criteria increases the confidence in the diagnosis of constrictive pericarditis, but with only moderate increase in diagnostic sensitivity and specificity. Two new dynamic hemodynamic criteria, respiratory discordance in right and left ventricular pressures and early diastolic pulmonary capillary wedge to left ventricular end-diastolic pressure as proposed by Hurrell et al. [6], appears to advance our accuracy with regard to establishing the diagnosis of constrictive pericardial disease. Following the review and case examples of Higano et al. [7], we present two additional patients with abnormal hemodynamics who illustrate several of the diagnostic dilemmas in the hemodynamic diagnosis of constrictive pericarditis.

CASE REPORT
Case 1

A 58-year-old female who had atrial septal defect repair with pulmonary valvulotomy 10 years ago reported increasing abdominal girth and nocturnal chest discomfort lasting for hours at a time over the past 2 months. Evaluation showed hepatomegaly by both physical examination and CT scanning. Two-dimensional echocardiography demonstrated normal left ventricular systolic function, right ventricular enlargement, moderate tricuspid regurgitation, pulmonary hypertension, and mild mitral regurgitation.

Physical examination showed a well-appearing woman with a blood pressure of 137/90 mm Hg, heart rate 47 beats/min, and respiratory rate 16/min. There was no neck vein distension or carotid bruits. The lungs were clear. Heart examination demonstrated quiet precordial impulse, a II/VI systolic murmur along the high left sternal border, a II/VI diastolic murmur at the base of the left sternal border, and a fixed S_2. There was no abdominal distension or palpable hepatosplenomegaly at this examination. The extremities were without edema or cyanosis. The electrocardiogram showed sinus bradycardia with right bundle branch block. The patient was referred to cardiac catheterization to determine the etiology of symptom presentation.

Right and left heart catheterization was performed in a routine fashion using the Seldinger technique from the right femoral artery and vein with 7 Fr and 8 Fr fluid-filled catheters. Mean right atrial pressure (Fig. 1) was 13 mm Hg. There was a blunted X- and prominent Y-descent with a markedly positive Kussmaul's sign (Fig. 1, right). The mean pulmonary capillary wedge pressure was 17 mm Hg with giant V-waves to 36 mm Hg. The prominent A-waves reached 20 mm Hg (Fig. 2, left). The pulmonary artery pressure was 55/16 mm Hg (Fig. 2, far right). The aortic pressure was 108/40 mm Hg with a left ventricular pressure of 108/18 mm Hg. There was diastolic equilibration of right atrial, pulmonary capillary wedge, and left ventricular diastolic pressures (Fig. 3). The dynamic changes in left ventricular-pulmonary capillary wedge gradient were not recorded. Simultaneous right and left ventricular pressures demonstrated diastolic equalization with an early dip with a diastolic plateau configuration (Fig. 4). The respiratory variation of right

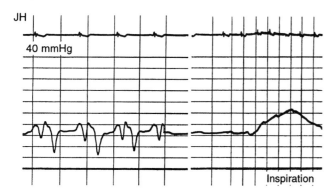

Fig. 1. Hemodynamic tracings of right atrial pressure on a 0–40-mm Hg scale. Note the bradycardia and the M configuration with blunted X- and exaggerated Y-descent. Kussmaul's sign is positive as shown by the increase in mean right atrial pressure during inspiration.

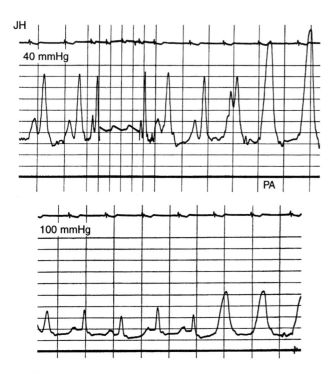

Fig. 2. Pulmonary capillary wedge pressure on a 0–40-mm Hg scale (top left) and on a 0–100-mm Hg scale (bottom left). The pulmonary capillary wedge balloon is deflated, yielding the pullback to the pulmonary artery pressure (top and bottom right).

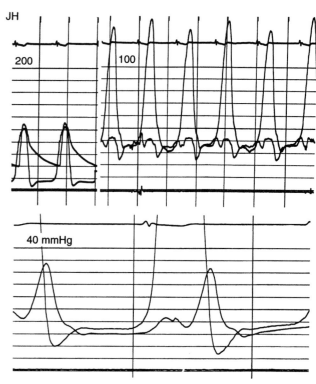

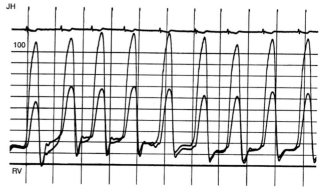

Fig. 3. Top left: Aortic and left ventricular pressures on a 0–200-mm Hg scale. Top right: Right ventricular and right atrial pressures on a 0–100-mm Hg scale. Bottom: Left ventricular and pulmonary capillary wedge pressure on a 0–40-mm Hg scale.

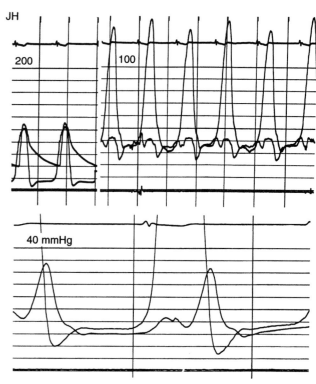

Fig. 4. Simultaneous right and left ventricular pressures over an inspiratory cycle period. Peak end expiration is beat 5 from the left and end inspiration is beat 7.

and left ventricular systolic pressures demonstrated concordance with end inspiration. Left and right ventricular systolic pressures (Fig. 4, beat 5) both increased (130 and 68 mm Hg). End expiratory pressures were 110 and 54 mm Hg, respectively (Fig. 4, beat 7). Cardiac output was 2.2 L/min by thermodilution technique. No intracardiac shunt was noted by oximetry with oxygen saturations of 64% in the right atrium and pulmonary artery.

Left ventriculography was normal with an ejection fraction of 66% and mild mitral regurgitation. Right

ventriculography performed with a 7 Fr Berman catheter was also normal with a mildly dilated right ventricular chamber. There was mild to moderate tricuspid regurgitation. By angiography, the pulmonic valve had a thickened leaflet as a residual of the prior pulmonary valvuloplasty with good leaflet excursion. There was significant pulmonary insufficiency demonstrated by angiography as well. Coronary arteriography was normal. Based on traditional hemodynamics, clinical findings, and noninvasive data, the patient was recommended for pericardial stripping. The operation was performed with only modest relief of symptoms.

Case 2

A 71-year-old female with heart murmur and enlarged heart since childhood was admitted with a chest pain syndrome. A permanent pacemaker was inserted 5 years ago for a sick sinus syndrome. She complained of dyspnea on exertion increasing over the past several months. The patient had 3–4 hr of left-sided chest pain at rest, which was relieved by sublingual nitroglycerin in the emergency department. In the coronary care unit, acute myocardial infarction was excluded. Two-dimensional and Doppler echocardiography demonstrated normal left ventricular function and transvalvular flow velocities. A dipyridamole cardiolyte study revealed a small reversible apical defect.

On physical examination, there was no neck vein distension at 45° elevation. The lungs were clear. There were no carotid bruits. Heart examination showed a regular rate and rhythm with a fixed split S_2 and a normal S_1. There was a II/VI holosystolic murmur across the left precordium. The abdominal and extremity examinations were unremarkable. The electrocardiogram demonstrated a pacemaker rhythm. Medications at the time of catheterization were diltiazem, Heparin, Lasix, and sublingual nitroglycerin.

Right and left heart cardiac catheterization was performed from the right femoral artery and vein using 6 Fr and 8 Fr catheters and fluid-filled transducers in the standard fashion. Mean right atrial pressure was mildly elevated at 18 mm Hg (Fig. 5) with a blunted Y-descent. Pulmonary artery pressure was 55/20 mm Hg (Fig. 5, top right). Aortic pressure was 150/70 mm Hg and left ventricular pressure was 150/22 (Fig. 5, bottom). Pulmonary capillary wedge was elevated with a mean of 30 mm Hg with V-waves to 50 mm Hg. A prominent C-notch was also noted in the pulmonary capillary wedge pressure waveform. There was minimal left ventricular-pulmonary capillary wedge diastolic pressure gradient without respiratory variation (Fig. 6). The simultaneous measurement of right and left ventricular pressures (Fig. 7) showed an early diastolic dip with a blunted diastolic filling pattern and diastolic pressure equalization without respiratory discordance. Note the timing delay of left ventricular contraction by the paced rhythm with the right ventricular pressure upstroke is superimposed on the left ventricular pressure upstroke (Fig. 7). There was respiratory concordance of right and left ventricular systolic pressures.

Left ventriculography was normal (ejection fraction of 75%) with mild mitral regurgitation. Coronary arteriogra-

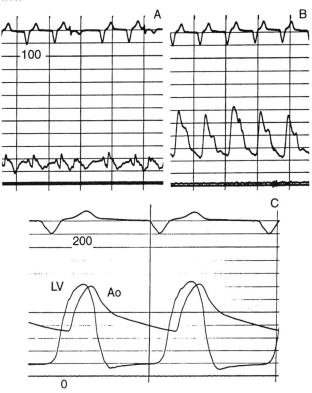

Fig. 5. A: Right atrial pressure on a 0–100-mm Hg scale. B: Pulmonary artery pressure on a 0–100-mm Hg. C: Left ventricular and aortic pressures on a 0–200-mm Hg scale.

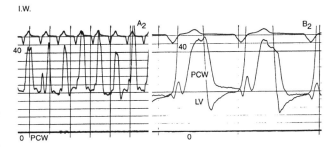

Fig. 6. Left: Pulmonary capillary wedge pressure on a 0–40-mm Hg scale. Right: Pulmonary capillary wedge and simultaneous left ventricular pressure on a 0–40-mm Hg scale.

phy was normal. These findings suggested restrictive cardiac physiology with mild pulmonary hypertension. The patient was continued on medical therapy. The hemodynamic data for the two patients are summarized on Table I.

DISCUSSION

These case examples highlight the continuing difficulty in using traditional static hemodynamic criteria for the diagnosis of constrictive pericarditis. Both patients were

I.W.

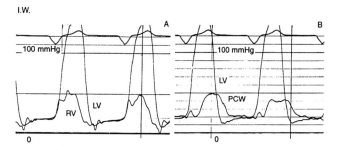

Fig. 7. A: Right and left ventricular pressures on a 0–100-mm Hg scale. B: Left ventricular and pulmonary capillary wedge pressures on a 0–100-mm Hg scale. RA = mean right atrial pressure (mm Hg); RV = right ventricular pressure (mm Hg); PA = pulmonary artery pressure (mm Hg); PCW = mean pulmonary capillary wedge pressure (mm Hg); Ao = aortic pressure (mm Hg); CO = cardiac output (L/min); PVR = pulmonary vascular resistance (dynes·sec/cm⁵); SVR = systolic vascular resistance (dynes·sec/cm⁵); Art = arterial.

symptomatic with elevation and diastolic equalization of right and left ventricular pressures with abrupt cessation of early ventricular filling. As noted earlier [2], classic hemodynamic criteria for the diagnosis of constrictive pericarditis included left ventricular end-diastolic minus right ventricular end-diastolic pressure ≤5 mm Hg, pulmonary artery systolic pressure <55 mm Hg, ratio of right ventricular end-diastolic pressure to right ventricular systolic pressure >1/3, and a "dip and plateau" diastolic filling pattern (also noted by echocardiographic findings an increase in the height of the left ventricular rapid filling wave), and finally, lack of respiratory variation in the mean right atrial pressure [8–11]. Table II shows the presence and absence of these criteria in the two patient examples presented here.

The static end-diastolic pressure relationships appear to be limited in predicting the presence of pericardial constriction [1,2,12]. In constrictive pericarditis, Doppler echocardiographic findings characteristically demonstrate increased transvalvular flow velocity variations with respiration. Dynamic respiratory changes in ventricular pressures, the hemodynamic equivalent of the long-accepted Doppler echocardiographic criteria, should also be used to increase the diagnostic accuracy of the traditional hemodynamic data and demonstrate the degree of ventricular interdependence [8,9]. Hurrell et al. [6] were the first to demonstrate the value of dynamic respiratory changes in left and right ventricular pressures for the diagnosis of constrictive pericarditis. Dynamic respiratory changes in hemodynamics were assessed at end inspiration and end expiration. Ventricular interdependence was examined with high fidelity left and right ventricular pressure waveforms during respiration. To compute the degree of pressure concordance, at the onset of inspiration the peak left and right ventricular systolic

pressures were measured for each of the beats throughout one respiratory cycle. The maximum systolic pressure differences were then assigned a value of 100% and the lowest value 0%. The remaining beats were assigned percentage of the maximum difference [6]. Although the mean right atrial pressure, left ventricular rapid filling wave, and right and left ventricular end-diastolic pressures were significantly different between patients with constrictive pericarditis and congestive heart failure, the five traditional criteria for constrictive pericarditis yielded significant overlap between patient groups. The investigators identified respiratory changes in the early diastolic transmitral gradient, as estimated by pulmonary capillary wedge and left ventricular minimum pressures. Patients with constrictive pericarditis had significant variation as compared to those with congestive heart failure. Increased ventricular interdependence in the constrictive pericardial group was demonstrated during peak inspiration with an increase in right ventricular systolic pressure when left ventricular systolic pressure decreased. In contrast, in patients with congestive heart failure during peak inspiration, there was a concordant decrease in both right and left ventricular systolic pressures. Ventricular pressure disconcordance was 100% sensitive and 95% specific for the diagnosis of constrictive pericarditis. As noted in the two cases presented, although static hemodynamics initially suggested constrictive physiology, patient 1 had little benefit after pericardial stripping, whereas patient 2 was characterized as having a restrictive cardiomyopathy. The sensitivity, specificity, and predictive positive and negative values are summarized in Table III.

The mechanisms of the dynamic respiratory criteria for constrictive pericarditis are described by Higano et al. [7]. In normal individuals, an inspiratory decrease in intrathoracic pressure is transmitted to the cardiac chambers. Transmitral filling pressure during early diastole is unchanged over the respiratory cycle. Left ventricular filling is also unchanged. In constricting physiology, the encasing pericardium does not transmit the inspiratory decrease in pulmonary venous and intrathoracic pressure into the cardiac chambers. The failure to transmit the inspiratory decrease in pulmonary venous and thoracic pressure results in a phasically transmitral pressure gradient and delayed left ventricular filling. The constricting pericardium decreases left ventricular volume out of phase with the corresponding increase in right ventricular volume [6].

The two patients described here had none of the other conditions that may result in dynamic ventricular respiratory variations producing Doppler and hemodynamic findings resembling constrictive pericarditis. For example, severe lung disease with marked respiratory changes and intrathoracic pressure can cause changes in mitral flow velocity mimicking those reported previously

TABLE I. Hemodynamic Data[a]

Patient number	RA	RV	PA	PCW	LV	Ao	CO	PVR	SVR	Oxygen saturations (%)		
										RA	PA	Art
1	13	65/16	65/16	17	108/18	108/40	2.2	291	1855	64	64	97
2	18	55/10	55/20	30	150/22	150/70	4.3	93	1340	55	55	92

[a]RA = mean right atrial pressure (mm Hg); RV = right ventricular pressure (mm Hg); PA = pulmonary artery pressure (mm Hg); PCW = mean pulmonary capillary wedge pressure (mm Hg); Ao = aortic pressure (mm Hg); CO = cardiac output (L/min); PVR = pulmonary vascular resistance (dynes · sec/cm^5); SVR = systolic vascular resistance (dynes · sec/cm^5); Art = arterial.

TABLE II. Hemodynamic Criteria of Constrictive Pericarditis[a]

	Case 1	Case 2
LVEDP − RVEDP ≤5 mm Hg	+	+
PAS <55 mm Hg	−	−
RVS/RVED >1/3	−	+
Dip plateau	+	+
No RA respiratory variation	+	−

[a]LVEDP − RVEDP = left and right ventricular end-diastolic pressure; PAS = pulmonary artery systolic pressure; RVS = right ventricular systolic; RVED = right ventricular end-diastolic; RA = right atrial; + = present; − = absent.

TABLE III. Sensitivities, Specificities, Positive Predictive Value, and Negative Predictive Values as a Function of Criteria[a]

Criteria	Sensitivity (%)	Specificity (%)	PPV (%)	NPV (%)
Conventional				
LVEDP − RVEDP ≤5 mm Hg	60	38	4	57
RVEDP/RVSP >1/3	93	38	52	89
PASP <55 mm Hg	93	24	47	25
LV RFW ≥7 mm Hg	93	57	61	92
Respiratory change in RAP <3 mm Hg	93	48	58	92
Dynamic respiratory				
PCWP/LV respiratory gradient ≥5 mm Hg	93	81	78	94
LV/RV interdependence	100	95	94	100

[a]LVEDP − RVEDP = left and right ventricular end-diastolic pressure; RVSP = right ventricular systolic pressure; PASP = pulmonary artery systolic pressure; PPV = positive predictive value; NPV = negative predictive value; RFW = rapid filling wave; RAP = right atrial pressure; PCWP = pulmonary capillary wedge pressure; RV = right ventricular. From Hurrell et al. [6].

[13]. Increased left atrial pressure may also mask Doppler respiratory variations. Irregular heart rhythms, including atrial fibrillation, may obscure the significance of initial mitral valve flow velocity alterations.

The conventional static hemodynamic diagnostic criteria appear insensitive and nonspecific for constrictive pericarditis. The dynamic respiratory changes in left and right ventricular pressures and early transmittal pressure gradient augment the sensitivity and specificity of the diagnosis and should be used to provide more reliable hemodynamic criteria for distinguishing patients with constrictive pericarditis.

ACKNOWLEDGMENTS

The authors thank the J.G. Mudd Cardiac Catheterization Laboratory Team and Donna Sander for manuscript preparation.

REFERENCES

1. Lorell BH, Grossman W. Profiles in constrictive pericarditis, restrictive cardiomyopathy, and cardiac-tamponade. In: Grossman W, editor. Cardiac catheterization and angiography, 3rd ed. Philadelphia: Lea & Febiger; 1986. p 427–445.
2. Shabetai R. Pathophysiology and differential diagnosis of restrictive cardiomyopathy. Cardiovasc Clin 1988;19:123–132.
3. Benotti JR, Grossman W, Cohn PF. Clinical profile of restrictive cardiomyopathy. Circulation 1980;61:1206–1212.
4. Vaitkus PT, Kussmaul WG. Constrictive pericarditis versus restrictive cardiomyopathy: a reappraisal and update of diagnostic criteria. Am Heart J 1991;122:1431–1441.
5. Shabetai R, Fowler NO, Guntheroth WG. The hemodynamics of cardiac tamponade and constrictive pericarditis. Am J Cardiol 1970;26:480–489.
6. Hurrell DG, Nishimura RA, Higano ST, Appleton CP, Danielson GK, Holmes Jr DR, Tajik AJ. Value of dynamic respiratory changes in left and right ventricular pressures for the diagnosis of constrictive pericarditis. Circulation 1996;93:2007–2013.
7. Higano ST, Azrak E, Tahirkheli NK, Kern MJ. Hemodynamic rounds, series II: hemodynamics of constrictive physiology: influence of respiratory dynamics in ventricular pressures. Cathet Cardiovasc Intervent 1999; in press.
8. Appleton CP, Hatle LK, Popp RL. Central venous flow velocity patterns can differentiate constrictive pericarditis from restrictive cardiomyopathy. J Am Coll Cardiol 1987;9:119A.
9. Fowler NO. Constrictive pericarditis: new aspects. Am J Cardiol 1982;50:1014–1017.
10. Hirschmann JV. Pericardial constriction. Am Heart J 1978;97:110–122.
11. Kesteloot H, Denef B. Value of reference tracings in diagnosis and assessment of constrictive epi- and pericarditis. Br Heart J 1970;32:675–682.
12. Appleton CP, Hatle LK, Popp RL. Demonstration of restrictive ventricular physiology by Doppler echocardiography. J Am Coll Cardiol 1988;11:757–768.
13. Oh JK, Hatle LK, Seward JB, Danielson GK, Schaff HV, Reeder GS, Tajik AJ. Diagnostic role of Doppler echocardiography in constrictive pericarditis. J Am Coll Cardiol 1994;23:154–162.

Chapter 24

Hemodynamics of Constrictive Physiology—Section VI:
Hemodynamics of Cardiac Tamponade in a Patient With AIDS-Related Non-Hodgkin's Lymphoma

Elie Azrak, MD, Morton J. Kern, MD, and Richard G. Bach MD

Although cardiac involvement has been commonly described in HIV-infected patients, cardiac tamponade is an unusual feature of AIDS-related non-Hodgkin's lymphoma. We describe an AIDS patient with undiagnosed non-Hodgkin's lymphoma presenting with hemodynamics of pericardial tamponade. *Cathet. Cardiovasc. Diagn. 45:287–291, 1998.*

INTRODUCTION

Since cardiac involvement in HIV was first reported in 1983 by Antran et al. [1], the relatively high prevalence of pericardial disease in AIDS has been commonly described. Although the manifestations of pericardial disease in this patient population include those of asymptomatic effusion, nonspecific or infectious pericarditis, and pericardial tamponade, the finding of pericardial tamponade is an unusual, often unanticipated, yet potentially fatal feature of AIDS-related non-Hodgkin's lymphoma (NHL). The nonspecific nature of the associated symptoms, physical signs, and electrocardiographic and radiographic findings renders the prompt diagnosis of pericardial tamponade in AIDS-related non-Hodgkin's lymphoma (NHL) difficult to establish. A high index of suspicion during evaluation of these patients is particularly appropriate in the presence of poor prognostic features, such as a history of AIDS prior to diagnosis of NHL, a CD4+ count of <200 cells/µl, bone marrow involvement, or a poor performance status.

The diagnosis of pericardial tamponade is usually suggested by classical clinical findings such as hypotension, elevated jugular venous pressure, and clear lungs, along with the presence of pulsus paradoxus exceeding 10 mm Hg. Tamponade physiology is confirmed with noninvasive two-dimensional echocardiography, which would demonstrate pericardial effusion and evidence of right atrial and right ventricular diastolic collapse. On Doppler echocardiography, the presence of exaggerated respiratory variation in mitral and tricuspid inflow velocities exceeding 15% is highly suggestive of the diagnosis.

Although AIDS-related NHL is a systemic disease involving extranodal organs such as the heart, central nervous system, bone marrow, and bowel, the finding of pericardial tamponade as a sentinel sign has only rarely been described.

CASE PRESENTATION

A 52-year-old bisexual man with hepatitis B and AIDS presented to the emergency department with a 1-wk history of progressive dyspnea, chills, night sweats, and increased abdominal girth. His medications on admission included clarithromycin, didanosine, stavudine, nelfinavir, acyclovir, and Septra DS. Six months prior to admission he had had a negative intradermal Purified Protein Derivative (PPD) test.

On physical examination he was dyspneic. Blood pressure was 160/100, pulse 100 beats/min, and respiratory rate 24/min. There was jugular venous pulsation at the angle of the jaw and bilateral submandibular lymphadenopathy. The lungs were clear. The heart sounds were distant, without gallop or rub. There was shifting abdominal dullness and bilateral inguinal lymphadenopathy. The lower extremities were without edema.

The admission electrocardiogram revealed sinus tachycardia and low-voltage QRS. The admission chest radiograph showed cardiomegaly and a possible mediastinal mass. Creatinine was 1.2 mg/dl, total leukocyte count 3,200 cells/µl, and serum LDH 1,532 U/l.

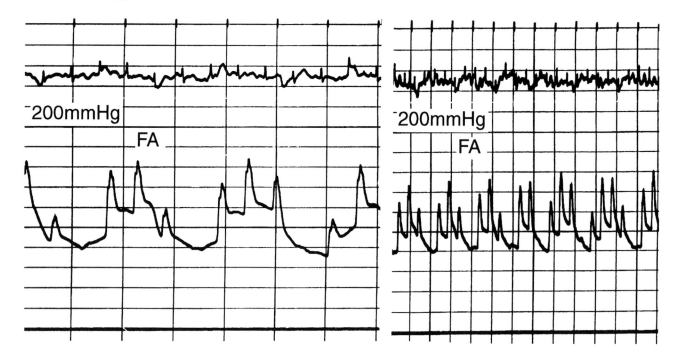

B.C. 53y M

Fig. 1.   Aortic pressure on a 0–200 mm Hg scale, demonstrating marked pulsus paradoxus and obliteration of the aortic pulse during inspiration. Left: Pressure waveform at 25 mm/sec. Right: Pressure waveform at 10 mm/sec. Note the cyclical variation and marked respiratory difference between systolic pressures during the inspiratory cycle.

Computerized tomography of the chest revealed bilateral axillary, mediastinal, deep pelvic, and inguinal adenopathy, a large pericardial effusion, bilateral pleural effusions, and ascites. A transthoracic echocardiogram confirmed the presence of a large pericardial effusion with right atrial and ventricular collapse. There was marked respiratory variation in the aortic and mitral valve velocities.

The patient was taken to the cardiac catheterization laboratory and underwent pericardiocentesis. Initial hemodynamics prior to pericardiocentesis showed that the arterial pressure was 120/80, but was associated with >80 mm Hg pulsus paradoxus, with complete loss of femoral arterial upstroke periodically during inspiration (Fig. 1). Mean right atrial pressure was 40 mm Hg, with striking respiratory variation and obliteration of phasic waveforms (Fig. 2). Pulmonary artery and right ventricular systolic pressures matched peak expiratory right atrial pressure. The mean pulmonary artery wedge, right atrial, and mean intrapericardial pressures were elevated and equal. Right ventricular pressure was 62/20 mm Hg, pulmonary artery pressure 64/40 mm Hg, mean pulmonary artery pressure 48 mm Hg, mean pulmonary capillary wedge pressure 40 mm Hg, mean pericardial pressure 40 mm Hg, and arterial pressure 160/100 mm Hg.

After removal of 420 cc hemorrhagic pericardial fluid, the hemodynamics were repeated, with a decrease in mean right atrial pressure to 22 mm Hg, mean pulmonary artery capillary wedge pressure to 24 mm Hg, pulmonary artery pressure to 58/28 mm Hg, mean pulmonary artery pressure to 38 mm Hg, and mean pericardial pressure to 14–16 mm Hg. Following removal of a total 1,450 ml of pericardial fluid, mean right atrial pressure declined to 22 mm Hg with reinstitution of phasic waveforms and a prominent "Y" descent. Mean intrapericardial pressure was 16 mm Hg, with no evidence of residual pericardial fluid (Fig. 3). After pericardiocentesis, pulsus paradoxus was alleviated, with return of near-normal right ventricular pressure (Fig. 4). The patient tolerated the procedure well.

Pericardial fluid analysis revealed an LDH concentration of 17,760 U/l, and a total leukocyte count of 200 cells/μl. Microscopic examination revealed lymphocytosis without evidence of opportunistic infection, and flow cytometric analysis revealed 76% of cells within the monocyte region expressing a monoclonal B-cell immunophenotype. These data, along with cytomorphological examination, were diagnostic of involvement of the

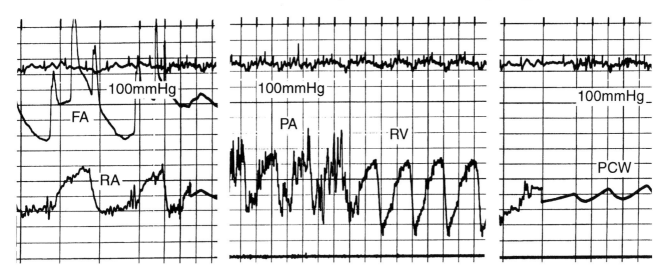

B.C. 53y M

Fig. 2.   Left: Aortic and right atrial pressure on a 0–100 mm Hg scale. Mean right atrial pressure is approximately 40 mm Hg, with obliteration of phasic waveforms of "A" and "V" waves. Note the marked inspiratory and expiratory variation of the right atrial pressure. Middle: Pulmonary artery and right ventricular pressure during catheter pullback, demonstrating the high filling pressures of right ventricular pressure. Right: Mean pulmonary capillary wedge pressure of 40 mm Hg on a 0–100 mm Hg scale.

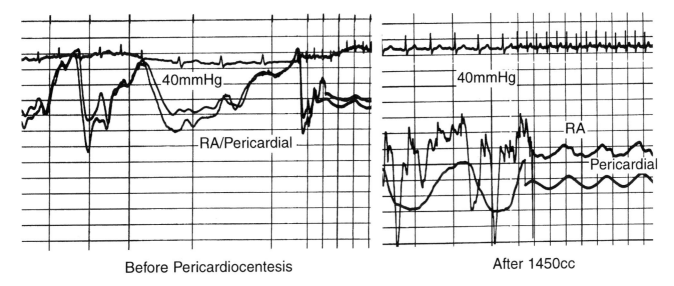

Before Pericardiocentesis   After 1450cc

Fig. 3.   Right atrial and pericardial pressure on a 0–40 mm Hg scale before pericardiocentesis (left) and after pericardiocentesis (right). Note the reduction in right atrial and pericardial pressure with return of some "A" wave, and the phasic nature of the right atrial pressure. Mean right atrial pressure is 22 mm Hg and pericardial pressure 14 mm Hg.

pericardial fluid by malignant lymphoma, non-Hodgkin's, small noncleaved cell (Burkitt's lymphoma).

DISCUSSION

This case demonstrates the finding of pericardial tamponade, an unusual complication of AIDS-related malignant lymphoma, as a sentinel sign for the diagnosis of this entity. Furthermore, the hemodynamic features associated with pericardial tamponade were also remarkable for the severity of pulsus paradoxus and elevated and equilibrated right heart pressures.

Malignant Pericardial Effusions

In patients with cancer, autopsy series reveal that pericardial effusions are present in up to 20% of individu-

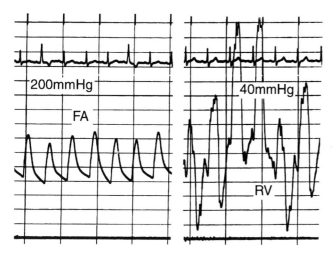

Fig. 4.   Left: Femoral artery pressure after pericardiocentesis. Right: Right ventricular pressure after pericardiocentesis. Note the absence of pulsus paradoxus, the regularization of the arterial pressure waveform, and the return of the right ventricular end-diastolic pressure notch, consistent with right atrial pressure.

als [2,3]. Primary tumors associated with pericardial effusions include lung (40%), breast (23%), lymphoma (11%), and leukemia (5%) [2–6]. Pericardial effusions are malignant in approximately 50% of cases, with nonmalignant causes being secondary to radiation-induced pericarditis and infections [3]. The common presentations of dyspnea, cough, orthopnea, and chest pain are present in approximately 85%, 30%, 25%, and 20% of patients, respectively, with a paradoxic pulse associated with pericardial effusion in 45% of patients also noting tachypnea, tachycardia, hypotension, and peripheral edema. As in the case example, however, cardiac tamponade, requires prompt treatment to eliminate dyspnea, congestion, and hypotension.

Non-Hodgkin's Lymphoma

Burkitt's lymphoma is an unusual subtype of malignant small-cell, noncleaved lymphomas. Burkitt's lymphoma is usually manifest in children, young adults, and immunocompromised patients such as those with HIV. There is a male-to-female predominance, and frequent extranodal involvement has been noted. Bone marrow involvement similar to that in ALL-L3 has been reported. The diffuse lymph node involvement contains a monotonous morphology of cells of uniform size and shape, with scanty cytoplasm. The round or slightly irregular nucleus is laced with coarse chromatin and several nucleoli. Frequent mitotic figures are common. A starry sky appearance under the microscope with scattered macrophages is not a hallmark, but may be observed in other highly proliferative lymphomas. The nomenclature of "Burkitt-like lymphoma" has been suggested for those lymphomas

in which cell size and nuclear morphology are intermediate between large-cell and Burkitt's lymphomas [7,8]. A listing of tumors of the pericardium is provided in Table I and indicates the infrequency of Burkitt's type. General clinical manifestations of cardiac tumors are listed in Table II and demonstrate the wide variety of pathologic involvement of this rare entity.

Therapeutic Approaches

The decision to treat a patient with malignant pericardial effusion is more often based on physiologic and symptomatic parameters rather than on the size or appearance of the pericardial effusion. The standard management of malignant pericardial effusion is ill-defined. Current recommendations derived from small series of patient cases treated prospectively and large retrospective reviews reveal that techniques of pericardial drainage and installation of sclerosing agents (bleomycin, doxycycline, minocycline, or radioisotopes) have had varied results [9,10]. Pericardial windows either surgically or with balloon catheter may permit fluid drainage successfully in many cases. Pericardial stripping is also a therapeutic option. Systemic chemotherapy and radiotherapy to the pericardium have been effective in controlling some malignant pericardial effusions [10]. Catheter drainage of malignant pericardial effusions has been reported to control fluid reaccumulation for more than 30 days in >90% of patients. The sclerosing agents noted above, in a single prospective study of 27 patients comparing doxycycline and bleomycin, demonstrated similar efficacy but shorter hospitalization with bleomycin than with doxycycline [6]. Tetracycline, commonly used for pleural and pericardial effusions, is not commercially available. Surgical or balloon pericardiotomy for malignant pericardial effusions controls the effusion in 85–90% of patients. The advantage of a percutaneous subxyphoid balloon pericardiotomy is the reduction in need for general anesthesia.

Hemodynamics of Pericardial Tamponade

The striking pulsus paradoxus with obliteration of the arterial waveform at end inspiration is rarely observed [11–13]. The "group beating" changing over the respiratory cycle can be appreciated with the arterial pressure recorded at a slower paper speed (Fig. 1, right). The presentation of tamponade-related hypotension was modified by the large respiratory variation, resulting in a mean arterial pressure of approximately 80 mm Hg. The narrow pulse pressure and tachycardia were consistent with a reduced cardiac output of the compromised left ventricle. The marked elevation and equilibration of the right heart pressures were also noteworthy. The right ventricular, pulmonary artery, and systolic pressures were only slightly higher than the expiratory mean right atrial pressure,

TABLE I. Tumors of the Pericardium

Primary		Secondary
Benign	Malignant	
Pericardial (coelomic) cyst (15.49%) (pericardial diverticulum)	Mesothelioma (3.6%) (diffuse type or, rarely, solitary type)	Carcinomas of the lung Carcinomas of the breast
Angiomas (hemangioma, lymphangioma, vascular hamartoma)	Sarcomas (3%): angiosarcoma, fibrosarcoma, other	Malignant melanoma Leukemias
Mesothelioma (solitary type)	Tertoma	Other malignant neoplasms
Heterotopic tissue origin (bronchial cyst, dermoid cyst, teratoma (2.6%), thymoma, thyroid adenoma)		
Miscellaneous: lipoma, fibroma, leiomyoma, neurilemoma, neurofibroma		

TABLE II. General Clinical Manifestations of Cardiac (and Pericardial) Tumors

Pericardial involvement
  Chest pain
  Pericarditis
  Pericardial effusion
  Abnormal cardiac silhouette on chest roentgenogram
  Arrhythmias, usually atrial
  Cardiac compression/constriction
  Cardiac tamponade
Myocardial involvement
  Arrhythmias, ventricular and atrial
  Electrocardiographic changes
  Abnormal cardiac silhouette on chest roentgenogram
    Generalized cardiac enlargement
    Localized cardiac enlargement
  Conduction disturbances and heart block
  Congestive heart failure
  Coronary involvement
    Angina pectoris
    Myocardial infarction
Intracavity tumor
  Cavity obliteration
  Valve obstruction and valve damage
  Embolic phenomena: systemic, neurological, coronary
  Constitutional manifestations

consistent with severe tamponade physiology. The right atrial waveform was also unusual in the dramatic obliteration of its phasic components, a feature which improved on relief of the tamponade. The final right atrial and pericardial pressures remained elevated but separate, despite complete pericardial drainage. These postprocedural hemodynamics are not unusual for effusive-constrictive pericardial effusions [14].

CONCLUSIONS

Patients with HIV may have pericardial involvement presenting as NHL. Clinical signs of cardiac tamponade should prompt rapid evaluation and treatment.

REFERENCES

1. Antran BR, Gorin I, Leibowitch M, Laroche L, Escande JP, Hewitt J, March CL: AIDS in a Haitian woman with cardiac Kaposi's sarcoma and Whipple's disease. Lancet 1:767–768, 1983.
2. Maher EA, Shepherd FA, Todd TJ: Pericardial sclerosis as the primary management of malignant pericardial effusion and cardiac tamponade. J Thorac Cardiovasc Surg 112:637–643, 1996.
3. Pass HI: Malignant pleural and pericardial effusions. In DeVita VT, Hellman S, Rosenberg SA (eds): "Cancer: Principles and Practice of Oncology," 5th ed. Philadelphia: J.B. Lippincott Co., 1997, pp 2586–2598.
4. Wilkes JD, Fidias P, Vaickus L, Perez RP: Malignancy-related pericardial effusion: 127 cases from the Roswell Park Cancer Institute. Cancer 76:1377–1387, 1995.
5. Laham RJ, Cohen DJ, Kuntz RE, Baim DS, Lorell BH, Simons M: Pericardial effusion in patients with cancer: Outcome with contemporary management strategies. Heart 75:67–71, 1996.
6. Liu G, Crump M, Goss PE, Dancey J, Shepherd FA: Prospective comparison of the sclerosing agents doxycycline and bleomycin for the primary management of malignant pericardial effusion and cardiac tamponade. J Clin Oncol 14:3141–3147, 1996.
7. Yano T, van Krieken JH, Magrath IT, Longo DL, Jaffe ES, Raffeld M: Histogenetic correlations between subcategories of small non-cleaved cell lymphomas. Blood 79:1282–1290, 1992.
8. Pavlova Z, Parker JW, Taylor CR, Levine AM, Feinstein DI, Lukes RJ: Small non-cleaved follicular center cell lymphoma: Burkitt's and non-Burkitt's variant in the US. II. Pathologic and immunologic features. Cancer 59:1892–1902, 1987.
9. Lashevsky I, Ben Yosef R, Rinkevich D, Reisner S, Markiewicz W: Intrapericardial minocycline sclerosis for malignant pericardial effusion. Chest 109:1452–1454, 1996.
10. Vaitkus PT, Herrmann HC, LeWinter MM: Treatment of malignant pericardial effusion. JAMA 272:59–64, 1994.
11. Shabetai R, Fowler NO, Fenton JC, Massangkay M: Pulsus paradoxus. J Clin Invest 44:1882—1898, 1965.
12. Reddy PS, Curtiss EI, Uretsky BF: Spectrum of hemodynamic changes in cardiac tamponade. Am J Cardiol 66:1487–1491, 1990.
13. Ramsey HW, Sbar S, Elliott LP, Eliot RS: The differential diagnosis of restrictive myocardiopathy and chronic constrictive pericarditis with calcification: Value of coronary arteriography. Am J Cardiol 25:635–638, 1970.
14. Hancock EW: Subacute effusive-constrictive pericarditis. Circulation 43:183–192, 1971.

PART IV: ARRHYTHMIAS

Cardiac arrhythmias continue to be the major source of obscured and bizarre pressure waveforms. The clinician interpreting pressure waveforms should always be vigilant to the changing electrocardiogram and cardiac rhythm. His attention to the rhythm and alterations often explains the apparent physiologic consequences. Understanding the sequence of chamber activation and its influence on the pressure waveforms is truly of great clinical value and well demonstrated by close scrutiny of the pressure waveforms.

Morton J. Kern, MD

Chapter 25

Cardiac Arrhythmias

Morton J. Kern, MD, Thomas Donohue, MD, Richard Bach, MD, and Frank V. Aguirre, MD

INTRODUCTION

Physiologic pressure waveforms are determined by the underlying cardiac rhythm. Normal sinus rhythm produces the characteristic atrial and ventricular filling patterns, which are further influenced by the cardiac cycle length, chamber compliance, resting circulating volume, and extrinsic factors of pericardial restraint, pulmonary resistance, and ventricular-aorto and ventricular-ventricular interactions [1,2]. Further compounding the interpretation of pressure waves, disturbances of normal impulse conduction will distort or obliterate these waveforms or initiate unique pressure patterns. Some of the most obvious examples of altered hemodynamic pressure patterns occur during cardiac arrhythmias induced during normal pacemaker function, as previously described [3]. Even more unusual rhythms can be observed in patients who are cardiac transplant recipients with the native or donor heart rhythm at times interfering with or, in the case of heterotopic transplantation, potentiating normal pressure waves [4]. This rounds will review several examples of common arrhythmias and associated hemodynamics that can be observed during routine diagnostic or interventional cardiac catheterization procedures.

PREMATURE CONTRACTIONS

The most commonly observed cardiac arrhythmia is a premature ventricular contraction (PVC). A naturally occurring or mechanically (catheter) induced PVC causes a systole which generally ejects a substantially reduced stroke volume, often limiting the arterial pressure pulse and resetting the sinus rhythm with a prolonged, compensatory pause (Fig. 1). The post PVC beat generally is stronger than the normal beat due to both enhanced filling (Frank-Starling mechanism) and an enhanced contractile state. In general, the hemodynamic result of the PVC is of little clinical importance, but may serve a diagnostic purpose in the hemodynamic assessment of hypertrophic cardiomyopathy (recall the Brockenbrough-Braunwald sign) (Fig. 2) [5]. PVCs have also been used to assess contractile reserve and viability of ischemic hypokinetic myocardial segments [6]. In the absence of mechanical stimulation, frequent PVCs may portend serious and life-threatening events, and must be considered a treatable risk factor during diagnostic and therapeutic catheterization laboratory procedures.

Consider the hemodynamics of a 54-year-old woman with a rumbling apical systolic murmur (Fig. 3). Simultaneous left ventricular and pulmonary capillary wedge pressures were measured with fluid-filled catheters. The pulmonary capillary wedge tracing demonstrated large V waves, consistent with clinically significant mitral regurgitation. Intermittent PVCs produce characteristic changes in the magnitude of both the left ventricular pressure and V wave. The systolic left ventricular pressure of one sinus beat (#2) is 146 mm Hg with a large V wave (60 mm Hg). The PVC (beat #3) has a left ventricular systolic pressure of 120 mm Hg with a smaller (<40 mm Hg) and delayed V wave. Note also that the V wave peak falls outside the left ventricular downstroke. The post PVC beat (#4) systole is augmented (152 mm Hg) with a V wave of 44 mm Hg. Of interest is the timing of the PVCs in this example. These beats are late-cycle escape-type PVCs. The speed of the recording

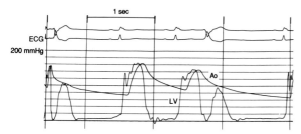

Fig. 1.   Left ventricular (LV) and aortic (Ao) pressures during a premature ventricular contraction. Note the minimal change in aortic pressure and large post-PVC arterial pressure.

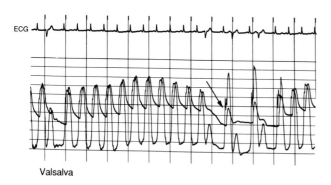

Valsalva

Fig. 2.   Premature ventricular contraction (arrow) in a patient with hypertrophic cardiomyopathy. Note post-PVC reduction of pulse pressure.

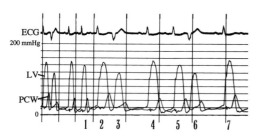

Fig. 3.   Left ventricular (LV) and pulmonary capillary wedge pressure (PCW) in a patient with mitral regurgitation. Left ventricular pressures vary with the cardiac rhythm. Why is the V wave larger on beat #2? See text for details.

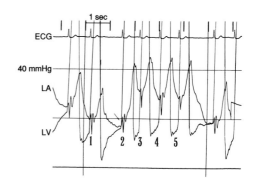

Fig. 4.   Left atrial (LA) and left ventricular (LV) pressures in a patient with an irregular rhythm. Identify A, C, and V waves. See text for details.

changes from 10 mm/sec to 25 mm/sec, but the rhythm and associated pressures demonstrate features of grouped beats. The PR interval prolongs with a regular frequency followed by a pause with a PVC. Mobitz type I (Wenckebach) rhythm is present with period 3:2 and 4:3 beats. The P wave without its QRS is likely to be obscured by the late PVC. The influence of a longer ventricular filling period during the sinus arrhythmia (between beats #1 and 2) may account for the larger V wave.

IRREGULAR RHYTHMS

PVCs are often characterized by compensatory pauses and distorted QRS complexes. However, the QRS complex may not be easily distinguishable from a normal beat on physiologic monitors with reduced or poor quality electrocardiographic waveforms due to loose electrocardiographic leads. This fact often requires scrutiny of the pressure waves when the electrocardiographic artifacts cause loss of the audible beep of the regular rhythm. This audible rhythm is important to appreciate, especially at the beginning of a procedure during catheter and sheath placement. The changing, slowing audible beeps may be the only warning or evidence of a vagal reaction. Early treatment with atropine (0.6 mg intravenous) can save time and extra procedures (e.g. temporary pacemaker, leg raising, etc.)

Because the electrocardiographic monitor complex is not always detailed enough to see each part of the entire PQRST complex, interpretation of the rhythm can be difficult. Examine the hemodynamic left atrial and left ventricular waveforms obtained in a 39-year-old woman with mixed mitral stenosis and regurgitation (Fig. 4). Left atrial pressure was obtained by the transseptal technique prior to consideration of mitral valvuloplasty. The rhythm is irregularly irregular without grouped beats, and no P waves are evident on the electrocardiographic tracing and no A waves on left ventricular and left atrial pressures. The absence of an A wave is especially evident on beat #2 with a long pause before the next systole. This rhythm is obviously atrial fibrillation and demonstrates that equilibration of left atrial-left ventricular pressure occurs with long cardiac cycles (>900 msec). A run of short RR cycles, shown on beats #3–5, is associated with a substantial left atrial-left ventricular gradient, resulting in the appearance of symptoms during periods of tachycardia (e.g., exercise). With proper heart rate control, valve repair or valvuloplasty may be delayed.

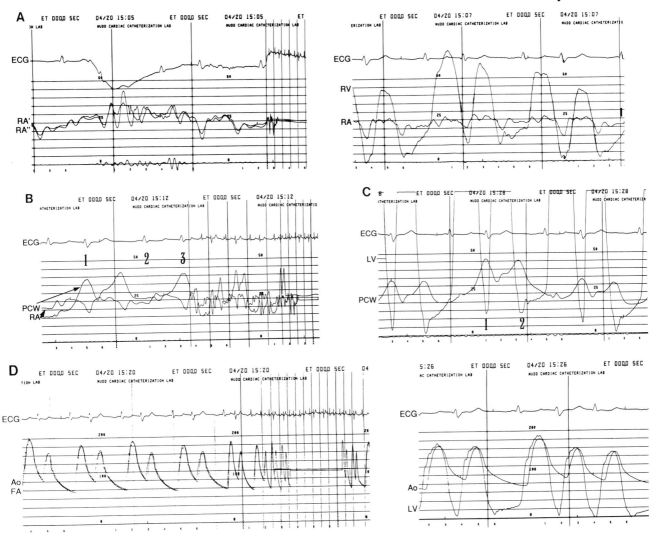

Fig. 5. A: Left panel: Simultaneous 2-catheter measurement of right (RA′, RA″) pressure in preparation to assess tricuspid stenosis. Pressures match during the irregular rhythm. Right panel: Right ventricular (RV) and right atrial (RA) pressures in the same patient. Note grouped beating of right ventricular pressure. The magnitude of pressures varies due to respiratory activity. See text for details. B: Simultaneous pulmonary capillary wedge (PCW) and right atrial (RA) pressures. Note that the right atrial waveform has X and Y descents with smaller A and V waves. Does the pulmonary capillary wedge pressure wave- form have large A and V waves? C: Left ventricular (LV) and pulmonary capillary wedge (PCW) pressures (0–50 mm Hg scale) demonstrating a coupled rhythm. Note the bigeminal pat- tern with V waves and no A waves. See text for details. D: Left: Femoral (FA) and central aortic (Ao) pressures (0–200 mm Hg scale) demonstrating coupled beats during the bigeminal rhythm. Right: The rhythm is atrial fibrillation with periods of coupled beats. LV = left ventricular pressure. See text for de- tails.

MISLEADING ATRIAL WAVEFORMS DURING ARRHYTHMIAS

A 53-year-old woman presented with increasing dys- pnea 6 years after tricuspid and mitral valve replace- ments. She had a childhood history of rheumatic fever. Consider the right heart hemodynamics with attention to the cardiac rhythm (Fig. 5A). Because of suspected tri- cuspid stenosis, one catheter was positioned in the right atrium and one in the right ventricle to measure the gra- dient. Before crossing the tricuspid valve, the pressures

from both catheters were matched to verify the equiva- lency of the transducers (Fig. 5A, left panel). The matched and elevated right atrial pressures show attenu- ation of the normal A and V waves. The right ventricu- lar-right atrial tracing demonstrates significant tricuspid stenosis with an irregular rhythm and grouped beats with systolic pressures varying with respiration (Fig. 5A, right panel). The pulmonary capillary wedge and right atrial pressures are displayed at 50 mm/sec paper speed, with the pulmonary capillary wedge pressure showing a

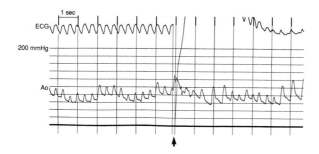

Fig. 6. Wide complex QRS tachycardia with mild arterial hypotension. Note the pattern changes at the arrow. See text for details.

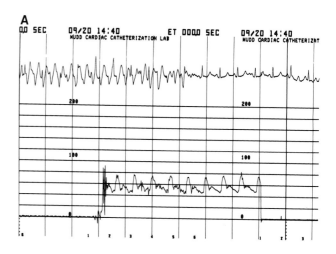

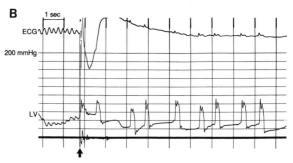

Fig. 7. A: Electrocardiogram showing ventricular fibrillation with preserved arterial pressure? B: Electrocardiogram showing ventricular fibrillation with gradual restoration of a sinus mechanism after electrocardioversion. See text for details.

distinct A and V wave (Fig. 5B, beat #1). The electrocardiographic complex has a first-degree AV block with a presumed PR interval of nearly 50% of the RR interval. Consider beat #2. No such A and V waves are present. The QRS is different with a short PR interval. Note that the right atrial pressure on beat #1 does not show the same striking A or V waves of the pulmonary capillary wedge pressure but has a distinct X and Y descent (X>Y). This pattern repeats itself over the remaining beats.

Further clarification of these findings occurs on examination of the left ventricular-pulmonary capillary wedge pressure tracings (Fig. 5C). The paired beats are now more clearly displayed with an abbreviated left ventricular diastolic period (beat #1) and a coupled beat with a longer filling period (beat #2). Beat #1 can now be easily identified as a PVC and beat #2 as a junctional beat (no A wave). The biphasic waveform previously assumed to be A and V waves on the right atrial-pulmonary capillary wedge tracings (Fig. 5B) can now be seen to be a V wave of an ectopic ventricular beat with the coupled V wave of the underlying predominant junctional beat. No A wave is present either on the left ventricular or pulmonary capillary wedge tracings. This rhythm is then a junctional rhythm with ventricular bigeminy. The patient was receiving digoxin for atrial fibrillation and had developed transient periods of a regular rhythm with coupled beats. Arterial and left ventricular pressures (Fig. 5D) clearly demonstrate the predominate patterns of this rhythm. This case is an example of how reliance on pressure waves of the pulmonary capillary wedge alone (or any single pressure) may be confusing, resulting in a misinterpretation of the cardiac events.

RHYTHM WITH WIDE QRS PATTERNS

Many patients undergoing cardiac catheterization have abnormal electrocardiographic complexes from prior myocardial infarction, bundle branch block or left ven-

tricular hypertrophy. Wide QRS complexes can also be generated by unusual lead placement in some situations. The most important features to observe with wide complex rhythms are the heart rate and arterial pressure. Consider the rhythm and arterial pressure obtained in a 64-year-old man during diagnostic evaluation for coronary artery disease. On entry into the laboratory, his pressure was 135/70 mm Hg, with a rate of 95 beats/min and a wide complex upright QRS. A wider QRS complex and faster heart rate developed before left ventricular catheter placement (Fig. 6, left side). Arterial pressure was maintained fluctuating with respirations around 90/72 mm Hg. Is this a satisfactory situation? Because of the increased heart rate (>130 beats/min) with the QRS change and the decrease of arterial pressure, the rhythm diagnosed as ventricular tachycardia was immediately treated. Since no right or left ventricular catheters were in place to stimulate a PVC, which can occasionally be useful in breaking a ventricular tachycardia, cardioversion with 50 joules was performed with restoration of a sinus rhythm in 5 sec (Fig. 6, far right side). The baseline upright QRS returned, producing an arterial pressure of 120/70 mm Hg (Fig. 6, last beat). This patient had a prior

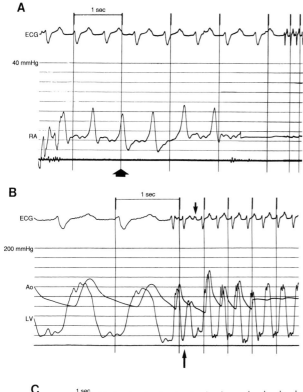

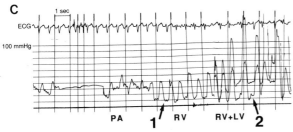

Fig. 8. A: Right atrial (RA) pressure with wide complex QRS rhythm. Are the sharp peaks (arrow) V waves? See text for details. B: Simultaneous left ventricular (LV) and aortic (Ao) pressures. A PVC (bottom arrow) produces a change in the electrocardiogram to reveal a P wave (top arrow). C: Right heart catheter pullback from pulmonary artery (PA) to right ventricle (RV) and then simultaneous left ventricle (LV) to right ventricle (0–100 mm Hg scale). Note the rhythm change after right ventricular beat #1.

myocardial infarction with syncope due to recurrent ventricular tachycardia and was undergoing diagnostic study prior to electrophysiologic evaluation and treatment.

Occasionally an electrocardiographic tracing will look like ventricular fibrillation due to patient movement or a loose lead. Immediately check the patient, "Are you okay, Mr. Jones?" and the pressure (Fig. 7A). In some patients it may be artifact, in others this may be real (Fig. 7B). Treatment of ventricular fibrillation may be delayed if the operator is not monitoring arterial pressure and assuming the electrocardiographic changes to be an artifact.

Wide complex QRS rhythms also include accelerated junctional rhythms with or without atrial dissociation. Examine the right atrial pressure in a 65-year-old man with dyspnea and coronary artery disease (Fig. 8A). The rhythm is regular. The peaked waves occur at the T-wave downstroke (arrow). Are these sharp V waves? Review the rhythm again. A P wave may be conducted retrograde to generate a notched T wave and a cannon A wave. Another clue to this rhythm is the response to a PVC. Figure 8B shows the left ventricular and aortic pressures during a PVC (bottom arrow), which separates the P wave from the QRST complex (top arrow). This rhythm was also exposed as a junctional rhythm during right heart catheter pullback, which produced a transient right bundle branch block and separated the P waves, demonstrating a brief period of sinus rhythm. Of interest, the right and left ventricular A waves also reflect the changing rhythm, with retrograde P waves contributing notching to right ventricular filling. Compare right ventricular beat #1 to right ventricular beat #3 (Fig. 8C) and the diastolic portion of the left ventricular beat #2 (Fig. 8C) with that on Fig. 8B.

SUMMARY

Various arrhythmias can produce distorted pressure waveforms, which may be confused with benign physiologic events. Delay in the management of serious arrhythmias can be avoided by vigilant monitoring of systemic pressures.

ACKNOWLEDGMENT

This authors wish to thank the J.G. Mudd Cardiac Catheterization Laboratory team and Donna Sander for manuscript preparation.

REFERENCES

1. Meisner JS, McQueen DM, Ishida Y, Vetter HO, Bortolotti U, Strom JA, Peskin CS, Yellin El: Effects of timing of atrial systole on ventricular filling and mitral valve closure: computer and dog studies. Am J Physiol 249 (Heart Circ Physiol):H604–H619, 1985.
2. O'Rourke MF: Pressure and flow waves in systemic arteries and the anatomical design of the arterial system. J Appl Physiol 23:139–149, 1967.
3. Kern MJ, Deligonul U: Hemodynamic rounds: interpretation of cardiac pathophysiology from pressure waveform analysis. Pacemaker hemodynamics. Cathet Cardiovasc Diagn 24:22–27, 1991.
4. Kern MJ, Deligonul U, Miller L: Hemodynamic rounds: interpretation of cardiac pathophysiology from pressure waveform analysis. IV. Extra hearts: Part I. Cathet Cardiovasc Diagn 22:197–201, 1990.
5. Brockenbrough EC, Braunwald E, Morrow AG: A hemodynamic technique for the detection of hypertrophic subaortic stenosis. Circulation 23:189–194, 1961.

6. Popio KA, Gorlin R, Bechtel DJ, Levine JA: Post-extrasystolic potentiation as a predictor of potential myocardial viability: preoperative analyses compared with studies after coronary bypass surgery. Am J Cardiol 39:944, 1977.

Chapter 26

Pacemaker Hemodynamics

Morton J. Kern, MD, and Ubeydullah Deligonul, MD

INTRODUCTION

Many patients coming into the cardiac catheterization laboratory will have temporary or permanent pacemakers implanted for myocardial diseases related to conduction disturbances. The normal timing of physiologic events is disturbed with corresponding abnormalities in pressure waveforms. The hemodynamic consequences of sequential atrial ventricular contraction is of interesting and often clinical importance relative to the generation of regurgitant waves, arterial pressure and optimal left ventricular filling. As will be seen, the influence of atrial systole principally influences, through the Frank-Starling mechanism [1], the end diastolic pressure-volume relationship of both the right and left ventricles. The hemodynamic tracings presented in this "Rounds" will illustrate several altered sequences of atrial-ventricular activation and their hemodynamic consequences.

CASE PRESENTATION AND DISCUSSION
Atrial Waves During Pacemaker Activity

A 63-yr-old woman had a pacemaker implanted for syncope and heart failure 2 yrs prior to the onset of vague atypical chest pains with increasing dyspnea. Right and left heart cardiac catheterization was performed using fluid-filled catheters. Right atrial pressure was recorded during a period of pacemaker activity (Fig. 1). Examine the rhythm and waveforms of right atrial pressure. Two waveforms are evident. On the left panel of Figure 1, atrial pacing is not present. Ventricular activation without associated atrial pacing produces indistinct wave-

forms which may be confused with artifact and offer no organized transport of atrial blood to the right ventricle. On the right panel of Figure 1, AV sequential pacing generates distinct A waves (the smaller wave is the V wave) which augment atrial transport and increase right ventricular performance [2–4]. The mean pressure of both atrial wave patterns is equal. In this patient, the right heart filling pressures were low and tricuspid regurgitation or right ventricular volume overload were not considered important. In the same study, the pulmonary capillary wedge pressure was obtained with a balloon flotation pulmonary artery catheter (Fig. 2). The pacemaker spike artifact on the electrocardiographic signal shows only ventricular activation. Explain how the distinct and equivalent A and V waves of pulmonary capillary wedge pressures are produced. The A–V sequential pacemaker with leads placed in the right atrial appendage and right ventricular apex senses P waves to suppress atrial pacing. Although atrial activity is not registering on the electrocardiographic tracing, a P wave is occurring, possibly from only the left atrium and produces a hemodynamic A wave without an electrical P wave or atrial spike seen on the electrocardiogram. This example serves to illustrate that although the pacemaker activity may *appear* to be functioning in only one mode, non-recorded atrial contraction can be detected on the hemodynamic tracings.

A more common abnormality of right atrial pressure would be that of dyssynchronous atrial activity producing atrial contraction against a closed mitral valve. In a patient with mild aortic stenosis, a pacemaker was implanted for lightheadedness and transient sinus arrest (Fig. 3). The right atrial pressure of this patient during a

197

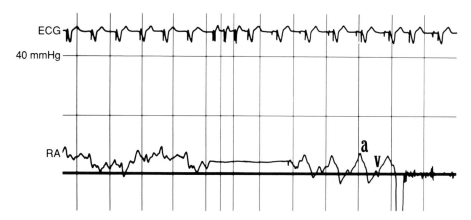

Fig. 1. Right atrial (RA) pressure in a patient with A-V sequential pacing (0–40 mm Hg scale). See text for details.

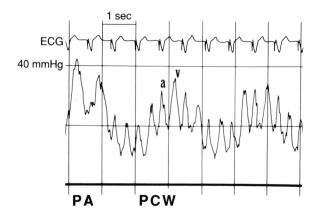

Fig. 2. Pulmonary capillary wedge (PCW) and pulmonary artery (PA) pressure tracings (0–40 mm Hg scale) in a patient with pacemaker for heart block. See text for details.

paced and sinus rhythm readily demonstrates an alteration in the right atrial pressure waveform. Large cannon waves (in the beats preceding the asterisk) show the effect of late or retrograde atrial contraction occurring after ventricular pacing. When the patient moves into sinus rhythm, the pressure waveform changes to a normal A and V wave configuration with the corresponding normal X and Y descents. Although the cannon waves are of no significance, the loss of atrial contraction to ventricular filling in this patient was important (see below Fig. 7).

Dissociated Atrial Activity and Hemodynamic Function

Pacemakers of a single pacing mode (e.g., VVI) often are associated with dyssynchronous atrial activity which may produce unusual hemodynamic findings. The influence of dissociated atrial contraction on the ventricular filling function is readily apparent when examining the pressure data collected from a 52-yr-old woman with a

pacemaker inserted for complete heart block. The VVI (ventricular sensed, paced, and inhibited) mode pacemaker was functioning normally. Right and left ventricular and pulmonary capillary wedge pressures were measured with fluid-filled catheters in a routine fashion (Figs. 4, 5). The hemodynamic results of atrial contraction can be readily seen on beat #1 (Fig. 4) as a large and early A wave on the left, as well as right ventricular pressure tracings. Note that the right ventricular pressure, normally enclosed entirely within the left ventricular pressure outline, has an earlier and more rapid upstroke than on the following beat #2 without an atrial contribution to ventricular filling. Peak right ventricular (and left ventricular) pressures are higher when atrial systole is appropriately timed. Compare peak right ventricular systolic pressure on beats #1 and #4 with beats #2 and #3. Also, a difference in the compliance (the pressure-volume relationship) of the two ventricular chambers can be appreciated on beat #2 by comparing the upslope of the diastolic pressures. The left ventricular diastolic pressure slope is steep. The right ventricular diastolic pressure slope is horizontal with slowed filling in the absence of the atrial contribution. The dissociated atrial activity influences ventricular filling pressures dependent on its timing relative to ventricular ejection. An optimal P-Q interval for ventricular function in experimental animal preparations of complete heart block was 85 to 125 msec [3]. Very early atrial activity with pressure wave deformity can be seen on beat #3 (Fig. 4) demonstrated by the notch in the early diastolic period of the right ventricular pressure tracing. Compare right and left ventricular minimal diastolic pressure waveforms. The P wave is located in the T wave and not readily appreciated on the electrocardiogram. Beat #4 shows atrial activity superimposed on the T wave, but has less of an effect on right and left ventricular pressures. However, the diastolic filling pattern of both ventricles show the effect of early atrial contraction with a continued rise

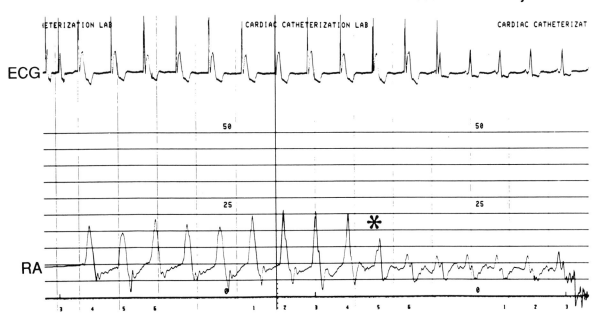

Fig. 3. Right atrial (RA) pressure in a patient with aortic stenosis and a pacemaker. Asterisk indicates a change in rhythm. See text for details.

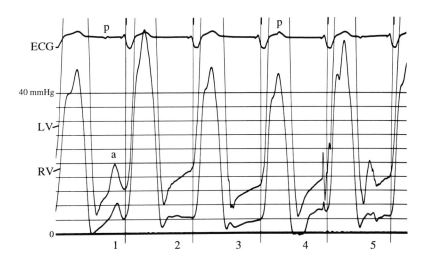

Fig. 4. Right (RV) and left ventricular (LV) pressures (0–40 mm Hg scale) demonstrating the influence of atrial activity on left ventricular filling. See text for details.

in diastolic pressure and larger peak systolic pressure (beats #1 and #4). The P wave activity in beat #4 occurs earlier than in beat #5 with the pressure pattern repeating. This example demonstrates 2 points: the importance of atrial filling to ventricular pressure and differences in ventricular filling pattern between the 2 ventricles. These findings have been extensively studied and were confirmed in both experimental and clinical studies over 2 decades ago [4, 5].

A similar lesson can be obtained from the simultaneous left ventricular and pulmonary capillary wedge pressures (Fig. 5) in the patient described above. The

atrial and ventricular pacing activity are dyssynchronous. In beat #3 (Fig. 5), the P wave produces an atrial contraction occurring earlier in left ventricular diastole. The corresponding A wave on the pulmonary capillary wedge pressure is blunted and the V wave following the paced beat is large. In the next beat #4, the A wave occurs in normal sequential timing, the pulmonary capillary wedge A wave is small and the V wave is somewhat attenuated. The shape of the V wave downslope is more rapid than the preceding V wave. Does the A wave occurring in beat #3 occur early enough to account for the reduced height of the V wave relative to the following beats in

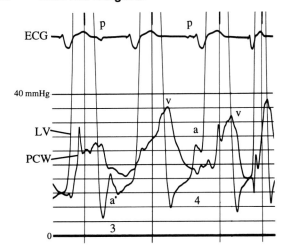

Fig. 5. Left ventricular (LV) and pulmonary capillary wedge (PCW) pressures (0–40 mm Hg scale) demonstrating the influence of atrial activity on pulmonary capillary wedge waveforms. See text for details.

which a more normal A-V synchrony is obtained? This question is difficult to answer from this tracing alone. An A wave superimposed on a V wave should generally increase not decrease the V wave size. Why this V wave is altered may be due to artifact.

Normal and Paced Atrial Systoles and Left Ventricular Pressure

AV sequential pacing usually produces effective atrial contractions. Simultaneous right and left ventricular pressures were measured during A-V sequential pacing (Fig. 6). However, normal atrial systole remains a more effective mechanism for augmenting left ventricular filling. Examine the rhythm and corresponding left ventricular pressure. Atrial pacing is inhibited in beat #1. The

left ventricular A wave is normal. On beats #2 and #3, the AV sequential pacing spikes can be observed with only minimal alteration in the left ventricular end diastolic pressure (arrow) upstroke. The atrial contraction in beat #3 produces more of a deformation of the left ventricular end diastolic pressure which, as the timing of normal atrial sysole supervenes (in beats #4 and #5), is even more pronounced. The normal P wave may not be well seen on the electrocardiogram during cardiac catheterization and the physiology of active atrial contraction only appreciated by noting alteration of the diastolic left ventricular pressure waveform. Two other features are of interest. First the atrial contraction does not produce the A wave on this right ventricular pressure tracing; the left ventricular compliance is usually different from the right ventricle. Compare the effect of atrial contraction on a stiffer right ventricle (see Fig. 4). The second finding of note is the artifact of distorted right ventricular pressure on beat #1 and last 40 msec of systole on beat #2. Right ventricular pressure is superimposed on the left ventricular pressure downslope. In beat #1, the sharp cutoff of systole indicates a non-physiologic artifact of the catheter tip touching the ventricular septum transiently blocking pressure transmission and producing an artifical matching of the left ventricular pressure decline. The normal right ventricular pressure pattern of right bundle branch block conduction includes only a slight delay of right ventricular pressure increase, but the decline should be within the left ventricular pressure decline.

Clinical Significance of Ventricular Pacemaker Hemodynamics

The clinical importance of pacemaker function is related to the ventricular compliance and need for the atrial contribution to filling. Normal sequential atrial-ventric-

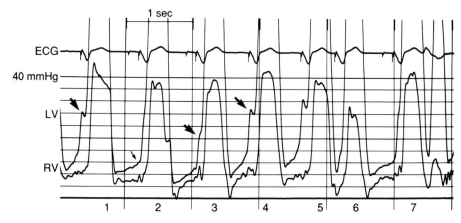

Fig. 6. Right (RV) and left ventricular (LV) pressures (0–40 mm Hg scale). A-V sequential pacing is occurring at variable times during this hemodynamic tracing. Why is the right ventricular morphology in beat #1 different from beats #3–5? See text for details.

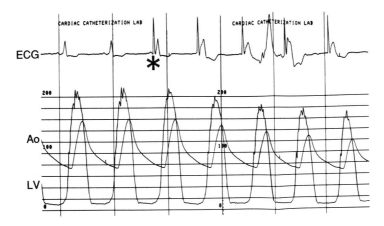

Fig. 7. Left ventricular (LV) and aortic (Ao) pressures in a patient with aortic stenosis with pacemaker. Asterisk indicates onset of pacemaker activity. See text for details.

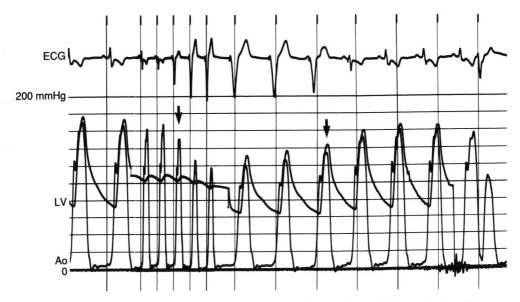

Fig. 8. Left ventricular (LV) and aortic (Ao) pressures in a patient with hypertension. Pacemaker onset is shown by the first arrow and return of sinus rhythm shown after the second arrow. Note the decline in systemic pressure. See text for details.

ular contraction is particularly important in patients with noncompliant left ventricles. In some patients, loss of atrial contraction has a dramatic influence on the systemic pressure and cardiac output [4, 5].

A 78-yr-old man had a VVI pacemaker placed for episodic third heart block with near syncope. Non-invasive evaluation suggested mild aortic stenosis. Because of persistent fatigue and vague periods of lighheadedness, hemodynamic evaluation was requested. Left ventricular and femoral artery pressures (matched with central aortic pressure) were recorded during a change in the cardiac rhythm (Fig. 7). The left ventricular-aortic gradient (200 mm Hg–160 mm Hg) was maintained while both systolic pressures fell after the pacing began (left

ventricular-aortic pressures, 140–100 mmHg). The decline in pressure during ventricular pacing produced mild symptoms while recumbent. It is interesting to note no change in aortic valve gradient, but a lower cardiac output due to reduced stroke volume (without the atrial contribution to filling) would yield a smaller calculated valve area. The low left ventricular compliance and abnormal relaxation is also suggested by the flat or slightly declining left ventricular diastolic pressure during left ventricular filling. This pattern has been associated with incomplete left ventricular relaxation as may occur in patients with hypertrophic cardiomyopathy. A similar example of the contribution of atrial filling to systemic pressure is also shown in Figure 8 without aortic stenosis. Both of these patients became asymptomatic with A-V sequential pacing.

As noted by Benchimol et al. [4], in patients with normal hearts, atrial and ventricular pacing results in nearly identical changes in cardiac output, stroke volume, systemic pressure, ventricular power, and stroke power at any given pacing rate. The contribution of atrial systole to cardiac function in normal man is small or relatively unimportant. Furthermore, in impaired ventricles, at any given rate of cardiac pacing, cardiac output, systemic pressure, ventricular power, stroke work, and systolic ejection rate are significantly higher with atrial pacing than ventricular pacing. These classic observations of over 2 decades ago are still applicable and evident in hemodynamics obtained in daily practice.

SUMMARY

The abnormal sequence of A-V contraction produces alteration of right and left heart hemodynamics reflecting the inappropriate timing of atrial contraction to ventricular filling. Some symptomatic patients may require A-V sequential pacing to improve cardiac output. The clinical effects of the atrial contribution to left ventricular func-

tion can be demonstrated by careful review of hemodynamic tracings in these individuals.

ACKNOWLEDGMENTS

The authors wish to thank the J.G. Mudd Cardiac Catheterization Team and Donna Sander for manuscript preparation.

REFERENCES

1. Linderer T, Chatterjee K, Parmley WW, Sievers RE, Glantz SA, Tyberg JV. Influence of atrial systole on the Frank-Starling relation and the end-diastolic pressure-diameter relation of the left ventricle. Circulation 67:1045–1053, 1983.
2. Samet P, Castillo C, Bernstein WH. Studies in P wave synchronization. Am J Cardiol 19:207–212, 1967.
3. Brockman SK, Manlove A. Cardiodynamics of complete heart block. Am J Cardiol 16:72–83, 1965.
4. Benchimol A, Ellis JG, Dimond EG. Hemodynamic consequences of atrial and ventricular pacing in patients with normal and abnormal hearts. Am J Med 39:911–922, 1965.
5. Samet P, Castillo C, Bernstein WH. Hemodynamic consequences of sequential atrioventricular pacing: Subjects with normal hearts. Am J Cardiol 21:207–212, 1968.

PART V: HYPERTROPHIC OBSTRUCTIVE CARDIOMYOPATHY

The treatment of hypertrophic obstructive cardiomyopathy (HOCM) in symptomatic patients despite maximal medication evolves to implantation of a DDD pacemaker, surgical myectomy, or most recently, alcohol-induced septal myocardial infarction producing a "medical" myomectomy in these individuals. New case studies in this section are illustrative. The classical hemodynamics of HOCM dramatically demonstrate the abnormal arterial waveforms and intra-ventricular gradients and the restoration to near normal pressures after alcohol-induced infarction of the hypertrophied septum. The hemodynamic findings of DDD pacing and alcohol septal infarction are detailed in Chapters 19 and 20. The understanding of the pressure waveforms of the HOCM patient is even more important now that novel therapeutic approaches are readily available.

Morton J. Kern, MD

Chapter 27

Intraventricular Pressure Gradients

Morton J. Kern, MD, and Ubeydullah Deligonul, MD

INTRODUCTION

Among the most interesting and unusual hemodynamic findings encountered in the cardiac catheterization laboratory are those of intraventricular pressure gradients, most commonly due to hypertrophic cardiomyopathy [1–3]. The following case examples will illustrate several important features of pressure measurements for the diagnosis of hypertrophic cardiomyopathy with or without resting intraventricular gradients.

DISAPPEARING AORTIC STENOSIS

A 44-year-old woman is admitted with episodic shortness of breath and loud systolic murmur thought to be aortic stenosis by her physician. There were occasional episodes of palpitations. Electrocardiogram revealed left ventricular hypertrophy. Chest x-ray was normal. Physical examination demonstrated a loud systolic murmur at rest. The echocardiogram demonstrated hypertrophy of the left ventricle and wide aortic valve excursion. Cardiac catheterization was performed for the non-invasive findings of aortic stenosis. With the aid of fluid-filled catheters, aortic (7 French pigtail catheter) and peripheral arterial (8 French sheath) simultaneous pressures were matched prior to crossing the aortic valve. Immediately after crossing the aortic valve, a large pressure gradient between the left ventricle and aorta was seen (Fig. 1). As the pigtail catheter was repositioned, the aortic-left ventricular gradient disappeared. On pullback of the pigtail catheter from the left ventricular apex, the intraventricular gradient is abolished (beats 5 and 6) and can be seen to reappear on slight advancement of the

catheter (beats 7 and 8) and is again fully absent when the catheter is moved to a more proximal left ventricular position (beats 9 and 10). The left ventricular-aortic gradient is due entirely to a gradient produced below the aortic valve within the deeper portion of the ventricle. Several features clearly distinguish this tracing from that of aortic stenosis. The most obvious finding is the loss of aortic-left ventricular gradient on catheter repositioning with the ventricle while still beneath the aortic valve, locating the gradient as truly subvalvular. Secondly, the upstroke of aortic pressure is nearly vertical with a very early peak. Compare this waveform and that of Figure 2 to the late and slow upstroke in aortic stenosis (Fig. 3). In hypertrophic myopathy the largest left ventricular-aortic pressure gradient occurs in mid systole; whereas in aortic stenosis, the largest gradient usually occurs in early systole. Other more subtle differences between valvular and subvalvular gradients, such as timing changes of left ventricular volume, velocity of left ventricular flow and characteristic aortic pressure waves are illustrated on Figures 3 and 4.

METHODS TO PROVOKE INTRACAVITARY PRESSURE DIFFERENCES

Three mechanisms augment intraventricular gradients: 1) decreasing ventricular end diastolic volume (i.e., lowering left atrial filling or reducing length of diastole [4]); 2) increasing force or duration of ventricular contraction; and 3) decreasing aortic outflow resistance. Whether these intraventricular gradients represent true flow obstruction has been the source of considerable controversy [5,6]. In human studies when no resting gradients are evident, use of isoproterenol infusions to produce hyper-

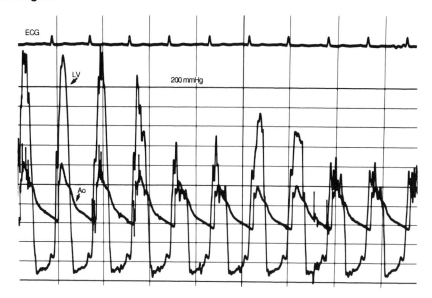

Fig. 1. Simultaneous left ventricular (LV) and aortic (Ao) pressures (200 mm Hg scale) in a patient with "disappearing aortic stenosis." See text for details.

contractile state has been proposed and applied by White et al. [4].

Four common maneuvers have been employed in the catheterization laboratory. The use of the Valsalva maneuver, nitroglycerin, and post-extra-systolic potentiation [1,6] or isoproterenol infusion [4].

A 72-year-old man presented with a history of increasing fatigue, vague chest pain, and mild shortness of breath. Electrocardiogram revealed mild left ventricular hypertrophy. There was an occasional and intermittent systolic ejection-type murmur. Echocardiogram revealed a hypertrophied left ventricle without marked resting aortic outflow tract gradient. Fluid-filled catheters were used to measure left ventricular and simultaneous aortic pressures (the aortic pressure is matched to the femoral artery pressure, Fig. 2). No left ventricular-aortic gradient was initially observed, but during bigeminy on the post-extra-systolic beat, a marked systolic gradient occurred. A diminution in the aortic pulse pressure on the beat following the extra-systolic beat is a common, if not hallmark, finding of hypertrophic cardiomyopathy (Brockenbrough-Braunwald sign) [1]. When the patient returns to normal sinus rhythm (right side of the tracing), the intraventricular gradient is no longer evident. Provoking the intraventricular gradient with extra-systolic beats may be the only evidence of obstructive hypertrophic myopathy in some patients.

Brockenbrough, Braunwald, and Morrow first described hemodynamic characteristics of patients with hypertrophic cardiomyopathies in 1961 [1], revealing striking differences between valvular aortic stenosis and discrete subvalvular stenosis (shown in Fig. 3 and 4). In patients with aortic stenosis, an increase in arterial pulse pressure accompanies a rise in peak left ventricular systolic pressure following premature ventricular contractions. In contrast, in patients with hypertrophic subaortic stenosis, premature ventricular contractions are followed by narrowing of the arterial pulse pressure in association with increasing left ventricular systolic pressure, the Brockenbrough-Braunwald sign. A characteristic change in left ventricular-aortic gradient with an alteration of the aortic pressure contour reflect early forceful left ventricular ejection (spike and dome pattern) is commonly seen during the Valsalva maneuver in these patients.

Although failure of the pulse pressure to increase in the post premature beat is often characteristic of hypertrophic cardiomyopathy, left ventricular ejection time may be a more sensitive and more specific finding [2].

PRELOAD ALTERATIONS AND INTRAVENTRICULAR GRADIENTS

A 47-year-old woman was admitted with a recent history of increasing dyspnea. Left ventricular hypertrophy was documented by electrocardiography and echocardiography. No outflow tract flow disturbances were identified on Doppler echocardiogram. Simultaneous aortic and left ventricular pressures were obtained with a fluid-filled catheters (Fig. 5). A premature ventricular contraction also showed no gradient. To produce an intraventricular gradient, alteration of preload with several maneuvers was performed. During the Valsalva maneuver with the left ventricular diastolic pressure increasing with increasing intrathoracic pressure (after beat 7), the

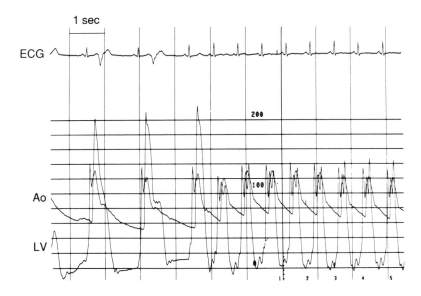

Fig. 2. Simultaneous aortic (Ao) and left ventricular (LV) pressures (200 mm Hg scale). Note the influence of premature ventricular contractions. See text for details.

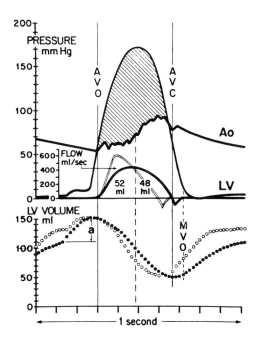

Fig. 3. Hemodynamic examples of a patient with discrete obstructive gradient with aortic stenosis. Ao = aorta; LV = left ventricle; MVO = mitral valve opening; AVC = aortic valve closure; AVO = aortic valve opening; a = atrial contribution to ventricular filling. See text for details. (Reproduced with permission from Criley [5].)

post-extra-systolic beats produce large intraventricular gradients and reduced aortic pulse pressure (see Brockenbrough-Braunwald discussion above). The magnitude of the intraventricular gradient is significantly reduced on termination of the Valsalva maneuver (beat 3 from

right). In distinction to the previous patient, premature ventricular contraction alone did not elicit an intraventricular gradient (beat 2, from left). After Valsalva, premature ventricular contractions provoked an intraventricular gradient for the diagnosis of hypertrophic myopathy.

In the same patient, to elucidate the response to decreases in left ventricular preloading conditions and intraventricular gradients, the hemodynamic responses to nitroglycerin were also examined (Fig. 6). Left ventricular-aortic pressures after nitroglycerin now demonstrated reduced systolic pressure and a small resting gradient (approximately 10 mmHg) not seen with Valsalva alone (Fig. 5). Systolic aortic and left ventricular pressures before nitroglycerin (Fig. 5) averaged around 140 mmHg; after nitroglycerin, the left ventricular systolic pressure is 100 mmHg and aortic pressure 90 mmHg. A Valsalva maneuver was then performed. During the initial phases of the Valsalva maneuver, a run of 4 premature ventricular contractions produces a striking aortic-left ventricular gradient. After Valsalva, the arterial pressure temporarily rises above resting levels. Later premature ventricular contractions also demonstrate an intraventricular gradient with nitroglycerin. Sustained preload reduction with nitroglycerin or transient reduction with Valsalva maneuver can elicit important changes in intraventricular gradients in these patients.

The Valsalva maneuver increases the intraventricular gradient by the progressive reduction in stroke volume. Increasing intrathoracic pressure progressively increases the magnitude of pressure gradient immediately on increase of thoracic pressure. Reflex increase in contractility during Valsalva maneuver does not appear to con-

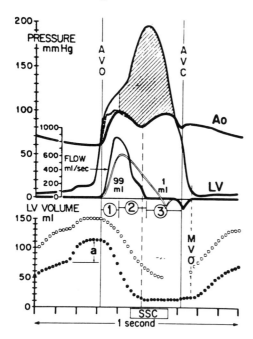

Fig. 4. Dynamic gradient in hypertrophic cardiomyopathy. Ao = aorta; LV = left ventricle; MVO = mitral valve opening; AVC = aortic valve closure; AVO = aortic valve opening; a = atrial contribution to ventricular filling; SSC = onset of septal anterior leaflet motion and septal contact. Numbers in circles 1, 2, and 3 identify the three phases of ejection from the left ventricle and discrete alterations in pressure and waveform due to motion and obstruction with intraventricular pressure gradient development. (See text for details. Reproduced with permission from Criley [5].)

tribute to this gradient change since increases in heart rate and peripheral vascular resistance occur only at the end of the Valsalva maneuver. Valsalva maneuver reduces left ventricular inflow and preload to the ventricular chamber.

Nitroglycerin increases pressure gradients in hypertrophic myopathy, but decreases pressure gradient in patients with valvular aortic stenosis [1,4]. Reduction in venous return to the heart decreases left ventricular filling and decreases left ventricular outflow, increasing the intraventricular gradient.

Intraventricular pressure gradients can be noted in patients both with and without asymmetric and symmetric myocardial hypertrophy and in those without hypertrophy in whom angiographic left ventricular cavity obliteration is observed. The post-extra-systolic beat potentiation phenomenon may also be observed in patients with symmetric, as well as asymmetric septal hypertrophy, indicating that cavity obliteration by itself may have a hemodynamic significance. This contraction abnormality, hyperejection of blood from the left ventricle, is characteristic of *hypertrophic diseased states,* and it may be observed in patients with hypertension, aortic steno-

sis, and symmetric hypertrophy related to pathophysiologic pressure overload of ventricular function [3].

DYNAMIC GRADIENTS

Dynamic gradients between the body of the outflow tract and left ventricle may be recorded at rest or during provocation in patients with hypertrophic cardiomyopathy. A brisk aortic upstroke and *late systolic gradient* are characteristic of the intraventricular gradients. Dynamic gradients may be present in normal or hypertrophied ventricles without myopathy in which inotropic hypovolemic or vasodilator provocations occur [4,5,7]. The gradient may result from mid-cavity obstruction, mitral anterior leaflet-septal opposition, or catheter entrapment in the apical portion of the left ventricle. Three phases characterize the dynamic gradients in patients with hypertrophic myopathy (Fig. 4). Phase 1 occurs early in systole in which the impulse gradient is larger than normal since peak flow and acceleration velocity are markedly enhanced. Phase 2 is characterized by increasing left ventricular-aortic gradient with a decline in aortic flow to zero. The pressure gradient achieves its maximal dimension during phase 2. Left ventricular ejection ends as the ventricle realizes the smallest volume and a super normal ejection fraction. In phase 3, aortic outflow has ceased. The ventricle is isovolumetric at this point. A persistent decline in the pressure gradient occurs as the left ventricle relaxes and pressure falls. There is a secondary rise in outflow tract and aortic pressures at this time (accounting for the dome of the spike and dome of arterial pressure).

Dynamic left ventricular outflow tract obstruction can also be seen without hypertrophic cardiomyopathy, especially in situations with decreased left ventricular filling and increased contractility [8,9]. We recently observed hemodynamically significant left ventricular outflow tract obstruction during cardiac tamponade without hypertrophic myopathy, an association previously not described [10]. A 64-year-old woman underwent successful left anterior descending coronary angioplasty for unstable angina 5 days after acute anterior myocardial infarction. Eighteen hours after angioplasty, hypotension, nausea, and vomiting with ST segment elevation were noted. Dobutamine, dopamine, Levophed, and intubation was needed to maintain a systolic blood pressure of 80 mm Hg in the presence of a significant pericardial effusion. Coronary angiography revealed the left anterior descending angioplasty site to be intact. Simultaneous aortic (femoral artery) and left ventricular pressures are shown on Figure 7A, demonstrating a subaortic-left ventricular gradient prior to pericardiocentesis. The intraventricular gradient was documented on multiple catheter pullbacks. Akinesis of the apical septum was

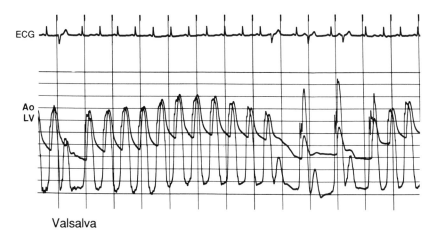

ECG

Ao
LV

Valsalva

Fig. 5.   Simultaneous aortic (Ao) and left ventricular (LV) pressures (200 mm Hg scale) during Valsalva maneuver. Note the influence of premature ventricular contractions before and during the maneuver. See text for details.

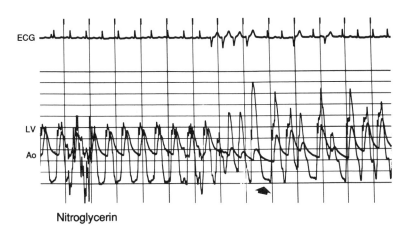

ECG

LV
Ao

Nitroglycerin

Fig. 6.   Simultaneous aortic (Ao) and left ventricular (LV) pressures (200 mm Hg scale) during nitroglycerin and Valsalva maneuver (same patient as in Fig. 5). Note the influence of premature ventricular contractions. See text for details.

observed on ventriculography and marked systolic obstruction of the outflow tract was documented with approximation of the septum and anterior mitral valve leaflet (Fig. 7B,C). There was no left ventricular septal or left ventricular free-wall hypertrophy. After pericardiocentesis, echocardiography confirmed absence of pericardial effusion and resolution of systolic anterior mitral leaflet motion with normalization of aortic flow velocity. The intraventricular gradient also disappeared (Fig. 7D). Dynamic left ventricular outflow tract obstruction without hypertrophic myopathy after acute myocardial infarction with pericardial effusion was due to a marked decline in left ventricular volume as a result of marked underfilling of the ventricle, increased catecholamines during tamponade, and additional inotropic effects of intravenous pharmacologic pressure support agents, all

contributing to the intraventricular gradient by increasing contractility while decreasing systolic volume. Pericardial tamponade is not previously known with the development of outflow tract obstruction in patients without hypertrophic myopathy, suggesting that systolic anterior motion of the mitral leaflet alone may contribute to some degree of intracavity dynamic pressure development. This unusual case highlights the importance of understanding cardiac hemodynamics for treatment of such complicated patients.

INTRAMYOCARDIAL PRESSURE AS CAUSE OF INTRAVENTRICULAR PRESSURE GRADIENT

An intraventricular pressure gradient may also be encountered in some patients, if the catheter becomes en-

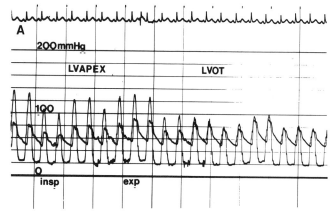

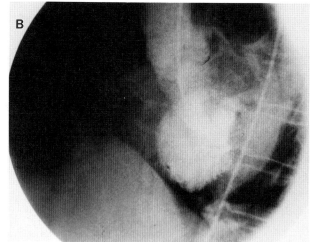

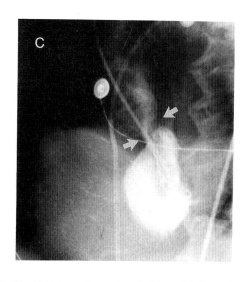

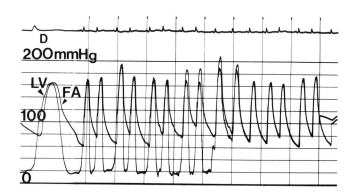

Fig. 7. A: Simultaneous femoral arterial and left ventricular pressures from the left ventricular apex and outflow tract document the subvalvular aortic gradient. The femoral arterial pressure showed pulsus paradoxus with a decrease in systolic pressure and narrowing of the pulse pressure during inspiration. **B,C:** End systolic frames from the left anterior oblique cranial left ventriculograms before PTCA (B) and during tamponade (C). A significant narrowing of the left ventricular outflow tract between the upper septum and the anterior mitral leaflet is clearly seen in C (arrows). The distal part of the septum was akinetic. **D:** Immediately after pericardiocentesis, the simultaneous femoral artery (FA) and left ventricular (LV) pressures indicate no pressure gradient.

trapped or embedded in the cardiac muscle. In late systole, a high left ventricular pressure would be recorded, reflecting subendocardial, intramyocardial tissue pressure. An entrapped catheter does not eject blood nor permit blood sampling through its lumen during systole. The initial inflow tract pressure as well as other intracavitary pressures would be equal to aortic systolic pressure. This type of pressure artifact must be identified before attributing intraventricular pressures to that of hypertrophic cardiomyopathy. The characteristic intramyocardial pressure usually has a very late peaking pressure which is *maximal at the aortic pressure of the dicrotic notch.* Catheter entrapment, producing this artifact, is most commonly present when using end hole catheters

deeply embedded from the transseptal or transvalvular aortic approach [11].

LEFT VENTRICULAR DIASTOLIC WAVEFORM ABNORMALITIES

The diastolic left ventricular waveform in Figure 1 shows a large "A" wave and high left ventricular end diastolic pressure. Beside increased "stiffness" (i.e., low compliance), other abnormalities of left ventricular diastolic pressure have been described in these patients. For example, in Figure 6 (black arrow), the diastolic left ventricular pressure after the fourth premature ventricular contraction has an abnormal relaxation pattern. This

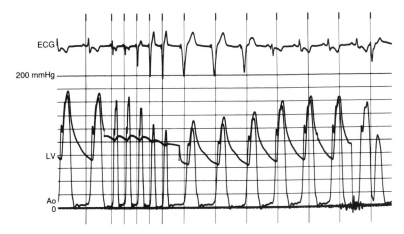

Fig. 8. Simultaneous left ventricular (LV) and aortic (Ao) pressures (200 mm Hg scale) in an elderly patient with hypertrophic cardiomyopathy and no resting intraventricular gradient who spontaneously goes into pacemaker rhythm. The contribution of atrial activity in a noncompliant left ventricle is evident by the marked drop in arterial pressure. See text for details.

waveform change should not be confused for artifact with pigtail catheter malposition partly in the aorta (the last 2 beats of Fig. 6). (The effect of pigtail catheter side holes positioned slightly outside the aortic valve markedly elevates early left ventricular diastole. Normally, left ventricular pressure is at its lowest level in early diastole. Nonetheless, the systolic aortic-left ventricular gradient can still be appreciated. A malposition of the pigtail catheter side holes usually reduces the aortic-left ventricular gradient.)

A normal ventricle should have a rising left ventricular pressure across the entire diastolic period. The characteristic abnormality of the left ventricular *diastolic* pressure, decreasing slowly in mid-diastole (black arrow Fig. 6), in hypertrophic myopathy has been reported to be due to abnormal left ventricular relaxation [12]. Although uncommon even for patients with hypertrophic cardiomyopathy, left ventricular diastolic pressure may continue to decline over the course of diastole, an abnormal relaxation pattern which may be abolished by calcium channel blockers [7]. In the patient described in Figure 6 in whom an intraventricular gradient was provoked during nitroglycerin, Valsalva, and extra-systoles, the left ventricular diastolic pressure contour following a premature ventricular contraction and long pause (black arrow, Fig. 6) can be seen to decline, suggesting intermittent abnormal relaxation on several of these post-systolic beats.

Although hypertrophic muscle may have an extraordinarily vigorous contraction, ventricular relaxation and compliance characteristics are markedly impaired. Consider the hemodynamics in a 75-year-old man with a hypertrophic cardiomyopathy (nonobstructive type) with no provokable gradient (Fig. 8). Simultaneous left ventricular and aortic pressures were measured during a spontaneous episode of pacemaker rhythm in which atrial synchrony was lost. This arrhythmia resulted in a 20–25% drop in systolic aortic pressure from 175 mm Hg to 130 mm Hg due to loss of the atrial contribution to left ventricular filling.

These phenomenon have been excellently reviewed by Criley and Segal [5] and Wigle [6,13,14] and greatly contribute to the differentiation and understanding of the different types of ventricular cavity pressure gradients. The spectrum of hypertrophic cardiomyopathy with its attendant morbidity and mortality and propensity for sudden death may be attributable to the derangement of cellular architecture. Whether obstruction occurs or is a functional result of ejection is related to the spectrum of myocardial muscle hyperdevelopment. Neither an intraventricular pressure gradient nor systolic anterior mitral valve motion are equated with the presence of ventricular obstruction. Examples of the controversial viewpoints between obstructive and nonobstructive cardiomyopathy presented in the hemodynamics and left ventricular function and filling patterns here should enhance the conceptualization of the mechanisms of hypertrophy myopathy.

ACKNOWLEDGMENTS

The authors wish to thank Donna Sander for manuscript preparation.

REFERENCES

1. Brockenbrough EC, Braunwald E, Morrow AG: A hemodynamic technic for the detection of hypertrophic subaortic stenosis. Circulation 23:189–194, 1961.

2. White CW, Zimmerman TJ: Prolonged left ventricular ejection time in the post-premature beat: a sensitive sign of idiopathic hypertrophic subaortic stenosis. Circulation 52:306–312, 1975.

3. Raizner AE, Chahine RA, Ishimori T, Awdeh M: Clinical correlates of left ventricular cavity obliteration. Am J Cardiol 40:303–309, 1977.

4. White RI, Criley M, Lewis KB, Ross RS: Experimental production of intracavity pressure differences. Am J Cardiol 19:806–817, 1967.

5. Criley JM, Siegel RJ: Has 'obstruction' hindered our understanding of hypertrophic cardiomyopathy? Circulation 72:1148–1154, 1985.

6. Wigle ED: Hypertrophic cardiomyopathy: a 1987 viewpoint. Circulation 2:311–322, 1987.

7. Wigle ED, Marquis Y, Auger P: Muscular subaortic stenosis: initial left ventricular inflow tract pressure in the assessment of intraventricular pressure differences in man. Circulation 35:1100–1117, 1967.

8. Come PC, Bulkley BH, Goodman ZD, Hutchins GM, Pitt B, Fortuin NJ: Hypercontractile cardiac states simulating hypertrophic cardiomyopathy. Circulation 55:901–908, 1977.

9. Erdin RA Jr, Abdulla AM, Stefadouros MA: Hypercontractile cardiac state mimicking hypertrophic subaortic stenosis. Cathet Cardiovasc Diagn 7:71–77, 1981.

10. Deligonul U, Uppstrom E, Penick D, Seacord L, Kern MJ: Dynamic left ventricular outflow tract obstruction induced by pericardial tamponade during acute anterior myocardial infarction. Am Heart J (In press, 1990).

11. Pasipoularides A: Clinical assessment of ventricular ejection dynamics with and without outflow obstruction. J Am Coll Cardiol 15:859–882, 1990.

12. Lorell BH, Paulus WJ, Grossman W, Wynne J, Cohn PF, Braunwald E: Improved diastolic function and systolic performance in hypertrophic cardiomyopathy after nifedipine. New Engl J Med 303:801–803, 1980.

13. Ross J Jr, Braunwald E, Gault JH, Mason DT, Morrow AG: The mechanism of the intraventricular pressure gradient in idiopathic hypertrophic subaortic stenosis. Circulation 34:558–578, 1966.

14. Murgo JP, Alter BR, Dorethy JR, Altobelli SA, McGranahan GM Jr: Dynamics of left ventricular ejection in obstructive and nonobstructive hypertrophic cardiomyopathy. J Clin Invest 66:1369–1382, 1980.

Chapter 28

Hemodynamics of Dual-Chamber Pacing and Valsalva Maneuver in a Patient With Hypertrophic Obstructive Cardiomyopathy

Morton J. Kern, MD, Sanjeev Puri, MD, Thomas J. Donohue, MD, and Richard G. Bach, MD

INTRODUCTION

Hypertrophic cardiomyopathy may present with disabling symptoms of exertional dyspnea, angina, and syncope. These symptoms have been variably ascribed to the associated obstructive left ventricular gradient resulting in high velocity left ventricular, outflow mitral regurgitation, and diastolic left ventricular dysfunction [1,2]. Although the treatment for hypertrophic myopathy has often been relegated to beta adrenergic and calcium channel blocking agents [3], those patients with refractory hemodynamic symptomatology may benefit from septal myectomy [4]. The morbidity and mortality associated with the procedure, however, may be excessive. Recent studies have suggested dual-chamber pacing as an alternative therapy [5–7]. A decrease in left ventricular outflow gradient as well as symptomatic improvement has been reported after implantation of a permanent dual-chamber pacemaker, thought to be due to alteration of septal activation from pacing at the right ventricular apex [8]. The effects have not been uniformly beneficial, and issues regarding diastolic dysfunction have suggested that AV sequential pacing may be superior to right ventricular pacing [5–7]. To examine the effects of AV pacing in a patient with obstructive hypertrophic cardiomyopathy, left ventricular outflow hemodynamics were recorded at rest, during provocative maneuvers–Valsalva and premature ventricular contractions (PVC)—and during AV sequential pacing. Characteristic hemodynamic waveforms are presented for discussion.

CASE HISTORY

A 36-yr-old woman had a 1-yr history of progressive exertional dyspnea, light headedness, and chest pain. She had frequent episodes of near syncope and one documented episode of syncope 1 mo prior to evaluation. The light headedness occurred with mild exertion, especially during activities of daily life, which include climbing one flight of stairs. Two-dimensional echocardiography revealed marked asymmetric septal hypertrophy (intraventricular septum markedly thickened at 3.5 cm) with a systolic left ventricular outflow tract gradient at rest estimated at 64 mmHg by Doppler. The patient also reported a brother who died suddenly at age 31 with infective mitral valve endocarditis. At autopsy he was noted to have a hypertrophic cardiomyopathy with a maximal septal thickness of 2.5 cm and myofiber disarray on histologic examination.

PHYSICAL EXAMINATION

The patient had a blood pressure of 110/80 mmHg with a heart rate of 80 beats/min. There was no neck vein distension or carotid bruit. The S_1 and S_2 heart sounds were normal. There was a III/VI late peaking crescendo/decrescendo systolic murmur along the left sternal border radiating to the apex, which increased with standing and Valsalva's maneuver and decreased with squatting. The remaining examination was unremarkable. The electrocardiogram showed normal sinus rhythm and left ventricular hypertrophy.

Left and right heart catheterization was performed from the right femoral artery approach in a standard fashion. Resting hemodynamics (Fig. 1) demonstrated a mean right atrial pressure of 3 mmHg, right ventricular

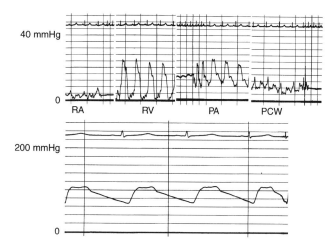

Fig. 1. Hemodynamics at rest. Right heart hemodynamics show right atrial (RA) pressure, right ventricular (RV) pressure, pulmonary artery (PA) pressure, pulmonary capillary wedge (PCW) pressure on a 0–40 mmHg scale and aortic (Ao) pressure on a 0–200 mmHg scale. Note the bisferiens arterial pulse at rest on the aortic pressure waveform.

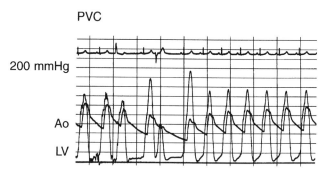

Fig. 2. Left ventricular (LV) and aortic (Ao) pressures during premature ventricular contractions (PVC) on a 0–200 mmHg scale.

pressure of 24/4 mmHg, pulmonary artery pressure of 24/10 mmHg with a mean of 14 mmHg, and a mean pulmonary capillary wedge pressure of 8 mmHg. Aortic pressure was 110/70 mmHg with a waveform that demonstrated two systolic peaks characterizing pulsus bisferiens. Simultaneous left ventricular and aortic pressures (Fig. 2) were 156/18 mmHg and 120/70 mmHg, respectively. There was a 34 mmHg resting intraventricular pressure gradient. Left ventricular systolic pressure increased to 190 mmHg and aortic pressure fell to 90/50 mmHg with the left ventricular outflow tract gradient increasing to 100 mmHg during postpremature ventricular contraction. The left ventricular outflow tract gradient also increased to ~80 mmHg during Valsalva's maneuver within the first several beats of the strain phase (Fig. 3). Following these maneuvers, atrial and ventricular pacemakers were placed in the right heart chambers. During AV pacing at 85 beats/min with an AV delay of 75 msec

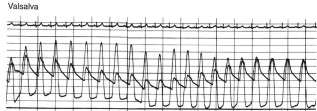

Fig. 3. Left ventricular (LV) and aortic (Ao) pressures during Valsalva maneuver on a 0–200 mmHg scale.

(Fig. 4), the left ventricular pressure fell slightly (150/14 mmHg), but with a concomitant fall in aortic pressure (120/70 to 105/75 mmHg). The left ventricular outflow tract gradient remained ~50 mmHg. At a paced heart rate of 100 beats/min with an AV delay of 75 msec, hemodynamics were largely unaffected with the left ventricular outflow tract gradient remaining at 50–60 mmHg. With an increase of the AV delay to 100 msec at the paced rate of 100 beats/min, findings were unchanged. Left ventriculography demonstrated normal systolic function with midchamber obliteration and ejection fraction > 70%. The coronary arteries were normal. The patient was treated with metoprolol without improvement and is currently on a calcium channel blocker. Following discharge from the hospital, she wore an event monitor for 30 d. She continued to remain symptomatic with frequent episodes of chest discomfort, light headedness, and near syncope. The event monitor revealed normal sinus rhythm during all episodes, which decreased the suspicion of ventricular arrhythmias playing any role in her symptomatology.

To contrast the hemodynamic responses in the case presented above, Steely and colleagues [9] have provide an example of a different response to dual-chamber pacing in a 58-yr-old woman with exertional dyspnea and chest discomfort ascribed to hypertrophic cardiomyopathy. The resting left ventricular outflow gradient was minimal with left ventricular pressure at rest of 150/10 mmHg, aortic pressure 156/66 mmHg. With Valsalva maneuver, a significant increase in left ventricular outflow gradient was noted (Fig. 5, left). PVCs provoked a further decrease in pulse pressure and increase in the postextra systolic gradient demonstrating the Brockenbrough-Braunwald-Morrow sign. Temporary dual-chamber atrial and ventricular pacing was performed, which reduced the left ventricular and aortic pressures and eliminated the left ventricular outflow tract gradient during Valsalva maneuver (Fig. 6).

DISCUSSION

The cases demonstrate alterations in left ventricular outflow tract gradient in patients with hypertrophic

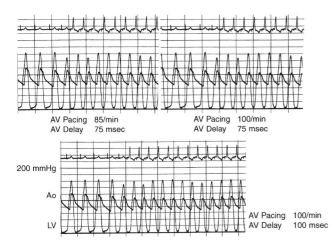

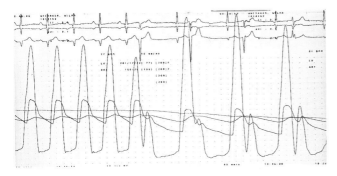

Fig. 4. Left ventricular (LV) and aortic (Ao) pressures during AV sequential pacing at 85 and 100 beats/min with AV delay 75 and 100 msec. Scale 0–200 mmHg.

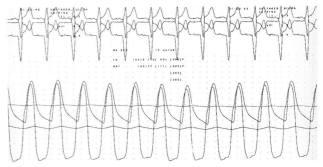

Fig. 6. Dual-chamber atrioventricular pacemaker hemodynamics demonstrating abolishment of left ventricular outflow tract gradient during Valsalva maneuver. Pressure scale is 0–200 mmHg. (Reproduced with permission from Steely D, Javier JJ, Bissett JK, Talley JD. It Fits! (Intelligence Transfer: From Images to Solutions): Pacemaker therapy in patients with hypertrophic obstructive cardiomyopathy. J Interven Cardiol 10:385–386, 1997.)

Fig. 5. Increase in left ventricular outflow tract gradient induced by Valsalva maneuver with PVCs inducing an increase in gradient and decrease in pulse pressure. Pressure scale is 0–200 mmHg. (Reproduced with permission from Steely D, Javier JJ, Bissett JK, Talley JD. It Fits! (Intelligence Transfer: From Images to Solutions): Pacemaker therapy in patients with hypertrophic obstructive cardiomyopathy. J Interven Cardiol 10:385–386, 1997.)

cardiomyopathy during Valsalva, PVC, and AV sequential pacing maneuvers. The decrease in left ventricular outflow gradient and hypertrophic obstructive cardiomyopathy with pacemaker therapy has been proposed to be due to three mechanisms: (1) a decrease in paradoxic septal motion, (2) late activation of septal contraction due to right ventricular pacing, and (3) decrease in left ventricular global contractility. Nishimura et al. [7] reported the effects of dual-chamber pacing on systolic and diastolic function in patients with cardiomyopathy. In 29 patients with hypertrophic cardiomyopathy, high fidelity pressure measurements of left ventricular outflow and left atrial pressures, ascending aortic pressure, cardiac output, and Doppler mitral flow velocity curves were obtained to evaluate cardiac function. During AV sequen-

tial pacing with an AV delay of 60 msec, there was significant decrease in cardiac output, positive dP/dt, and increase in mean left atrial pressure. There was also a prolongation of Tau, the time constant of left ventricular relaxation. During AV sequential pacing with an optimal AV delay (identified as the longest AV interval with pre-excitation), deterioration in both systolic and diastolic function variables occurred with lesser magnitude than during pacing with the shortest AV intervals. In 21 patients with and 8 patients without resting left ventricular outflow obstruction, this alteration of systolic and diastolic function was characterized by a modest decrease in left ventricular outflow tract gradient from 73 ± 45 to 61 ± 41 mmHg ($P < 0.03$) with dual-chamber pacing at the optimal AV delay compared to sinus rhythm. The investigators [7] concluded that the acute effect of pacing the right atrium and ventricle may be detrimental to both systolic and diastolic left ventricular function, particularly at the shorter AV intervals, and that further randomized studies to identify the benefits of dual-chamber pacing were required.

Previous studies [5,6] have demonstrated a reduction in the left ventricular outflow gradient in patients with obstructive hypertrophic myopathy undergoing dual-chamber pacing. The hypertrophied septum projecting into the left ventricular outflow tract produced high velocity blood flow and resultant anterior motion of the mitral valve, which were deemed responsible for the obstruction. With altered contraction of the septum, a reduction in the displacement of the mitral valve apparatus as well as improved cross-sectional area of the outflow tract was identified. A uniform response of the left ventricular outflow tract gradient to dual-chamber pacing was not present. Although a statistically significant decrease in gradient was noted with dual-chamber pacing, some patients had no change, where others had a significant reduction. The short AV intervals may have contributed to inadequate filling of the left ventricle from ineffective atrial contraction and thus may account for this lack of efficacy in some patients.

As suggested in this patient, there is a question whether the acute change in left ventricular outflow tract gradient in patients with hypertrophic obstructive cardiomyopathy can be used as a reliable indicator of a response to therapy [10]. Since the left ventricular outflow tract gradient is dependent on contractility as well as loading conditions, alterations in either of these two variables may produce a variation in the outflow tract gradient in the absence of mechanical intervention. The abnormal ventricular relaxation, typical of patients with hypertrophic obstructive cardiomyopathy, contributes to increased filling pressures. Whereas diastolic function can be altered by dual-chamber pacing, left atrial pressure may elevate further during pacing at short AV intervals [7]. The increase in left atrial pressure was probably related to both ventricular relaxation as well as interruption of the optimal AV synchrony for left ventricular emptying. Nishimura et al. [7] report that the mean Tau for all patients was longer during dual-chamber pacing than normal sinus rhythm, suggesting a potentially detrimental effect of pacing on left ventricular diastolic function and relaxation. Pacing at short AV intervals results in the most marked impairment of left ventricular relaxation and is related to a primary decrease in systolic contraction.

Others have suggested that there is a difference in the hemodynamic change between acute and chronic DDD pacing [6]. Most of the subjective and objective improvement as a result of DDD pacing probably is related to myocardial, hemodynamic, and electric adaptive changes after chronic therapy. A considerable difference was noted in left ventricular outflow tract gradients during cardiac catheterization studies at 3 and 16 mo after pacemaker implantation, attributed to myocardial adaptive changes [6]. Maron [10] stated in an editorial regarding the use of dual-chamber pacing that a continued examination of this modality for hypertrophic cardiomyopathy is warranted, especially in patients with both marked obstruction to left ventricular outflow and symptoms of congestive heart failure who are refractory to medical therapy. This subset of patients probably comprised only 5–10% of all patients with this clinical syndrome. Caution must be exercised in applying dual-chamber pacing as a treatment for the complex disease characterized by an abnormally hypertrophied, noncompliant left ventricle. Maron [10] also noted that pacing has no defined role in diminishing the risk for sudden cardiac death nor in relieving symptoms of patients with nonobstructive hypertrophic myopathy. Until the uncertainty regarding the role of efficacy of DDD pacing is resolved, clinicians should be aware of potentially deleterious effects or a lack of clinical benefit that may occur with DDD pacing in a patient with hypertrophic obstructive cardiomyopathy. However, some patient subgroups may derive substantial benefit from this technique and thus further studies are warranted.

This patient is of particular interest given her completely normal diastolic filling pressures. Her symptoms are clearly related to outflow problems and not to diastolic compliance abnormalities with elevated left heart filling pressures or ventricular arrhythmias. Patients with predominant complaints related to elevated outflow gradients should most benefit from septal ablative procedures.

Recent therapies may eliminate the need to consider the complex clinical and hemodynamic questions regarding dual-chamber pacing as therapy for patients with hypertrophic obstructive cardiomyopathy. Septal ablation with installation of intraseptal arterial alcohol [12] and controlled myocardial infarction in patients with hypertrophic myopathies demolishing or abolishing the left ventricular outflow tract gradient has been associated with favorable short-term clinical outcomes. Future studies may reveal the value of this approach as compared to other pharmacologic, mechanical, or pacing therapies for this difficult patient population.

ACKNOWLEDGMENTS

The authors thank the J.G. Mudd Cardiac Catheterization Laboratory team for technical support, Dr. J. David Talley for hemodynamic figures, and Donna Sander for manuscript preparation.

REFERENCES

1. Braunwald E, Morrow AG, Cornell WP, Aygen MM, Hilbish TF: Idiopathic hypertrophic subaortic stenosis: Clinical, hemodynamic and angiographic manifestations. Am J Med 29:924–945, 1960.
2. Wigle ED, Sasson Z, Henderson MA, Ruddy TD, Fulop J, Rakowski H, Williams WG: Hypertrophic cardiomyopathy: The importance of the site and the extent of hypertrophy: A review. Prog Cardiovasc Dis 28:1–83, 1985.
3. Goodwin JF: Treatment of the cardiomyopathies. Am J Cardiol 32:341–351, 1973.
4. Krajcer Z, Leachman RD, Cooley DA, Coronado R: Septal myotomy-myomectomy versus mitral valve replacement in hypertrophic cardiomyopathy: Ten-year follow-up in 185 patients. Circulation 80 (suppl I):I-57–I-64, 1989.
5. Jeanrenaud X, Goy JJ, Kappenberger L: Effects of dual-chamber pacing in hypertrophic obstructive cardiomyopathy. Eur Heart J 339:1318–1323, 1992.
6. Fananapazir L, Cannon RO III, Tripodi D, Panza JA: Impact of dual-chamber permanent pacing in patients with obstructive hypertrophic cardiomyopathy with symptoms refractory to verapamil and beta-adrenergic blocker therapy. Circulation 85:2149–2161, 1992.

7. Nishimura RA, Hayes DL, Ilstrup DM, Holmes DR Jr, Tajik AJ. Effect of dual-chamber pacing on systolic and diastolic function in patients with hypertrophic cardiomyopathy: Acute Doppler echocardiographic and catheterization hemodynamic study. J Am Coll Cardiol 27:421–430,1996.

8. McDonald KM, Maurer B: Permanent pacing as treatment for hypertrophic cardiomyopathy. Am J Cardiol 68:108–110, 1991.

9. Steely D, Javier JJ, Bissett JK, Talley JD. It Fits! (Intelligence Transfer: From Images to Solutions): Pacemaker therapy in patients with hypertrophic obstructive cardiomyopathy. J Interven Cardiol 10:385–386, 1997.

10. Maron BJ: Appraisal of dual-chamber pacing therapy in hypertrophic cardiomyopathy: Too soon for a rush to judgment? J Am Coll Cardiol 27:431–432, 1996.

11. Nishimura RA, Tajek AJ: Valsalva maneuver and response revisited. Mayo Clinic Proc 61:211–217, 1986.

12. Knight C, Kurbaan AS, Seggewiss H, Henein M, Gunning M, Harrington D, Fassbender D, Gleichmann U, Sigwart U: Nonsurgical septal reduction for hypertrophic obstructive cardiomyopathy: Outcome in the first series of patients. Circulation 95:2075–2081, 1997.

Chapter 29

Hemodynamic Effects of Alcohol-Induced Septal Infarction for Hypertrophic Obstructive Cardiomyopathy

Morton J. Kern, MD, Hassan Rajjoub, MD, and Richard G. Bach MD

INTRODUCTION

Patients with hypertrophic obstructive cardiomyopathy (HOCM) may demonstrate symptoms due to the outflow obstruction produced by hyperdynamic left ventricular contraction [1]. Unlike patients with ischemic cardiomyopathy, treating these symptoms often requires paradoxic therapy directed at reducing the adverse effects of the hypercontractile myocardium. Although beneficial in many types of ischemic heart disease or congestive heart failure, digitalis, sympathomimetic amines, and preload-reducing pharmacologic therapy are detrimental in this setting, often exacerbating symptoms, in patients with hypertrophic myopathy. Therapy that reduces myocardial contractility, such as beta-adrenergic blockers, calcium channel blockers, and other negative inotropic agents, have demonstrated symptomatic benefit in the HOCM patient [2]. When medical therapy fails, mechanically altering the sequence or degree of left ventricular contraction by DDD pacing or surgically reducing the hypertrophied muscle segment in the outflow tract has been advocated [3–7]. A new method of nonsurgical septal mass reduction by controlled septal infarction using alcohol for the symptomatic patient with HOCM has been reported [8–10].

We present the hemodynamics of two patients undergoing alcohol septal ablation for medically refractory symptomatic hypertrophic myopathy. In this hemodynamic rounds we examine the method and effects of induced septal infarction and review the available literature on this new approach to treating symptomatic HOCM patients.

CASE REPORT
Case 1

A 68-year-old man with HOCM diagnosed 7 years ago had increasing dyspnea and near syncope. Persistent dyspnea and near syncope on minimal exertion were occurring with daily frequency. The patient was treated with multiple medications, including tenormin with no symptomatic relief. On physical examination, the blood pressure was 120/80 mm Hg, pulse 65/min. There was no neck vein distension. A systolic murmur was well heard over the left precordium consistent with mitral regurgitation and a harsh systolic murmur that increased with Valsalva maneuver was noted at the left sternal border consistent with dynamic outflow tract obstruction. The electrocardiogram demonstrated normal sinus rhythm and left ventricular hypertrophy with nonspecific ST-T wave changes. Two-dimensional and Doppler echocardiography demonstrated a significantly increased left ventricular outflow tract velocity consistent with a substantial intraventricular pressure gradient and severe mitral regurgitation with an enlarged left atrium. The intraventricular septum was $\geq$2.2-cm thick at the level of the mitral valve.

Recent cardiac catheterization demonstrated significant resting intraventricular gradient of 60 mm Hg, normal coronary arteries, and normal right heart hemodynamic with a hypertrophied left ventricular and normal function. After discussing alternative therapies, the patient elected to undergo the alcohol septal ablation procedure. The patient gave consent to participate in the clinical research protocol, which was approved by the Human Subjects Committee of our Institutional Review Board.

The technique for the alcohol-induced septal infarction was performed as follows. The right and left femoral arteries and veins were cannulated using 6 and 8 Fr sheaths, respectively. A 5 Fr (Halo Angiodynamics, Inc., Minneapolis, MN) angiographic catheter was inserted into the left ventricle. A 5 Fr balloon-tipped pacemaker was inserted through the right femoral vein to the right ventricle. A 6 Fr multipurpose catheter was also positioned in the right ventricle from the left femoral vein. An 8 Fr JL4 coronary guide catheter was inserted through the left femoral artery.

Following positioning of the catheters, coronary arteriography identified a single large septal artery from the proximal left anterior descending artery (Fig. 1, patient J.H.). Weight-adjusted intravenous heparin (100 U/kg) was given.

Prior to septal ablation, demerol 50 mg iv was given. The first large septal artery was cannulated using a large double 45° bend on an 0.014″ angioplasty guidewire over which a short angioplasty balloon (2.5 × 10 mm Bandit, SCIMED, Minneapolis, MN) was completely advanced into the first septal artery. The septal artery balloon catheter was inflated and radiographic contrast was instilled into the occluding balloon to demonstrate the correct positioning of the balloon catheter without contrast reflux (Fig. 1, top middle). Simultaneous two-dimensional transthoracic echocardiography was performed. For contrast opacification of the hypertrophied septum, Optison (Mallinckrodt, St.Louis, MO) echo contrast (3 cc) was diluted 1:10 and instilled via the septal balloon lumen. The echo contrast opacified the protruding septum at the site of the highest velocity in the left ventricular outflow tract. Following echocardiographic confirmation of correct septal branch occlusion, 3 cc of 98% dehydrated alcohol was delivered slowly into the septal artery over 5 min, followed by a 5-min waiting period.

Hemodynamics were continuously measured before, during, and after alcohol septal ablation (Fig. 2). After the 5-min period following alcohol administration, the occluding balloon catheter was deflated and withdrawn. The patient had a junctional escape rhythm requiring temporary pacing. The classic "spike and dome" configuration of the arterial pressure (Fig. 2A), especially prominent on the potentiated postpremature ventricular contraction (PVC) beats, was eliminated, as were the potentiated PVC gradients and the Brockenbrough-Braunwald sign of reduced arterial pulse pressure after PVC. The junctional rhythm and, to some degree, the infarcted septal activity likely accounted for the reduction in arterial pressure from 140/78 to 100/76 mm Hg. There was no significant change in the left ventricular end-diastolic pressure (28 to 32 mm Hg, pre- vs. postalcohol). Note the

significant reduction of the resting left ventricular outflow tract gradient and loss of the PVC provocable gradient after septal ablation (Fig. 3). There was no significant change in right ventricular pressures after septal infarction. Coronary arteriography and coronary flow reserve were repeated (Table I). The temporary pacemaker and the vascular sheaths were secured in place. The patient was transferred to the coronary care unit for observation. The peak CPK was approximately 2,000 units with MB fraction of 53 units. The electrocardiogram showed minimal ST elevation in leads V_1 and V_2. At the end of 18 hr, the patient had no requirement for pacing and the pacemaker was removed.

With elimination of the left ventricular outflow tract gradient (Fig. 3), the patient noted dramatic symptomatic improvement within hours after the procedure and by the next morning was noted to be markedly improved. That afternoon the patient could, for the first time, walk the hallway without symptoms. He has been stable for 6 months.

Case 2

A 60-year-old male had dyspnea on exertional since 1990. Recently, near syncopal symptoms, as well as atypical chest pain, occurred frequently. An echocardiogram demonstrated severe left ventricular hypertrophy, an abnormal left ventricular outflow tract velocity and contour consistent with HOCM, and moderate, eccentric mitral regurgitation. On physical examination, the blood pressure was 140/70 mm Hg, heart rate 80/min. No bruits or jugular venous distension were noted. The S_1 and S_2 were normal. There was a III/VI systolic ejection murmur at the base and a II/VI holosystolic murmur at the apex radiating to the axilla. The abdomen and remainder of the examination was unremarkable. Electrocardiogram showed normal sinus rhythm with severe left ventricular hypertrophy.

After discussion of the alternative therapies for hypertrophic obstructive cardiomyopathy, the patient and family elected to participate in the alcohol septal ablation protocol. At cardiac catheterization, the left ventricle was hypercontractile. The left ventricular outflow tract gradient was 60 mm Hg at rest and 130 mm Hg with provocable maneuvers (Fig. 4). The arterial waveform showed classic features of the "spike and dome" pattern and the Brockenbrough-Braunwald sign after a PVC. To demonstrate the full extent of the left ventricular outflow tract obstruction, hemodynamics during the Valsalva maneuver with a PVC showed a left ventricular outflow tract gradient of 110 mm Hg, which increased to nearly 200 mm Hg with a PVC (Fig. 5). The arterial pressure on this beat was 62/48 mm Hg. Following positioning of a

J.H.   Before   After

J.B.   Before   After #1

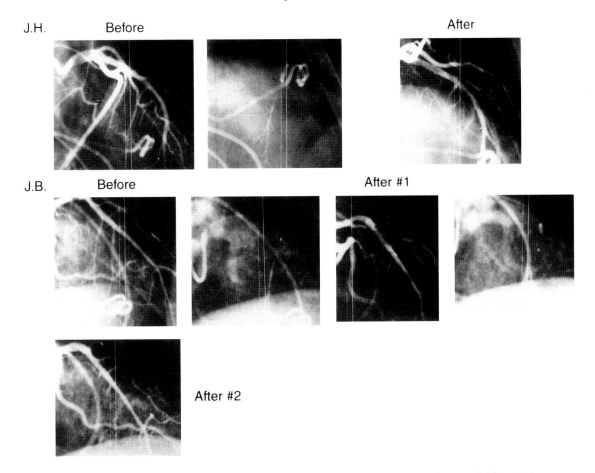

After #2

Fig. 1. Top: Patient 1, J.H. Angiographic frames showing first large septal artery (left), septal balloon occlusion (middle), and occluded septal artery after procedure (right). Middle: Patient 2, J.B. Angiography of two large septal arteries (middle left) and sequential balloon occlusion and alcohol ablation (middle left, right, and far right). Bottom: Angiogram of part 2 showing two occluded septal arteries.

left ventricular and pacing catheters, coronary arteriography demonstrated normal arteries and two large septal arteries (Fig. 1, patient J.B., left panel). Weight-adjusted intravenous heparin was administered. Left ventricular descending coronary flow reserve was also measured as in the first patient. A 2.0 × 9.0 mm balloon was positioned into the first septal artery branch. Radiographic contrast, given through the occluded balloon catheter, demonstrated the totally occlusive positioning of the balloon catheter in the first septal artery (Fig. 1, patient J.B., middle panels). Echo contrast (3 cc Optison, diluted 1:10) opacified only the top part of the obstructing septal muscle. Following echo contrast imaging, 3 cc of 98% dehydrated alcohol was delivered into the first septal artery over 5 min with a 5-min waiting period following alcohol administration. Hemodynamics were continuously measured. Following the waiting period, the balloon catheter was withdrawn, coronary arteriography was repeated, and coronary flow reserve of the left anterior descending coronary artery was repeated. Because of a

residual 40 mm Hg provokable left ventricular outflow tract gradient, the septal occlusion and ablation procedure was repeated in the second septal artery (Fig. 1, patient J.B., lower panel). After the two septal arteries were ablated, the left ventricular outflow tract gradient was <10 mm Hg at rest without a PVC provocable gradient. During Valsalva and PVCs, the largest resting gradient was 30 mm Hg without PVC augmentation (Fig. 6). Only at maximal Valsalva (Fig. 5, bottom, beat 7) was the arterial "spike and dome" waveform demonstrated. The paced rhythm was associated with complete heart block and A-V dissociation. A-waves can be seen on the left ventricular diastolic pressure wave (Fig. 6, top, beats 5–7 and 9). It is interesting to note the increased arterial pressure (130/70 to 150/80 mm Hg) after septal ablation.

Regarding coronary flow reserve, unlike in the first patient, coronary flow reserve in the left anterior descending artery increased from 1.5 before to 2.7 after septal ablation. Systolic flow reversal demonstrated prior to septal ablation was not seen afterward.

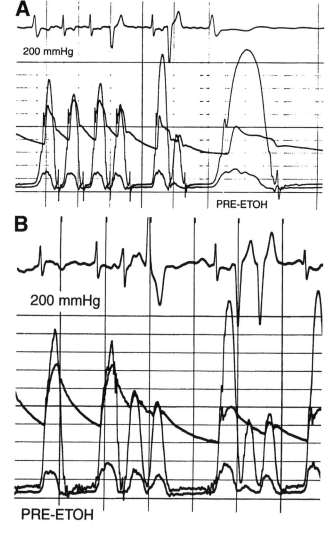

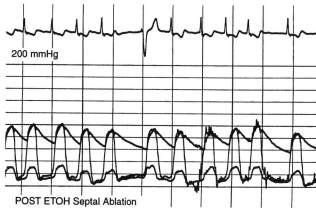

Fig. 3. Hemodynamics following alcohol septal ablation in patient 1. Left ventricular (LV), aortic (Ao), and right ventricular (RV) pressures now show a 0-mm Hg gradient at rest with loss of the "spike and dome" configuration of the aortic pressure. There is no post-PVC provocation of LV outflow tract gradient. Also note that the rhythm is not paced.

Fig. 2. A: Left ventricular (LV), aortic (Ao), and right ventricular (RV) pressures on a 0–200-mm Hg scale in patient 1 before alcohol septal ablation (ETOH). Note the large post-PVC gradient of 120 mm Hg peak-to-peak with a "spike and dome" configuration of the aortic pressure wave on beat at far right fast recording speed. B: Left ventricular (LV), aortic (Ao), and right ventricular (RV) pressures on a 0–200-mm Hg scale demonstrating the effect of a couplet on the post-PVC LV outflow tract gradient before septal ablation.

At the conclusion of the procedure, the vascular sheaths and temporary pacemaker were secured in place. The patient was transferred to the coronary care unit. Peak CPK was approximately 1,800 units with MB fraction of 59. The electrocardiogram showed junctional rhythm with minor ST elevation in leads V_1 and V_2. After 48 hr, the patient had persistent junctional bradycardia and episodes of complete heart block, for which he received a DDD pacemaker. He was discharged asymptomatic on hospital day 5. A summary of the hemodynamic and echocardiographic data is shown on Table I.

DISCUSSION

The hemodynamic findings in the two HOCM patients were among the most dramatic changes that one may observe in this condition. These pressure waveforms also emphasized the role of the obstructing septum in contributing to the outflow tract gradient and distinct arterial pressure waveform (i.e., "spike and dome" pattern). The pathophysiology of hypertrophic cardiomyopathy suggests that four therapeutic approaches may provide important symptomatic benefit. These methods include negative inotropic pharmacologic therapy, DDD pacing, surgical septal myomectomy with or without mitral valve replacement, and, most recently, alcohol septal ablation [11,12].

Dual-Chamber Pacing

Dual-chamber pacing shortens the AV conduction interval, altering the left ventricular depolarization and contraction sequence. The alteration of contractile events minimizes the obstructing septal contraction reducing the narrowing of the left ventricular outflow tract. DDD pacing, in some cases, provides substantial hemodynamic benefit [13,14]. The duration of symptomatic benefit of dual-chamber pacing has been reported to extend over a 5-year follow-up period [15].

Although dual-chamber pacing has been shown to reduce left ventricular outflow obstruction, diminish mitral regurgitation, and improve exercise performance, several reports of DDD pacing indicate that the acute and early cardiac changes may not be maintained over the long term. Prolonged pacing alters the electrical and hemodynamic properties of the myocardium [16]. Long-term DDD pacing results in adaptive left ventricular

TABLE I. Hemodynamic Data Before and After Alcohol Septal Ablation

	Patient 1		Patient 2	
	Pre	Post	Pre	Post
Right ventricular pressure (mm Hg)	30/10	30/10	40/8	
Aortic pressure (mm Hg)	125/74	100/70	130/70	150/80
Left ventricular pressure (mm Hg)	165/16	100/25	180/20	150/20
PVC gradient (mm Hg)	100	0	130 (160 with Valsalva)	0 (20 with Valsalva)
Resting gradient (mm Hg)	60	0	70	0
CVR_{LAD}	3.3	3.2	1.5	2.7
CVR_{ref}		2.5		2.2
Septal thickness (cm)	2.2	1.5	2.1	1.4
LVOT velocity (m/sec)	3.4	1.6	4.3	2.4
Intraventricular gradient (mm Hg)	46	20	70	23
Mitral regurgitation	Moderate	Moderate	Moderate	Moderate
Ejection fraction (%)	75	58	74	67

J.B.

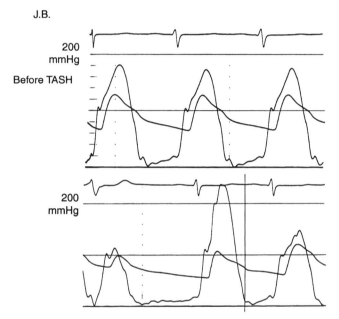

J.B.

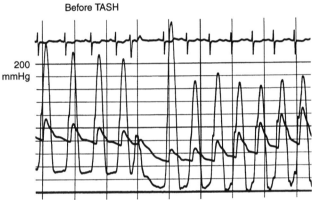

Fig. 5. Hemodynamic in patient 2 during Valsalva maneuver. The LV outflow tract gradient increases to 120 mm Hg with a post-PVC gradient of 160 mm Hg and dramatic Brockenbrough-Braunwald sign.

Fig. 4. Hemodynamic tracing in patient 2 before septal ablation. There is an 80-mm Hg resting left ventricular outflow tract (LVOT) gradient (top) and 130-mm Hg post-PVC gradient between the aortic and left ventricular pressures (lower, beat 2). Note the "spike and dome" configuration of aortic pressure waveform.

changes, reduction in left ventricular pressure, and late left ventricular remodeling. These alterations are associated with reduced angina and improved myocardial perfusion by stress imaging with reduction in left ventricular cavity dilatation [17]. Although the adaptive changes contribute to the success of dual-chamber pacemaker therapy for HOCM, the correlation between acute and chronic effects does not permit identification of an individual patient who may receive benefit from this mode of therapy. Dual-chamber pacing may not relieve left ventricular outflow tract obstruction due to the dependence on AV delay and ventricular capture poten-

tially interfering with left atrial emptying. Sixty percent of HOCM patients so treated also require drug therapy for continued symptoms at rest. DDD pacing has been used in patients who fail medical therapy. DDD pacing is ineffective in patients with atrial arrhythmias. Left ventricular myomectomy may be recommended in patients failing DDD therapy or in those needing other cardiac procedures such as coronary artery bypass surgery or valve replacement. Possible explanations for failure of dual-chamber pacing as reported by Fananapazir et al. [18] are summarized in Table II.

Surgical Septal Myectomy

Although effective in enlarging the left ventricular outflow tract and altering the left ventricular contractile sequence, septal myectomy is a complicated, open-chest surgical procedure with a mortality risk approaching 5% and a high incidence of intraventricular conduction block

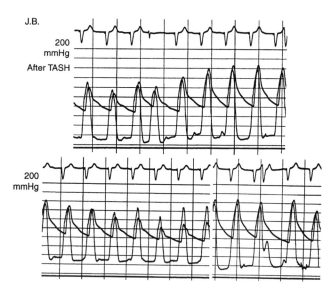

J.B.

200
mmHg

After TASH

200
mmHg

Fig. 6. Hemodynamics following alcohol septal ablation in patient 2. The rhythm is paced. There is no significant resting or post-PVC tract gradient (top and bottom right). Bottom middle: During Valsalva maneuver, there is a minimal 20-mm Hg increase in the resting gradient.

TABLE II. Failure of DDD Pacing to Reduce Symptoms or Left Ventricular Obstruction[a]

Inappropriate pacemaker programming
    Inadequate ventricular preexcitation: AV delay too long
    Interference with left atrial emptying: AV delay too short
Inadequate duration of trial of pacemaker therapy
Other associated abnormalities
    Proximal or high septal ventricular lead position
    Aberrant papillary muscle obstructing LV outflow
    Primary mitral valve regurgitation[b]
    Midcavity LV obstruction[c]
    Atrial and/or ventricular tachyarrhythmias
    LV diastolic dysfunction
    Myocardial ischemia
Inappropriate drug therapy
    Diuretic drugs
    Vasodilators
    Inotropic drugs
Symptoms unrelated to LV outflow obstruction
    LV diastolic dysfunction
    Arrhythmias
    Myocardial ischemia

[a]From Fananapazir et al. [18]. AV = atrioventricular; LV = left ventricular.
[b]Mitral valve regurgitation in obstructive hypertrophic cardiomyopathy may be primary and difficult to distinguish from severe mitral regurgitation due to septal anterior motion of the mitral valve when the outflow obstruction is relieved.
[c]Pacing may relieve midcavity obstruction if the ventricular lead is placed below the level of the obstruction.

requiring a permanent pacemaker [3–5]. Additionally, in some patients, the development of severe mitral regurgitation due to HOCM has required mitral valve replacement, a difficult and at times suboptimal therapy because of the reduced left ventricular cavity dimensions, which may interfere with prosthetic valve occluder motion. The long-term anticoagulation and its late prosthetic valve dysfunction makes this an option of last resort.

Induced Septal Infarction

The most recent technique, the induced septal infarction of the subaortic portion of the intraventricular septum by balloon occlusion with instillation of alcohol, as in our two patients, has been demonstrated to be a hemodynamically effective method of reducing left ventricular outflow tract obstruction. This procedure was first performed in 1995 by Sigwart [8], who noted that a brief septal artery balloon occlusion caused transient reduction in the outflow pressure gradient and that localized septal infarction with ethanol in three patients was effective over a longer follow-up.

In 1997, the clinical outcome of the first series of patients undergoing nonsurgical septal reduction for HOCM was reported by Knight et al. [9]. Eighteen patients underwent selective intraseptal alcohol injection to reduce left ventricular outflow obstruction. Doppler echo evaluation of left ventricular outflow gradients was performed before the procedure on the first postoperative day and at 3-month follow-up. Exercise testing and degree of symptom reduction 3 months after the procedure were also evaluated. Following the procedure, there

was a significant reduction in the left ventricular outflow obstruction gradient (67 to 25 mm Hg; $P < 0.0006$). At 3 months, the left ventricular outflow tract gradient stabilized at 22 mm Hg. The reduction in left ventricular outflow obstruction was associated with marked improvement in symptoms but an insignificant increase in exercise capacity in 10 patients of 25% time to symptoms. Left ventricular dimensions were not altered by alcohol septal ablation.

The complications in the first 18 patients included chest discomfort lasting from 1 to 2 min, which was treated with intravenous opiate analgesia. Four patients had complete heart block, although in none did the heart block remain permanent. Two patients had ventricular arrhythmias, one secondary to severe bradycardia during sheath removal. Ventricular tachycardia occurred in one patients as a consequence of alcohol leakage down the main lumen of the left anterior descending artery causing transient impairment of flow, marked ST elevation, and a large cardiac enzyme release. Arterial patency was restored by the following day without any long-term adverse events. The left ventricle appeared normal at follow-up. This complication was attributed to inadequate balloon occlusion of the first septal artery. This event led the investigators to caution operators that the balloon should not be positioned too proximally and should be of adequate size to prevent leakage. Injection of contrast into the septal artery through the balloon will ensure appropriate sealing of the septal artery prior to alcohol instillation, thus eliminating this complication.

In 1998, Seggewiss et al. [10] presented the acute and 3-month follow-up results of alcohol septal ablation in 25 patients. The mean age was 55 ± 15 years and 1.4 ± 0.6 septal branches were occluded with 4.1 ± 2.6 mL of 96% alcohol. Three-month follow-up of the left ventricular outflow tract gradient in 22 of 25 patients demonstrated a reduction from 62 ± 30 mm Hg (range, 4–152) to 19 ± 21 mm Hg (range, 0–74). The postextra systolic pressure gradient reduction was 141 ± 45 to 61 ± 40 mm Hg. Maximal CPK enzyme increase was 780 ± 436 units after 11 hr. In 13 of 25 patients, trifascicular block was present for 5 min to 8 days. Temporary and permanent pacing was required in 8 and 5 patients, respectively. One patient, an 86-year-old woman, died 8 days after alcohol septal ablation for ventricular fibrillation with beta-sympathomimetics for chronic obstructive pulmonary disease. All patients were discharged 11 days (range, 5–24) after the procedure. At 3-month follow-up, there were no late complications. Twenty-one patients decreased their New York Heart Association functional class from 3.01 ± 1.0 to 1.4 ± 1.1. A further reduction in left ventricular outflow tract gradient occurred in 14 patients.

In the short-term and initial series of patients undergoing the nonsurgical septal reduction technique, clinical outcomes have been uniformly beneficial. While it is clear that a large number of patients have not been studied in the United States, the initial 200 patients reported in the North American and European experience appear to support the application of this technique. This new method deserves serious consideration as an alternative to myomectomy for patients with HOCM.

Cautionary Notes

Fananapazir and McAreavey [18] have reviewed therapeutic options in patients with HOCM and severe drug-refractory symptoms. They note that patients with HOCM remain prone to arrhythmias and sudden death independent of the presence or degree of relief of left ventricular outflow tract obstruction. It has also been noted that hypertrophic left ventricular outflow tract obstruction is a highly variable condition [19] and may be induced by alterations of preload and intrathoracic pressures (cough, Valsalva maneuver). Functional mitral regurgitation due to increasing and adverse hemodynamic effects of systolic anterior motion of the mitral valve with increasing left ventricular outflow tract obstruction may also be the cause of disabling symptoms. Mid left ventricular cavity obstruction or complex forms of HOCM involving the apex, left ventricular, or right ventricular outflow tract may represent additional contributions to the symptoms

and adverse outcome [20,21]. Mechanically treating or chemically infarcting a hypertrophic septum may not necessarily alter impaired left ventricular diastolic and systolic function, subendocardial myocardial ischemia, or arrhythmias, all of which may coexist and result in the symptomatic incapacitation that has been attributed to the obstructive component of HOCM alone.

Nonetheless, in many cases of HOCM, left ventricular outflow obstruction appears linked to symptomatic status [6]. Therapies that reduce intraventricular pressure gradients appear to improve myocardial perfusion and reduce clinical symptoms [22,23]. As shown in the two case examples, septal ablation using ethanol infused into one or more of the septal perforators at the site of outflow obstruction produces significant reduction in left ventricular pressure and can improve clinical symptoms.

Complications of Alcohol Septal Ablation

Several authorities have expressed concern over the potential early and late complications of alcohol septal ablation [12,18]. Alcohol-induced septal infarction is a controlled myocardial infarction with its attendant complications, which may include conduction abnormalities, some requiring permanent pacemaker implantation in approximately 20%–30% of patients [9,10]. Ventricular arrhythmias and sudden death have been noted. Late complications of the procedure remain unknown. Conduction abnormalities resulting from septal infarction may increase the propensity for late complete heart block. Ventricular arrhythmias in patients with HOCM secondary to myocardial fiber disarray and fibrosis may be exacerbated by a segmentally infarcted myocardium leading to sustained ventricular arrhythmia or foci of arrhythmogenic ventricular myocardium.

Induced septal infarction may theoretically aggravate left ventricular dysfunction in the late course. Left ventricular hypertrophy eventually results in left ventricular remodeling with impairment of contractility despite an increased left ventricular wall thickness. Low wall stress and small left ventricular volume, although associated with a hypercontractile left ventricle, may obscure impaired systolic left ventricular function. In the late phase, alteration of myocytes, generation of fibrosis, myocardial cellular energy depletion, and diastolic dysfunction ultimately result in cardiac failure with left ventricular thinning. Whether the reduction in left ventricular pressure gradient at the time of septal ablation results in reduced left ventricular filling and improved myocardial perfusion with a delay of adverse events associated with left ventricular remodeling remains to be seen.

Contraindications to myomectomy, either surgical or alcohol septal ablation, include inadequate septal thickness (<18 mm), intrinsic mitral valve disease, or right bundle branch block. Relative contraindications may include significant left ventricular dysfunction or right bundle branch block.

Based on available data, it appears that alcohol septal ablation for HOCM is a promising nonsurgical catheter-based technique with significant immediate hemodynamic and clinical benefit. Long-term observations in large patient series are necessary to determine the durable therapeutic significance of this technique.

ACKNOWLEDGMENTS

The authors thank Dr. William Spencer and his associates of Baylor College of Medicine for their assistance and guidance in initiating the alcohol septal ablation program at Saint Louis University. The authors also thank the J.G. Mudd Cardiac Catheterization Laboratory Team and Donna Sander for manuscript preparation.

REFERENCES

1. Braunwald E, Lambrew CT, Rickoff SD, Ross J Jr, Morrow AG. Idiopathic hypertrophic subaortic stenosis. I. A description of the disease based upon an analysis of 64 patients. Circulation 1964; 30(suppl 4):3–119.
2. Rosing DR, Idanpaan-Heikkila U, Maron BJ, Bonow RO, Epstein SE. Use of calcium-blocking drugs in hypertrophic cardiomyopathy. Am J Cardiol 1985;55:185B–195B.
3. Morrow AG, Reitz BA, Epstein SE, Henry WL, Conkle DM, Itscoitz SB, Redwood DR. Operative treatment in hypertrophic subaortic stenosis: techniques and the results of pre- and post-operative assessment in 83 patients. Circulation 1975;52:88–102.
4. Mohr R, Schaff HV, Danielson GK, Puga FJ, Pluth JR, Tajik AJ. The outcome of surgical treatment of hypertrophic obstructive cardiomyopathy: experience over 15 years. J Thorac Cardiovasc Surg 1989;97:666–674.
5. Krajcer Z, Leachman R, Cooley D, Coronado R. Septal myotomy-myomectomy versus mitral valve replacement in hypertrophic cardiomyopathy: ten year follow-up in 185 patients. Circulation 1989;80(suppl 1):I57–I64.
6. Fananapazir L, Canon RO III, Tripodi D, Panza JA. Impact of dual chamber permanent pacing in patients with obstructive hypertrophic cardiomyopathy with symptoms refractory to verapamil and beta-adrenergic blocker therapy. Circulation 1992;85:2149–2161.
7. Jeanrenaud X, Goy J-J, Kappenberger L. Effects of dual-chamber pacing in hypertrophic obstructive cardiomyopathy. Lancet 1992; 339:1318–1323.
8. Sigwart U. Non-surgical myocardial reduction for hypertrophic obstructive cardiomyopathy. Lancet 1995;346:211–214.
9. Knight C, Kurbaan AS, Seggewiss H, Henein M, Gunning M, Harrington D, Fassbender D, Gleichmann U, Sigwart U. Nonsurgical septal reduction for hypertrophic obstructive cardiomyopathy: outcome in the first series of patients. Circulation 1997;95:2075–2081.
10. Seggewiss H, Gleichmann U, Faber L, Fassbender D, Schmidt HK, Strick S. Percutaneous transluminal septal myocardial ablation in hypertrophic obstructive cardiomyopathy: acute results and 3-month follow-up in 25 patients. J Am Coll Cardiol 1998;31:252–258.
11. Oakley CM. Non-surgical ablation of the ventricular septum for the treatment of hypertrophic cardiomyopathy. Lancet 1995;346:1624.
12. Braunwald E. Induced septal infarction: a new therapeutic strategy for hypertrophic obstructive cardiomyopathy. Circulation 1997;95:1981–1982.
13. Fananapazir L, Epstein ND, Panza A, Curiel R, Tripodi D, McAreavey D. Long-term results of dual chamber (DDD) pacing in obstructive hypertrophic cardiomyopathy: evidence for progressive symptomatic and hemodynamic improvement and reduction of left ventricular hypertrophy. Circulation 1994;90:2731–2742.
14. Simon JP, Sadoul N, de Chillou C, et al. Long-term dual chamber pacing improves hemodynamic function in patients with obstructive hypertrophic cardiomyopathy. PACE (Abstract) 1995;18:1769.
15. Sadoul N, Simon J-P, Bruntz J-F, Isaaz K, de Chillou C, Beurrier D, Dodinot B, Aliot E. Long-term dual chamber pacing reduces left ventricular mass in patients with obstructive hypertrophic cardiomyopathy. J Am Coll Cardiol 1993;21:94A.
16. McAreavey D, Fananapazir L. Altered cardiac hemodynamic and electrical state in normal sinus rhythm following chronic dual chamber pacing for relief of left ventricular outflow obstruction in hypertrophic cardiomyopathy. Am J Cardiol 1992;70:651–656.
17. Fananapazir L, Dilsizian V, Bonow RO. Dual chamber pacing relieves angina and improves myocardial perfusion abnormalities in patients with obstructive hypertrophic cardiomyopathy. Circulation 1992;86:I272.
18. Fananapazir L, McAreavey D. Therapeutic options in patients with obstructive hypertrophic cardiomyopathy and severe drug-refractory symptoms. J Am Coll Cardiol 1998;31:259–264.
19. Kizilbash AM, Heinle SK, Grayburn PA. Spontaneous variability of left ventricular outflow tract gradient in hypertrophic obstructive cardiomyopathy. Circulation 1998;97:461–466.
20. Spirito P, Chiarella F, Carratino L, Berisso MZ, Bellotti P, Vecchio C. Clinical course and prognosis of hypertrophic cardiomyopathy in an out-patient population. N Engl J Med 1989;320:749–755.
21. Maron BJ, Bonow RO, Cannon RO, Leon MB, Epstein SE. Hypertrophic cardiomyopathy: interrelations of clinical manifestations, pathophysiology, and therapy. N Engl J Med 1987;316:780–789, 844–852.
22. McCully RB, Nishimura RA, Tajik AJ, Schaff HV, Danielson GK. Extent of clinical improvement after surgical treatment of hypertrophic obstructive cardiomyopathy. Circulation 1996;94:467–471.
23. Heric B, Lytle BW, Miller DP, Rosenkranz ER, Lever HM, Cosgrove DM. Surgical management of hypertrophic obstructive cardiomyopathy: early and late results. J Thorac Cardiovasc Surg 1995;110:195–208.

PART VI: CORONARY HEMODYNAMICS

The practical applications of coronary physiology have had an impact among interventional cardiologists around the world. The use of coronary pressure and flow beyond research has matured to a clinical stage whereby absolute and relative coronary flow velocity reserve and pressure-derived fractional flow reserve (FFR, hyperemic distal to aortic pressure across a stenosis) can determine precisely the pressure-flow relationship and potential for myocardial ischemia of any given lesion. The detailed hemodynamic analysis of such lesions has led to improved decision making and outcomes for many patients with coronary artery disease. The description of coronary hemodynamics has been substantially enlarged and collated in a companion to this book entitled "Interventional Physiology Rounds: Case Studies in Coronary Pressure and Flow for Clinical Practice" (Wiley-Liss, 1996). Case studies for different applications of these specialized coronary hemodynamic data provide real work use of such measurements and highlight benefits as well as limitations.

The rationale to use coronary physiology arises from the goal of coronary interventions which, in most patients, is the relief of ischemic symptoms and myocardial dysfunction through the restoration of coronary blood flow. The search for suitable techniques to diagnose the flow-limiting nature of a coronary stenosis and assess procedural endpoints beyond angiography has been principally confined to noninvasive methods due to inadequate direct means to measure coronary blood flow in awake subjects in the catheterization laboratory.

Miniaturization of pressure and flow guidewire sensors for catheter-based interventions has extended the applications of both vessel imaging and physiology to the invasive investigation and treatment of coronary artery disease.

The newest use of translesional pressure, FFR, makes the concept of resting pressure gradients obsolete. Fractional flow reserve is defined as the maximum blood flow in the presence of a coronary stenosis, divided by normal maximum flow in the same artery. It is a lesion-specific index of the functional significance of the epicardial stenosis. It indicates the maximum perfusion of the myocardium supplied by that particular coronary artery. FFR has a number of unique features which enable clinical decision making in the catheterization laboratory. These features are listed in the table below and will be further discussed in the section chapters.

• FFRmyo is a lesion-specific index of epicardial stenosis severity.
• FFRmyo is independent of heart rate, blood pressure, and contractility.
• FFRmyo has an unequivocal normal value of 1.0 for every patient, every coronary artery, and every myocardial distribution.
• A value of FFRmyo of 0.75 distinguishes functionally significant and non-significant lesions with an accuracy of 95%.
• FFRmyo takes into account the contribution of collateral flow to myocardial perfusion.
• FFRmyo can be applied in single and multivessel disease. There is no need for a normal control artery to compare with.
• FFRmyo can be easily obtained, both at diagnostic and interventional procedures, by the ratio of mean hyperemic distal coronary pressure and aortic pressure:

• $FFRmyo = \dfrac{P_d}{P_a}$

Establishing objective indications for interventions is of critical importance for patient care. Particularly for questionable angiographic findings before or following angioplasty, the decisions for proceeding with treatment in the absence of other clinical data can now be augmented by objective physiologic data. Interventional physiology has provided new information about patient outcomes after cardiac catheterization and interventions. The table below lists current clinical applications of interventional physiology.

Clinical Applications of Interventional Physiology

Angioplasty
    Endpoint
    Monitoring complications
    Assessing additional lesions
    Collateral flow
    Stenting
    Atherectomy
Coronary vasodilatory reserve
    Chest pain, normal coronary arteries, syndrome X
    Transplant coronary arteriopathy
    Saphenous vein graft, internal mammary artery physiology
Coronary research
    Pharmacologic studies
    Intraaortic balloon pumping
    Coronary physiology of valvular disease
    Scintigraphic perfusion imaging correlation
    Endothelial function

Morton J. Kern, MD

Chapter 30

Coronary Hemodynamics—Section I:
Coronary Catheter Pressures

Morton J. Kern, MD

INTRODUCTION

The arterial pressure waveform from the tip of the catheter during coronary angiography is an important key to a safe procedure. One of the earliest clues to the presence of left main coronary stenosis is a characteristically abnormal arterial pressure immediately upon catheter engagement of the coronary ostium. The pressure waves in these patients are often referred to as ventricularized or damped. Ventricularization of coronary pressure has a recognized association with left main coronary stenosis by experienced angiographers over several decades [1–4]. It is critically important to identify and understand these coronary catheter waveforms. The significance of such an altered waveform during coronary angiography must be appreciated early in the angiographers career to avoid the catastrophic outcome after diagnostic angiography that has been associated with some patients with left main coronary stenosis.

CASE EXAMPLES
Pressure "Ventricularization"

A 60-yr-old woman had a 1 yr history of exertional chest pain with progressive pain over the past 3 months. In the past 1 month episodes of chest pain occurred with minimal exertion and at rest. An exercise test performed 1 day prior to coronary angiography revealed a reduced exercise tolerance (3 min, 40 sec) with 2 mm ST segment flattening in leads V_2–V_5, II, III and AVF (at 2 min) which accompanied anginal chest pain. Exercise testing was stopped after 2mm ST segment depression was iden-

tified. The ST segment depression persisted 8 min into recovery. The patient was admitted to the hospital and scheduled for cardiac catheterization the next day.

In the cardiac catheterization laboratory, coronary arteriography was performed in a routine (femoral) fashion using a 6 French Judkins diagnostic catheter. Catheter tip pressure from this patient during angiography is shown on Figure 1. On catheter tip engagement, arterial pressure dropped from 140 mm Hg to 60 mm Hg (systolic) with diastolic pressures dropping from 80 mm Hg to 35 mm Hg. A brief coronary injection was performed with immediate withdrawal of the catheter as evidenced by the rapid return of arterial pressure to normal. Note the wide pulse pressure, rapid diastolic decline and small positive deflection immediately before systolic upstroke. This pressure pattern, sometimes called ventricularized, is very commonly seen in patients with left main stenosis. To limit the time of impaired perfusion with the catheter partially obstructing the coronary ostium, the operator performed a "hit-and-run" maneuver with brief contrast injection and rapid removal of the catheter. Normal pressure and blood flow are resumed. Figure 2 is a frame from the shallow right anterior oblique coronary angiogram.

A similar hemodynamic tracing was obtained in a 65-yr-old man with chest pain following coronary artery bypass graft surgery. The left main coronary was previously known to be narrowed by 50%. On engagement of the coronary catheter (Fig. 3), the arterial pressure pattern showed characteristic changes of "ventricularization". Coronary arteriography was performed with immediate withdrawal of the catheter tip ("hit-and-run"

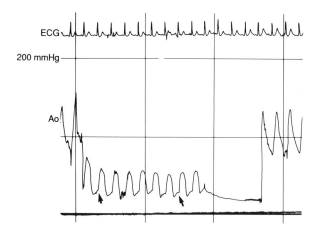

Fig. 1. Coronary catheter pressure before and during engagement of the left main coronary artery and during pullback of catheter immediately following injection. Arrow indicates presystolic positive deflection. See text for details.

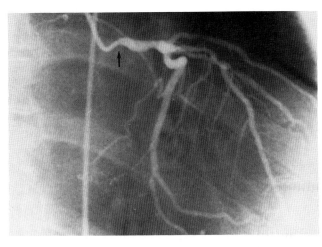

Fig. 2. Coronary angiogram (shallow right anterior oblique projection) showing left coronary ostial stenosis (arrow). Note the absence of contrast reflux into the aorta.

maneuver). In this patient, the arterial systolic presure dropped from 140 mm Hg to 100 mm Hg and diastolic pressure dropped from 75 mm Hg to 40 mm Hg (remember, left ventricular end-diastolic pressure is usually < 25 mm Hg, especially if clinical congestion is absent). Note the electrocardiogram which showed characteristic ST and T wave changes associated with contrast media injection. Should these "pseudoischemic" changes persist after angiography, myocardial ischemia should be suspected and immediate therapy be instituted to prevent the downward spiral of left ventricular ischemic decompensation with hypotension after contrast injection.

Pressure "Damping"

Significant pressure changes can also occur during angiography of the right coronary artery. In general, right coronary pressure alterations are more common due, in part, to a smaller artery, subselective conus branch engagement or catheter-induced coronary spasm. Ostial right coronary stenosis may give a "ventricularized" pattern. These changes carry less significant consequences unless left main or severe multivessel left coronary stenosis are also present.

The coronary pressure (Fig. 4) was recorded during injection of a right coronary artery in a patient with angina and positive exercise test. Thallium scintigraphic redistribution was present in the inferior and lateral regions. The coronary pressure damped on catheter tip engagement. Contrast was injected 15 sec after (rapid) positioning of the x-ray c-arm. The injector syringe pressure was recorded demonstrating the time, duration and intensity (pressure) of hand injection during the right coronary artery angiogram. The "hit-and-run" maneu-

ver also shows the immediate return of normal arterial pressure upon completion of contrast injection.

Ventricularization or Ventricular Pressure?

Simultaneous femoral artery 8 French femoral artery sheath and a 7 French Judkins coronary catheter pressures were recorded prior to left coronary angiography (Fig. 5). Pressure "ventricularization" was observed followed by transient asystole. The catheter was rapidly removed with return of sinus rhythm. Examine these tracings closely. Is this "ventricularization"? Why is there immediate asystole? From examination of the 2 pressures, the coronary pressure was actually left ventricular pressure. The catheter had fallen into the left ventricle. Coronary pressure "ventricularization" (on Fig. 3) differs from true left ventricular pressure in several important respects. Left ventricular pressure has equivalent systolic and aortic pressures and considerably lower end-diastolic pressure (in this example 20 mm Hg). The characteristic waveform pattern of true ventricular pressure is evident. This catheter had slipped into the left ventricle and prior to contrast injection, asystole occurred probably by stimulation of the left bundle creating transient left bundle block in the setting of a pre-existing right bundle branch block. On catheter removal, restoration of the left bundle conduction occurred and cardiac rhythm was restored with normal blood pressure. The morphology of "ventricularized" coronary pressure also has a distinct presystolic deflection resembling an 'a' wave. The upstroke is also slower than aortic pressure and down stroke steeper than aortic pressure. The pressure tracing of Figure 5 demonstrates that not all "ventricularization" is due to coronary pressure damping and

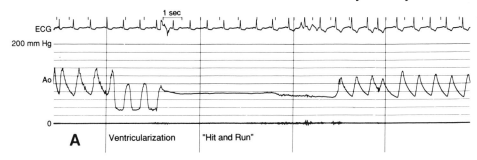

A   Ventricularization   "Hit and Run"

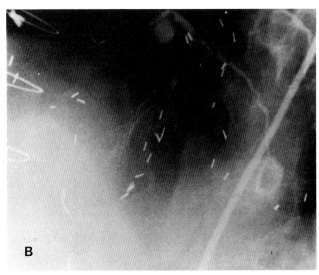

B

Fig. 3. A: Hemodynamic and electrocardiographic tracings during coronary angiography of a patient with left main coronary stenosis. On engagement of the left main coronary artery, ventricularization of the pressure waveform is noted. Contrast injection occurs during a brief "hit-and-run" period lasting approximately 5–7 sec with withdrawal of the catheter. Note the alterations of electrocardiogram immediately after contrast injection with marked T wave inversion. This contrast-induced ischemic pattern generally will revert to normal. See text for details. B: Left anterior oblique frame from cineangiogram demonstrating 80% left main coronary narrowing.

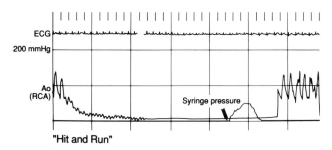

"Hit and Run"

Fig. 4. Right coronary pressure during contrast injection using a "hit-and-run" maneuver. Damping of pressure during right coronary artery does not show the ventricularization pattern. The technique of contrast injection is demonstrated by the injection syringe pressure (arrow) which was measured during this study. On immediate pullback of the catheter, aortic pressure is restored. There were no significant electrocardiographic abnormalities during this injection.

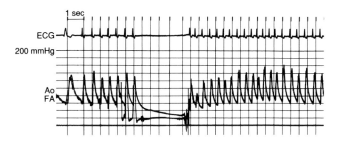

Fig. 5. Simultaneous aortic and femoral artery pressures measured prior to coronary angiography. Is this coronary "ventricularization"? See text for details.

that complications during coronary angiography may occur from causes other than catheters limiting coronary flow. The problem presented on Figure 5 is obvious during fluoroscopy and its identification immediately apparent. However, an inattentive operator may take several seconds to react promptly to limit asystole and hypotension.

Mechanisms of "Ventricularization"

The mechanisms of coronary pressure damping have been studied by Pacold et al. [5]. Variable degrees of intracoronary pressure changes upon cannulation of diseased left main coronary arteries were observed in 20 consecutive patients with ventricularization of coronary pressure. Confirmation of these pressure waveforms was obtained in an animal model by inserting a balloon-

tipped catheter and producing partial degrees of occlusion of the left main coronary artery.

The ventricularized pressure wave is derived from aortic pressure which is altered by its transmission across the narrowed left main coronary artery. Advancing a catheter into the ostium of a narrowed coronary artery reduces both systolic and diastolic pressures, as well as causing a steep decline of the pressure in diastole. A characteristic increase in pressure at end-diastole with a pre-systolic positive deflection was thought to be related to atrial contraction. This 'a' waveform (seen on Fig. 1, arrow), although at times inconspicuous, is more likely generated by the motion of the ascending aorta during systole [5]. The degree of pressure drop between the ascending aorta and stenosed left main coronary artery is variable depending on the degree of stenosis. Pacold et al. [5] also note that ventricularization may be seen in conditions other than left main coronary artery stenosis, such as matching diameters of the coronary artery and catheter or a deeply seated subselective position into a stenosed branch artery. Pressures from small right coronary arteries and stenosed proximal vein grafts may also demonstrate this phenomenon. The concept that "ventricularization" may occur by an unfavorable position of the catheter tip against an arterial wall without stenosis does not appear to be supported by the demonstration of Pacold et al. [5]. "Ventricularization" remains a critically important observation related to left main coronary artery stenosis. Appropriate special techniques to obtain safe angiograms for this situation should be employed [6].

Appropriate precautions in patients with suspected left main disease involve performing a non-selective aortic cusp flush, a brief "hit-and-run" injection in a shallow RAO or AP projection. Minimizing the number of contrast injections is important. Performance of ventriculography depends on a low risk/high benefit ratio. A low volume, digital subtraction ventriculogram may be a helpful "one-test" study for immediate surgical consultation. In patients with critical left main stenosis, insertion of an intra-aortic balloon pump and rapid transfer for emergency cardiac surgery may be required.

SUMMARY

The coronary pressure waveforms described in this rounds are an integral part of the angiographers approach to all patients, especially those with suspected left main coronary stenosis [7]. Patient management will differ according to the laboratory experience and training of the operators. Recognition and appreciation of abnormal coronary pressure waveforms may directly affect the life and death of these patients.

ACKNOWLEDGMENT

The author wishes to thank Donna Sander for manuscript preparation.

REFERENCES

1. Pritchard DO, Mudd JG, Barner HB: Coronary ostial stenosis. Circulation 52:46–48, 1975.
2. Baim DS, Grossman W: Coronary angiography. In: Grossman W, (ed) "Cardiac Catheterization and Angiography". Philadelphia: Lea & Febiger, 177–178, 1986.
3. Salem BI, Terasawa M, Mathur VS, Garcia E, deCastro CM, Hall RJ: Left main coronary artery ostial stenosis: Clinical markers, angiographic recognition and distinction from left main disease. Cathet Cardiovasc Diagn 5:125–134, 1979.
4. Cameron A, Kemp HG, Fisher LD, et al. Left main coronary artery stenosis: Angiographic determination. Circulation 68:484–489, 1983.
5. Pacold I, Hwang MH, Piao ZE, Scanlon PJ, Loeb HS: The mechanism and significance of ventricularization of intracoronary pressure during coronary angiography. Am Heart J 118:1160–1166, 1989.
6. Kern MJ: Approach to the patient with left main coronary artery stenosis. Cathet Cardiovasc Diagn 18:181–182, 1989.
7. Gordon PR, Abrams C, Gash AK, Carebello BA: Pericatheterization risk factors in left main coronary artery stenosis. Am J Cardiol 59:1080–1083, 1987.

Chapter 31

Coronary Hemodynamics—Section II:
Patterns of Coronary Flow Velocity

Morton J. Kern, MD

INTRODUCTION

The measurement of coronary blood flow in patients has been of interest to cardiologists since the beginning of cardiac catheterization. Until recently blood flow methodologies have been cumbersome and technically difficult. Indicator dilution and washout techniques had time constants too slow to measure rapid, precise changes in blood flow responses. Electromagnetic flow probes were limited to anesthetized patients in the operating suite. In the past decade, among the most successful methods was measurement of coronary venous efflux by the thermodilution technique as described by Ganz et al. [1] and refined by Pepine et al. [2]. This technique, estimating left ventricular myocardial flow, has been replaced by direct measurement of intra-arterial blood flow velocity using miniaturized Doppler crystals placed on small catheters [3,4]. With the use of the intracoronary Doppler technique, examination of coronary physiology under a variety of circumstances can be easily and safely obtained, offering new insights into coronary circulation in awake, unanesthetized patients. Although routinely studied in the early years of medical school, the responses of the coronary circulation as observed in patients in the cardiac catheterization laboratory are not generally familiar to cardiologists commonly performing the procedures. This ''rounds'' will examine patterns of coronary blood flow velocity signals that can be easily obtained with available catheters and will illustrate alterations occurring during common respiratory maneuvers and cardiac arrhythmias.

The use of coronary blood flow velocity measure-ments to determine the coronary vasodilatory reserve and the responses to hyperemic stimuli will be the subject of part III of coronary hemodynamics.

Techniques of Intracoronary Blood Flow Velocity Measurements

There are currently 3 Doppler catheters and one Doppler guide wire available to measure intracoronary blood flow velocity. One catheter is non-selective [5] and the other two catheters and guidewire measure sub-selective coronary velocity (Fig. 1). These tools employ the Doppler principle [6] and provide accurate measurement of red cell velocity moving down the coronary artery. The nonselective catheter technique is identical to standard Judkins catheter placement [5]. The subselective methods are nearly identical to placement of a coronary angioplasty balloon catheter [3,4,7]. An intracoronary 3 F Doppler catheter is advanced over a 0.014 in. very flexible angioplasty guidewire using a standard guiding catheter and Y connector. Intravenous heparin is required. The intracoronary Doppler catheter can be placed in any branch of the coronary tree. Once the Doppler catheter is positioned, the signal is adjusted moving the range of the sample volume 2–5 mm from the tip to optimize the waveform.

Consider the hemodynamic tracings obtained in the left anterior descending coronary artery in a 52-yr-old woman with an atypical chest pain syndrome (Fig. 2). Coronary flow velocity was measured to assess coronary vasodilatory reserve. Recall which points of aortic pressure demarcate the onset and cessation of coronary blood flow. Figure 1 shows the simultaneously recorded aortic

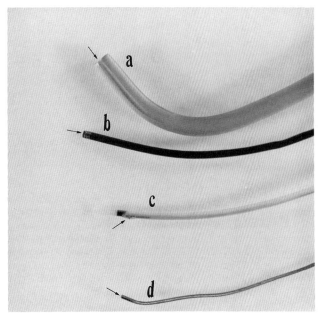

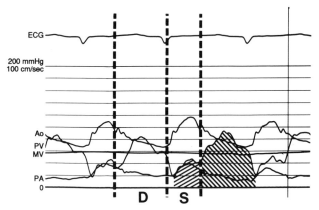

Fig. 2. Coronary flow velocity tracing with aortic and pulmonary artery pressures in a patient with normal coronary arteries. See text for details. Ao = aortic pressure; PV = phasic velocity; MV = mean velocity; PA = pulmonary artery pressure; S = systole; D = diastole. (Shaded areas correspond to flow integrals defined in Fig. 3).

Fig. 1. Coronary flow velocity catheters and guidewires. a: Judkins-style Doppler, b: Millar (end mounted crystal), c: Numed Doppler (side mounted crystal), d: Cardiometrics 0.018 in guidewire. Arrows indicate location and angle of Doppler beam.

and pulmonary artery pressure, phasic and mean coronary flow velocity signals, along with the electrocardiogram. The waveform of coronary flow velocity is typical, with the predominant flow velocity wave occurring in diastole. This normal waveform demonstrates a relatively rapid increase in diastolic flow velocity immediately following the aortic dicrotic notch and a rapid fall-off of the flow velocity signal just after the onset of systole. There is usually a small systolic component, approximately 25 to 50% of the diastolic flow velocity curve. The (electronic) mean velocity is computed from the integrated area of flow during both systole and diastole. The flow velocity signal is generally stable during respiratory maneuvers. If the ultrasound beam is directed into the arterial wall, the signal can be obscured, producing an artifactually low waveform. The waveform of flow velocity may be altered to various degrees of atherosclerotic disease within the coronary artery. In this example, the patient had normal coronary arteries with a normal flow velocity pattern. Figure 3 demonstrates several features of the flow velocity wave that can be quantitated.

Coronary Blood Flow Velocity During Respiratory Maneuvers

A 60-yr-old woman undergoing diagnostic coronary angiography has a 3 sec sinus arrest on injection of the right coronary artery. The operator asks the patient to cough vigorously. What does coughing do to coronary

blood flow? Although in the early years of angiography coughing was thought to clear contrast from the coronary arteries, we now know its only mechanism is maintenance of arterial pressure until normal cardiac rhythm is restored [8,9]. The effect of increased intrathoracic pressure on coronary blood flow velocity has been previously examined both echocardiographically [9] and by direct flow measurement [10] and demonstrates that neither coughing nor Valsalva augment coronary blood flow velocity. Examine the hemodynamic tracings in a patient with normal coronary arteries (Fig. 4). Cough increases both aortic pressure (> 240 mm Hg) and right atrial pressure (210 mm Hg) together producing a marked and parallel pressure increase. The pulse pressure (the difference between aortic diastolic and right atrial pressure, A) remains the same or decreases during cough (B'). The cough pulse pressure (B') is associated with a marked decrease in coronary flow velocity without any augmentation of either peak or mean flow on the subsequent beat(s). The limited and often reduced flow velocity is present whether single or multiple coughs are performed. With sustained increases of intrathoracic pressure that occurs with continuous coughing (Fig. 5), there is a prolonged and sustained decrease in coronary flow velocity.

The same physiology appears to apply for the coronary flow velocity changes occurring during the increased intrathoracic pressure of the Valsalva maneuver (Fig. 6). Although intrathoracic pressure is markedly increased during phase III, coronary blood flow velocity does not increase and, for most studies, declines slightly or remains unchanged [10–12].

Benign sinus arrhythmia and normal respiratory activity causes cyclical alterations in aortic pressure. Small changes in myocardial oxygen demand occur consistent

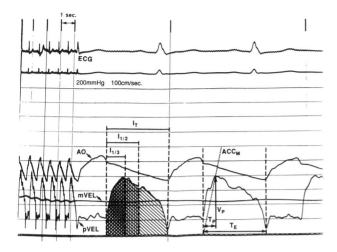

Fig. 3. Coronary flow velocity tracing and measurements made by analysis of the flow velocity waveform. I_T = diastolic flow velocity integral; T_P = time to peak; T_E = total duration of diastole; $I_{1/2}$ = first one-half of diastolic flow velocity integral; $I_{1/3}$ = first one-third of flow velocity integral; ACC_M = acceleration time to peak velocity; V_P = peak velocity; mVEL = mean velocity; pVEL = phasic velocity. With permission from Kern MJ, Deligonul U, Vandormael M, Lavovitz A, Gudipati R, Gabliani G, Bodet J, Shah Y, Kennedy HL: Impaired coronary vasodilatory reserve in the immediate post-coronary angioplasty period: Analysis of coronary arterial velocity flow indices and regional cardiac venous efflux. J Am Coll Cardiol 13:868–872, 1989.

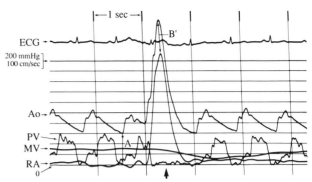

Fig. 4. Coronary flow velocity signals during cough (arrow). A = diastolic aortic pressure and right atrial pressure (RA); B′ = pulse pressure during cough. Arrow shows phasic flow velocity signal during diastolic period of cough. Reprinted with permission from Kern MJ, Gudipati G, Tatineni S, Aguirre F, Serota H, Deligonul U: Effect of abruptly increased intrathoracic pressure on coronary blood flow velocity in patients. Am Heart J 119: 863–870, 1990.

with the increasing and decreasing heart rate-pressure products. Examine the corresponding coronary flow velocity signal measured in a patient without coronary artery disease during sinus arrhythmia (Fig. 7). The mean and peak phasic flow velocity signals demonstrate parallel changes in response to alteration in arterial pressure during respiration. Coronary flow velocity, as shown in this patient, accurately reflects the autoregulatory response of the normal coronary circulation. With the appreciation of autoregulation and its effect on coronary flow velocity, can one predict what the result of loss of atrial activity would do to coronary flow velocity? Examine the data record in a patient who had temporary ventricular pacing for transient heart block during coronary arteriography (Fig. 8). Aortic pressure and mean and phasic coronary flow velocity were measured during a period of transition from sinus rhythm to paced rhythm and return to sinus rhythm. The coronary flow velocity remained nearly constant with a slight decline in the peak flow velocity during the period of ventricular pacing with loss of atrial activity. As the atrial contribution returns to the rhythm, flow velocity undergoes only an insignificant change. Although loss of atrial activity with decreased aortic pressure would likely reduce demand, the result on autoregulation in this patient was not reflected in a reduction in coronary flow velocity. Com-

pare this response with the marked changes seen in the patient in Figure 7 during sinus arrhythmia.

Coronary Flow Velocity During Atrial Fibrillation

Atrial fibrillation is a common arrhythmia in which very rapid ventricular depolarizations may cause ineffective arterial pressure generation. Although a loss of coronary flow during the pulse deficit might be anticipated, coronary flow velocity has not been commonly observed in these patients. Consider the systemic and pulmonary artery pressures and coronary flow velocity measured in a patient with atrial fibrillation and periods of rapid ventricular response (Fig. 9). During the cardiac cycles of different durations coronary flow, as measured by the flow-velocity area (time $\times$ flow = integral), varied in proportion to the RR cylce length with the mean flow remaining relatively constant. On beats #1 and #2, flow-velocity area was reduced from 23.7 to 13.0 units with reduced RR intervals of 933 to 667 msec. After beat #3 (Fig. 9) the ventricular rhythm exceeds 150 beats/ min (ventricular couplet). Coronary blood flow in beat #4 was abbreviated by the next early ventricular beat (flow integral = 5.8 units). Arterial pressure continued to decline and was not affected. The flow velocity was maintained during the subsequent rapid beats despite the loss of arterial pressure. A small arterial pressure wave, generated by beat #5, was associated with significant augmentation of the coronary blood flow integral (20.0 units), despite the minimal contribution to peripheral or coronary pressure.

Coronary Flow During Ventricular Tachycardia

Although rarely witnessed, as one might expect, coronary blood flow ceases during the disorganized rhythm

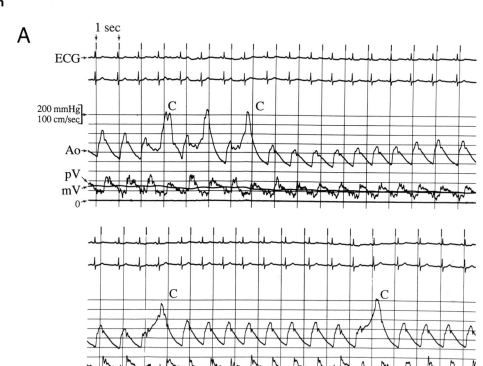

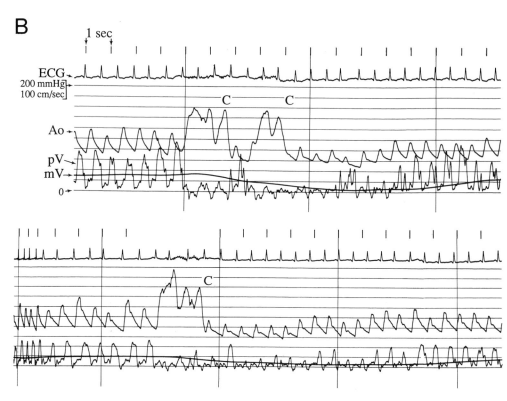

Fig. 5. Aortic and coronary flow velocity tracings during cough. Panel A shows single and multiple coughs (C). Panel B demonstrates sustained coughing reduced coronary flow velocity for a more prolonged period. These effects on coronary flow are present whether coronary flow velocity is measured proximally (top tracings of panels) or distally (bottom tracings of panels). Reprinted with permission from Kern, MJ, Gudipati C, Tatineni S, Aguirre F, Serota H, Deligonul U: Effect of abruptly increased intrathoracic pressure on coronary blood flow velocity in patients. Am Heart J 119:863–870, 1990.

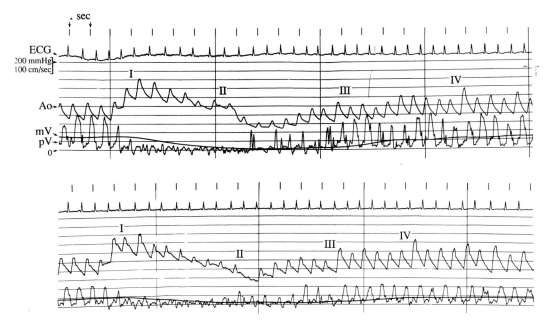

Fig. 6. Coronary flow velocity during Valsalva maneuver. Abbreviations as in Figure 2. Reprinted with permission from Kern MJ, Gudipati C, Tatineni S, Aguiree F, Serota H, Deligonul U: Effect of abruptly increased intrathoracic pressure on coronary blood flow velocity in patients. Am Heart J 119:863–870, 1990.

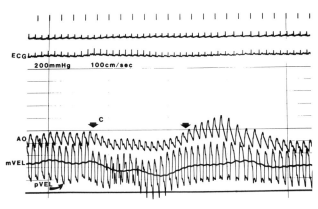

Fig. 7. Coronary flow velocity during sinus arrhythmia and respiratory variation. Note marked decline in arterial pressure (first arrow) with return on next respiratory cycle (second arrow). See text for details.

of ventricular tachycardia. Ineffective ventricular systole limits pressure generation and the markedly shortened diastole fails to permit ventricular relaxation curtailing coronary flow. Coronary flow velocity was measured in a patient undergoing diagnostic catheterization to determine coronary vasodilatory reserve (Fig. 10). Intracoronary papaverine (10 mg) was used as the hyperemic stimulus to produce maximal coronary flow. Intracoronary papaverine has been associated with prolongation of the QT interval and rare episodes of Torsade de Pointes and ventricular tachycardia [13]. Examine the hemodynamic

and coronary blood flow velocity tracings in Figure 10. Premature ventricular contractions preceded ventricular tachycardia. During ventricular tachycardia, when aortic pressure was not produced, coronary blood flow velocity rapidly fell to zero. Immediate defibrillation restored both rhythm and coronary flow with no residual adverse effects. Unlike ventricular fibrillation and depending on the rate, slow ventricular tachycardia (as seen on the couplet after beat #3, Fig. 9) could maintain some degree of coronary flow. Regardless of the coronary flow patterns, restoration of a normal rhythm for these patients is of obvious importance.

SUMMARY

These specialized tracings illustrate several important patterns of coronary blood flow velocity that may occur in patients during diagnostic cardiac catheterization. Recent advances in catheter methodologies [14] permit easy measurement of coronary blood flow during routine coronary angiography. At the current time, measurement of coronary blood flow velocity remains a research technique but is of continuing interest in clinical syndromes of atypical angina, myocardial hypertrophy and infarction, early transplant rejection, or premature (subangiographic) atherosclerosis in some patients.

A later hemodynamic rounds will examine the effects of coronary blood flow velocity and various hyperemic stimuli to assess coronary vasodilatory reserve.

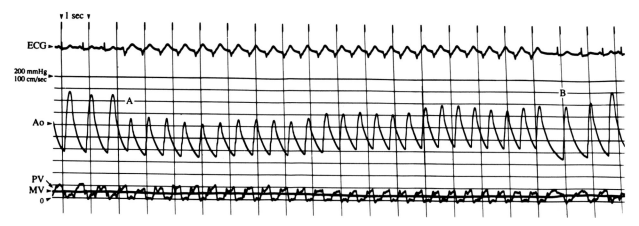

Fig. 8.   Arterial pressure and coronary flow velocity during temporary pacemaking. Pacemaker rhythm begins at beat #4 (A) and terminates 14 sec later at (B). See text for details.

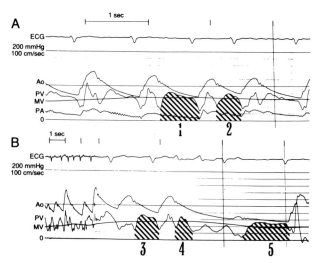

Fig. 9.   Coronary flow velocity during atrial fibrillation for long and short cardiac cycles. Cycle length during beats #1 and 2 is 933 and 667 msec with flow velocity integrals (23.7 and 13.0 units, shaded areas), respectively. During beat #5 coronary flow velocity is augmented over a long RR interval (1,000 msec) with flow velocity integral (20.0 units). See text for details.

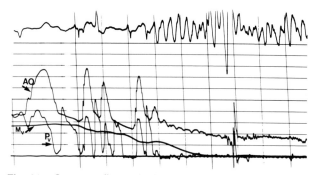

Fig. 10.   Coronary flow velocity during an episode of Torsade de Pointes and ventricular fibrillation. Abbreviations as in Figure 2. Reprinted from Kern MJ, Deligonul U, Serota H, Gudipati C, Buckingham T: Ventricular arrhythmia due to intracoronary papaverine: Analysis of clinical and hemodynamic data with coronary vasodilatory reserve. Cathet Cardiovasc Diagn 19: 229–236, 1990.

ACKNOWLEDGMENTS

The author thanks Donna Sander for manuscript preparation.

REFERENCES

1. Ganz W, Tamura K, Marcus HS, et al.: Measurement of coronary sinus blood flow by continuous thermodilution in man. Circulation 44:181–195, 1971.

2. Pepine CJ, Mehta J, Webster WW, Nichols WW: In vivo validation of a thermodilution method to determine regional left ventricular blood flow in patients with coronary disease. Circulation 58(5):795–802, 1978.

3. Wilson RF, Laughlin DE, Ackell PH, Chilian WM, Holida MD, Hartley CJ, Armstrong ML, Marcus ML, White CW: Transluminal, subselective measurement of coronary artery blood flow velocity and vasodilator reserve in man. Circulation 72:82, 1985.

4. Marcus ML, Wright C, Doty D, et al.: Measurement of coronary velocity and reactive hyperemia in the coronary circulation of humans. Circ Res 49:877–891, 1981.

5. Kern MJ, Courtois M, Ludbrook P: A simplified method to measure coronary blood flow velocity in patients: Validation and application of a Judkins-style Doppler-tipped angiographic catheter. Am Heart J 120:1202–1212, 1990.

6. Hatle L, Angelsen B: In "Doppler Ultrasound in Cardiology. Flow Velocity and Volumetric Principles." Philadelphia: Lea & Febiger, 1985, p 14.

7. Kern MJ, Deligonul U, Vandormael M, Lavoritz A, Gudipati R, Gabliani G, Bodet J, Shah Y, Kennedy HL: Impaired coronary vasodilatory reserve in the immediate post-coronary angioplasty period: Analysis of coronary arterial velocity flow indices and regional cardiac venous efflux. J Am Coll Cardiol 13:868–872, 1989.

8. Little WC, Reeves RC, Coughlan C, Rogers EW: Effect of cough on coronary perfusion pressure: Does coughing help clear the coronary arteries of angiographic contrast medium? Circulation 65:604, 1982.

9. Cohen A, Gottdiener J, Wish M, Fletcher R: Limitations of cough in maintaining blood flow during asystole: Assessment by two-dimensional and Doppler echocardiography. Am Heart J 118:474, 1989.

10. Kern MJ, Gudipati C, Tatineni S, Aguirre F, Serota H, Deligonul

U: Effect of abruptly increased intrathoracic pressure on coronary blood flow velocity in patients. Am Heart J 119:863–870, 1990.

11. Wilson RF, Marcus ML, White CW: Pulmonary inflation reflex: Its lack of physiological significance in coronary circulation of humans. Am J Physiol 255(Heart Circ Physiol 24):H866, 1988.

12. Benchimol A, Wang TF, Desser KB, Gartlan JL Jr: The Valsalva maneuver and coronary arterial blood flow velocity. Ann Intern Med 77:357, 1972.

13. Kern MJ, Deligonul U, Serota H, Gudipati C, Buckingham T: Ventricular arrhythmia due to intracoronary papaverine: Analysis of clinical and hemodynamic data with coronary vasodilatory reserve. Cathet Cardiovasc Diagn 19:229–236, 1990.

14. Kern MJ. Intracoronary flow velocity: current techniques and clinical applications of Doppler catheter methods. In Yock, P. (ed): "Coronary Ultrasound." (in press).

Chapter 32

Coronary Hemodynamics—Section III:
Coronary Hyperemia

Morton J. Kern, MD, Frank V. Aguirre, MD, Thomas J. Donohue, MD, and Richard G. Bach, MD

INTRODUCTION

With the advent of intracoronary flow velocity catheters, measurement of basal and hyperemic coronary flow velocities under a variety of research applications has become commonplace in university laboratories and may eventually be useful clinically in daily practice. In the previous hemodynamics rounds (1), we described the technique and patterns of coronary blood flow velocity measurements under a variety of clinical circumstances. In this hemodynamic rounds, we review coronary hyperemic responses and coronary vasodilatory reserve.

Coronary hyperemia is defined as a transient or permanent increase in coronary flow rate above the basal level in response to exercise, vasodilators, or relief of ischemia. Reactive (ischemic) hyperemia describes the flow response occurring after relaxation of transient arterial occlusion such as may be produced by coronary ligature release in animal models (Fig. 1) or during balloon deflation during coronary angioplasty in patients. Pharmacologic hyperemia can be induced with a number of common drugs such as papaverine, adenosine, dipyridamole, nitroglycerin, and radiographic contrast media. Coronary vasodilatory reserve, a ratio of basal to hyperemic flow, is considered to be the maximal increase in flow that can be achieved by the stimulated coronary bed. Coronary vasodilatory reserve is the result of several complex interrelating processes. Although measurements of coronary hyperemia can be easily obtained in the cardiac catheterization laboratory with coronary Doppler catheter techniques, the clinical application of this data currently remains in the research arena.

DOPPLER CATHETER TECHNIQUES

Current methodology and clinical applications of Doppler catheters have been reviewed in detail [1–3]. The earlier coronary hemodynamic rounds described the 2 types of available coronary Doppler catheters: the subselective or nonselective catheter [1]. Recall that the nonselective 8F Judkins-type Doppler catheter [4] uses the same technique as diagnostic angiographic catheterization for the left coronary artery and measures flow within the left main coronary artery only. A nonselective right coronary Doppler catheter remains under development. The subselective 3F Doppler catheter technique employs methods of coronary angioplasty using angioplasty guidewires (0.014″), guiding catheters (8F), and Y connectors to position the catheter deeply within the proximal and mid portions of the coronary arteries [5]. The most recent technical advance is a coronary Doppler angioplasty-type guidewire (0.018″, Cardiometrics, Inc. Flowire), which measures flow velocity with a 12 mhz transducer at its tip [6]. Because of its size, the Doppler flowire is the only technique that can measure both proximal and distal coronary flow velocity beyond atherosclerotic obstructions, including some total occlusions.

Coronary velocity signals are processed by 2 methods. The most common and least expensive is the zero-cross method. The velocimeter (Millar Instruments, Houston, TX; Triton Technology, San Diego, CA) detects the direction and rate at which the signal changes frequency (frequency shift) past a zero velocity point. The frequency shift is proportional to the velocity. The signals are easily acquired and recorded on a standard photographic oscilloscope recorder (Fig. 2). The zero-cross technique is used with most 20 mhz subselective and nonselective Doppler catheters.

The second method is spectral analysis. Time-averaged and instantaneous peak velocity values are processed by a computer using fast fourier transformation techniques that displays a gray scale depiction of all velocities recorded in the sample volume at one point in

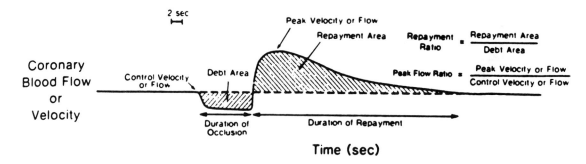

Standard Measurements Used to Analyze Reactive Hyperemic Responses

Fig. 1. Diagram of coronary blood flow velocity tracing demonstrating the reactive hyperemic response of transient coronary occlusion. Reprinted with permission from: Marcus ML, Wright C, Doty D, et al.: Measurement of coronary velocity and reactive hyperemia in the coronary circulation of humans. Circ Res 49:877–871, 1981.

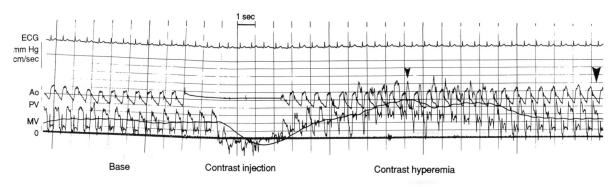

Base   Contrast injection   Contrast hyperemia

Fig. 2. Typical coronary hyperemic blood flow response during radiographic contrast media injection using the zero crossing signal analysis technique. The coronary flow velocity falls during contrast injection with reflux into the aorta. The peak hyperemic response occurs on the average of 10 seconds (first arrowhead) after injection and lasts for approximately 10 seconds (second arrowhead) thereafter. Ao=aortic pressure; PV=phasic velocity; MV=mean velocity (Velocity scale: 0–100 cm/second; pressure scale: 0–200 mmHg).

time. As with standard transthoracic echocardiographic technique, the more homogenous the velocity the more intense and uniform the velocity spectrum. Spectral analysis is applied to the 12 mhz signal obtained with the angioplasty Doppler flowire (Fig. 3).

CORONARY VASODILATORY RESERVE

Coronary vasodilatory reserve can be computed in several ways. First, coronary reserve can be calculated as the ratio of mean hyperemic to basal coronary flow velocity. Second, coronary vasodilatory reserve can be normalized for mean arterial pressure as follows: [(hyperemic flow velocity/mean arterial pressure at peak hyperemia)/(basal velocity/mean arterial pressure at basal pressure)]. A coronary resistance index may be computed as the ratio of mean arterial pressure and mean coronary flow velocity. A variety of factors influence basal and hyperemic flow responses, often limiting the

interpretation of a changing coronary vasodilatory reserve. The range of normal coronary vasodilatory reserve has been reported as low as 2.5, but > 3.0 (a threefold increase of the basal value) is widely considered the lower limit of normal. Pharmacologic hyperemic responses may be altered by metabolic, vascular, myocardial, and endothelial factors [7], specialized considerations beyond the scope of this discussion. However, in patients with normal left ventricular function, changes in the mean arterial pressure and left ventricular preload have a minimal influence on the reproducibility of measured coronary vasodilatory reserve. From an interstudy assessment of variability, when measured serially over an 11-month interval, the major changes in coronary vasodilatory reserve determinations appeared related to changes in heart rate more than other variables [8].

The determination of quantitative volumetric coronary blood flow is a well-known limitation of all Doppler catheter velocity techniques. The arterial cross-sectional

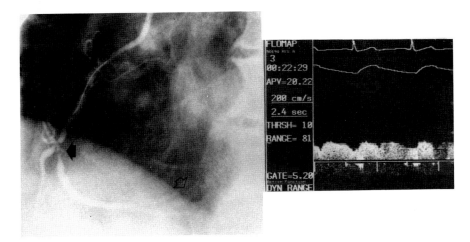

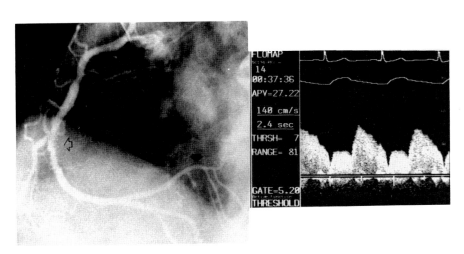

Fig. 3.   Doppler spectral flow velocity signals in right coronary artery obtained with a 0.018″ Doppler guidewire before (top) and after (bottom) coronary balloon angioplasty. Note systolic/ diastolic velocity integrals (areas) have normalized in the distal region after dilation. (Bottom flow signals.)

area (by quantitative angiography) can be used to compute volumetric flow by a formula in common use by echocardiographers where flow equals the product of the flow velocity integral (area under flow velocity curve)*heart rate*cross-sectional area of the vessel [9].

PHARMACOLOGIC AGENTS FOR CORONARY HYPEREMIA

In cardiac catheterization laboratory patients, coronary hyperemia is produced by intracoronary nitroglycerin [10], contrast media [11], intracoronary papaverine [12],

intravenous or intracoronary adenosine [13,14], or intravenous dipyridamole [15]. However, maximal hyperemia is achieved only with intracoronary papaverine or adenosine (intravenously or intracoronary). Nitroglycerin and contrast media do not produce maximal hyperemia. Intracoronary drugs are given directly into the coronary catheter after filling and flushing the guiding catheter or the Judkins-style Doppler catheter. Subselective delivery of the drug can be achieved through the 3F Doppler catheter with the guidewire removed. Care should be taken when manipulating the subselective Doppler catheter within the coronary artery when the guidewire has been removed to prevent vascular trauma.

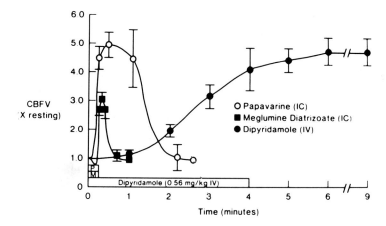

Fig. 4. The time course of the hyperemic responses of papaverine, meglumine diatrizoate, and dipyridamole. Reprinted with permission from: Wilson RF, White CW: Intracoronary papaverine: An ideal coronary vasodilator for studies of the coronary circulation in conscious humans. Circulation 73:444–451, 1986.

PAPAVERINE

Doses of 3–12 mg intracoronary papaverine markedly increases coronary blood flow within 30 seconds. Maximal hyperemia occurs 28 ± 15 seconds after intracoronary injection and returns to baseline within 128 ± 15 seconds [12]. Coronary flow velocity increases by an average of 3–5 times basal flow velocity in normal vessels (Fig. 4). Although the short duration of action and lack of major effects on systemic hemodynamics suggested papaverine was a near ideal agent for human studies, papaverine-induced QT interval prolongation and rare episodes of ventricular tachycardia [16] have been reported. Since low doses of papaverine may not elicit maximal hyperemia, an initial dose of 8–10 mg is administered with a second 12 mg dose to confirm a maximal vasodilatory response (Fig. 5).

ADENOSINE

Adenosine is regarded as the standard physiologic coronary vasodilator in animal and recently in human studies. Wilson et al. [13] determined that an intracoronary dose of 12 mcg produces reliable and safe maximal coronary hyperemia in 80% of patients. Intravenous adenosine (100–150 mcg/kg/min by continuous infusion or 2.5–5.0 mg intravenous bolus) has been found to be superior to intracoronary papaverine because of its exceptionally short duration of activity (time to peak 10–100 seconds, with return to baseline in 45–113 seconds) and lack of associated QT prolongation (Fig. 6) [14]. Angina-like chest pain and occasional transient bradycardia and/or asystole are observed with intravenous adenosine administration. High dose intravenous adenosine produces marked hypotension and reflex tachycardia. Intracoronary administration, in inappropriately high dosage, has been reported to produce maximal cor-

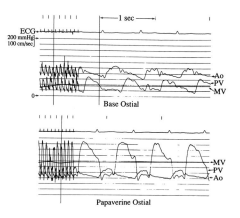

Fig. 5. Intracoronary papaverine (10 mg) induces maximal hyperemia for coronary vasodilatory reserve computation. Top: Baseline coronary flow velocity (mean 18 cm/sec) in left coronary artery. Bottom: After papaverine, hyperemia produces a 3-fold increase in mean velocity (60 cm/sec; CVR = 60/18 = 3.5). Ao = aortic pressure; MV = mean velocity; PV = phasic velocity.

onary vasodilation with heart block and a highly variable individual dose-response relationship [17]. However, specificity for single artery hyperemia coupled with a high safety profile when given in appropriate doses, and an ultrashort duration of activity of intracoronary adenosine make this the agent of choice for repetitive hyperemic studies.

DIPYRIDAMOLE

Intravenous dipyridamole, which acts by blocking uptake of adenosine, increases coronary blood flow velocity four to five times basal levels in normal subjects. Dipyridamole (0.56 mg/kg infused over 4 minutes) has been shown to increase flow velocity 4.8 ± 0.4 times

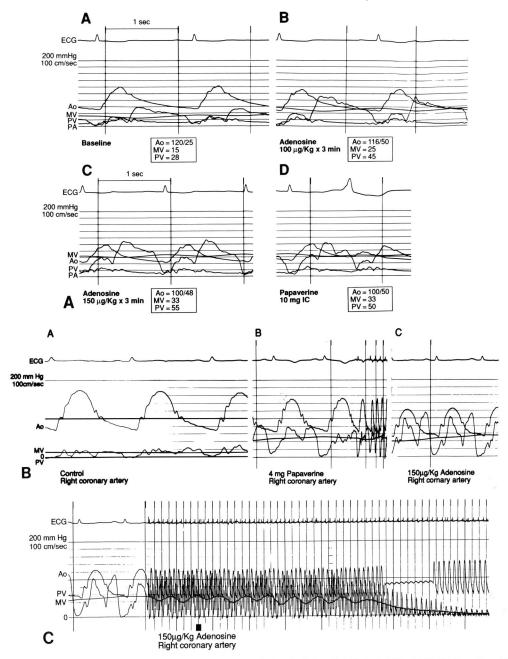

Fig. 6. **A.** Comparison of coronary hyperemia produced by intravenous infusion of adenosine and intracoronary papaverine. Intravenous adenosine in doses > 100 mcg/kg/min (panels B and C) produces similar degrees of coronary hyperemia compared to papaverine, but without QT prolongation. Note QT interval and ventricular premature contraction (2nd QRS complex) in panel D during papaverine hyperemia. Ao = aortic pressure; PV = phasic velocity; MV = mean velocity; PA = pulmonary artery pressure. Reproduced with permission from: Kern MJ, Deligonul U, Tatineni S, Serota H, Aguirre F, Hilton TC: Intravenous adenosine: Continuous infusion and low dose bolus administration for determination of coronary vasodilatory reserve in patients with and without coronary artery disease. J

Am Coll Cardiol 18:718–729, 1991. **B.** Baseline (A) and hyperemic responses in the right coronary artery with 4mg papaverine (B) and intravenous infusion of adenosine 150 mcg/kg/min (C). Note the electrocardiographic alteration with papaverine. The flow velocity pattern in the right coronary artery often has a lower systolic/diastolic peak velocity ratio compared to the left coronary artery flow velocity pattern. Mean velocity increased from 8 to 24 cm/sec. **C.** The offset (black mark) of coronary hyperemia is rapid, occurring within 30 seconds after cessation of intravenous adenosine infusion. Ao = aortic pressure; PV = phasic velocity; MV = mean velocity (from ref. 14 with permission).

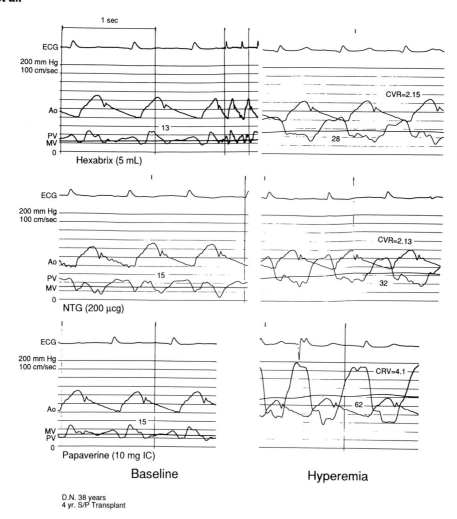

Fig. 7.   Nitroglycerin (middle panel) produces coronary hyperemia similar to that of contrast media (top panel). Hexabrix, nitroglycerin, and papaverine (bottom panel) demonstrate increases in mean coronary blood flow velocity of 28, 32, and 64 cm/second with coronary vasodilatory reserve (CVR) of 2.15, 2.13, and 4.1, respectively, in a 38-year-old woman 4 years after orthotopic cardiac transplantation. Ao = aortic pressure; PV = phasic velocity; MV = mean velocity.

basal flow velocity, a result that was significantly greater than contrast-induced hyperemia (meglumine diatrizoate, 3.1 ± 0.2, p < 0.01) [12,15]. Dipyridamole has a longer time to onset (6–10 minutes, see Fig. 4) than the other agents, with persistent effects for more than 20 minutes, making it unsuitable for repetitive studies. Patients receiving methylxanthines or similar drugs may have a markedly reduced effect from dipyridamole. Side effects from dipyridamle, including flushing, chest pain, and nausea, are rapidly reversed by theophylline administration.

NITROGLYCERIN

Neither intracoronary nitroglycerin nor contrast media (ionic, low osmolar, or nonionic) induced maximal hyperemia. These agents produce submaximal vasodilation

between 1.5 and 2.5 times basal flow velocity (Fig. 7). Intracoronary nitroglycerin in doses of 100–200 mcg produces vasodilation and doubles coronary venous efflux and arterial flow velocity [18]. Doses > 200 mcg are associated with significant decreases in mean arterial pressure and fall in coronary hyperemia. Nitroglycerin-induced hyperemic effects occur within 20 ± 5 seconds with a duration of up to 90–110 seconds. Coronary hyperemia after balloon deflation during angioplasty-induced ischemia is not attenuated by intracoronary nitroglycerin, producing hyperemia immediately prior to coronary occlusion [19].

RADIOGRAPHIC CONTRAST MEDIA

Radiographic contrast media produces transient coronary hyperemia with peak effect at 15 ± 7 seconds and

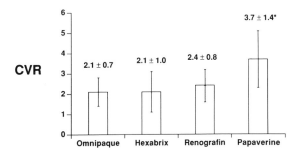

Fig. 8. Coronary vasodilatory reserve (CVR) for 3 radiographic contrast media was lower than the papaverine response (from ref. 20 with permission).

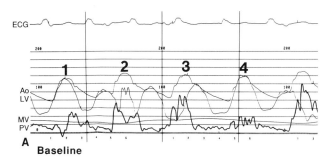

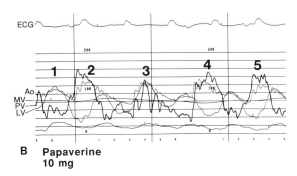

Fig. 9. A. Baseline coronary flow velocity measured in the native heart in a patient after heterotopic heart transplantation. Arterial pressure is produced by the donor heart. B. Papaverine hyperemia. Ao = aortic pressure; PV = phasic velocity; MV = mean velocity; LV = native left ventricular pressure.

duration of 30 ± 10 seconds (Fig. 2) [20]. Although some investigators suggest that reduced hyperemia may reflect reduced subendocardial ischemia with improved low osmolar or nonionic formulations, both types of contrast media in our laboratory produced similar submaximal coronary hyperemia (Fig. 8) [20].

CORONARY HYPEREMIA IN A PATIENT WITH TWO HEARTS

The hemodynamic findings of heterotopic heart transplanation, described in an earlier rounds [21], produce arterial waveforms generated by the vigorous donor heart, which may be altered by occasional strong ventricular contractions of the weakened native heart. We have had the opportunity to examine coronary flow in the native heart in such a patient during routine 1 year follow-up of the transplant status.

After diagnostic study, which included complete hemodynamics and angiography, left ventricular pressure in the native heart and systemic arterial pressure were measured with fluid-filled catheters from the right femoral artery. Native proximal left coronary artery flow velocity was measured with an 8F Judkins-Doppler catheter inserted from the left femoral artery. Baseline arterial and left ventricular pressure and mean and phasic coronary flow velocity signals are shown on Figure 9A. Remember arterial *systole* is produced by donor ventricular contractions. Coronary flow occurs in the native heart *diastole*. Native heart systole is documented by the rise in left ventricular pressure.

An analysis of the baseline data shows coronary flow velocity is maximal when 2 events coincide—arterial systole and left ventricular diastole. Note the increasing flow velocity from beats #1–3. On beat #4, flow velocity is impaired. Arterial systole is coincident with native left ventricular systolic pressure, resulting in reduced coronary inflow during native left ventricular systole. Flow velocity is markedly augmented on beat

#5 with the conjoint impact of heterotopic systole and native diastole.

To assess coronary vasodilatory reserve, intracoronary papaverine (10 mg) was given through the Judkins-Doppler catheter and coronary hyperemia measured 30 seconds later at peak response (Fig. 9B). Mean coronary velocity increased from 15 cm/sec to 42 cm/sec (coronary vasodilatory reserve = 2.8). However, again note the contribution to coronary flow augmentation of the heterotopic arterial systole with native left ventricular diastole beats #2, 4, and 5. This unusual example of augmented flow velocity during the "extra diastolic pressure" from a source external to the native heart coupled with native heart diastole is similar to that which has been observed during diastolic pressure augmentation of intra-aortic balloon counterpulsation (Fig. 10).

SUMMARY

Basal patterns (systolic/diastolic components) of coronary flow velocity as previously described are generally maintained during hyperemia and can be easily recorded in the catheterization laboratory during pharmacologic stimulation. The interpretation of the clinical significance of coronary vasodilatory reserve may be complicated by both coronary and myocardial diseases. Distal coronary artery hyperemic responses measured with ul-

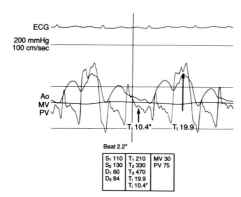

Fig. 10.   The effect of intra-aortic balloon pumping (2:1) on arterial pressure (Ao) and coronary blood flow velocity. MV = mean velocity; PV = phasic velocity. T$_i$ = total diastolic flow velocity integral (area); S$_1$, S$_2$, D$_1$, D$_2$ = systolic and diastolic pressures from onset of R wave. Arrows indicate mid point of T$_i$. Intra-aortic balloon pumping nearly doubles the diastolic flow velocity integral.

trasound Doppler-tipped guidewires will provide new information on traditional observations of coronary physiology in humans.

ACKNOWLEDGMENTS

The authors thank the J.G. Mudd Cardiac Catheterization Laboratory Team and Donna Sander for manuscript preparation.

REFERENCES

1. Kern MJ: Hemodynamic rounds: Interpretation of cardiac pathophysiology from pressure waveform analysis. Coronary hemodynamics, part II: Patterns of coronary flow velocity. Cathet Cardiovasc Diagn (in press), 1991.
2. Marcus, ML, Wright C, Doty D, et al: Measurement of coronary velocity and reactive hyperemia in the coronary circulation of humans. Circ Res 49:877–891, 1981.
3. Kern MJ: Intracoronary Doppler blood flow velocity catheters. In White CJ, Kamee SR (eds): "Interventional Cardiology; Clinical Application of New Technologies." Raven Press, NY, pp. 55–100, 1991.
4. Kern MJ, Courtois M, Ludbrook P: A simplified method to measure coronary blood flow velocity in patients: Validation and application of a Judkins-style Doppler-tipped angiographic catheter. Am Heart J 120:1202–1212, 1990.
5. Wilson RF, Laughlin DE, Ackell PH, Chilian WM, Holida MD, Hartley CJ, Armstrong ML, Marcus ML, White CW: Transluminal, subselective measurement of coronary artery blood flow velocity and vasodilator reserve in man. Circulation 72:82, 1985.
6. Doucette JW, Corl PD, Payne HM, et al: Validation of a Doppler guidewire for assessment of coronary arterial flow. Circulation 82:III–621, 1990.
7. Olsson RA: Myocardial reactive hyperemia. Cir Res 37:263–270, 1975.
8. McGinn AL, White CW, Wilson RF: Interstudy variability of coronary flow reserve: influence of heart rate, arterial pressure and ventricular preload. Circulation 81:1319, 1990.
9. Hatle L, Angelsen B: Doppler ultrasound in cardiology. In: "Flow Velocity and Volumetric Principles." Philadelphia: Lea & Febiger, 1985, p 14.
10. Kern MJ, Vandormael M, Deligonul U, Labovitz A, Gabliani G, Kennedy HL: Effects of nitroglycerin and nifedipine on regional coronary blood flow during transient myocardial ischemia in patients. Am Heart J 115:1164–1170, 1988.
11. Hodgson JM, Williams DO: Superiority of intracoronary papaverine to radiographic contrast for measuring coronary flow reserve in patients with ischemic heart disease. Am Heart J 114:704, 1987.
12. Wilson RF, White CW: Intracoronary papaverine: An ideal coronary vasodilator for studies of the coronary circulation in conscious humans. Circulation 73:444–451, 1986.
13. Wilson RF, Wyche K, Christensen BV, et al: Effects of adenosine on human coronary arterial circulation. Circulation 82:1595, 1990.
14. Kern MJ, Deligonul U, Tatineni S, Serota H, Aguirre F, Hilton TC: Intravenous adenosine: Continuous infusion and low dose bolus administration for determination of coronary vasodilatory reserve in patients with and without coronary artery disease. J Am Coll Cardiol 18:718–729, 1991.
15. Marchant E, Pichard A, Rodriguez JA, et al: Acute effect of systemic versus intracoronary dipyridamole on coronary circulation. Am J Cardiol 57:1401, 1986.
16. Kern MJ, Deligonul U, Serota H, Gudipati C, Buckingham T: Ventricular arrhythmia due to intracoronary papaverine: Analysis of clinical and hemodynamic data with coronary vasodilatory reserve. Cathet Cardiovasc Diagn 19:229–236, 1990.
17. Zijlstra F, Juilliere Y, Serruys PW, et al: Value and limitations of intracoronary adenosine for the assessment of coronary flow reserve. Cathet Cardiovasc Diagn 15:76, 1988.
18. Kern MJ, Deligonul U, Vandormael M, Labovitz A, Gudipati R, Gabliani G, Bodet J, Shah Y, Kennedy HL: Impaired coronary vasodilatory reserve in the immediate post-coronary angioplasty period: Analysis of coronary arterial velocity flow indices and regional cardiac venous efflux. J Am Coll Cardiol 13:868–872, 1989.
19. Kern MJ, Vandormael M, Deligonul U, Labovitz A, Harper M, Gibson P, Presant S, Kennedy HL: Intracoronary nitroglycerin and regional coronary blood flow responses during coronary angioplasty in patients. J Interven Cardiol 1:49–57, 1988.
20. Tatineni S, Kern MJ, Deligonul U, Aguirre F: The effects of ionic and non-ionic radiographic contrast media on coronary hyperemia in patients during coronary angiography. Am Heart J (in press), 1992.
21. Kern MJ, Deligonul U, Miller L: Hemodynamic rounds: Interpretation of cardiac pathophysiology from pressure waveform analysis. Extra hearts: Part I. Cathet Cardiovasc Diagn 22:197–201, 1990.

Chapter 33

Coronary Hemodynamics—Section IV:
Use of Absolute, Relative Coronary Velocity and Fractional Flow Reserve

Morton J. Kern, MD, Sanjeev Puri, MD, W. Randall Craig MD, Richard G. Bach, MD, and Thomas J. Donohue, MD

The application of absolute coronary velocity reserve, relative coronary velocity reserve, and pressure-derived fractional flow reserve of the myocardium may have influence on decision making for angioplasty and stenting in patients after myocardial infarction. This case highlights the use and limitations of these techniques in the setting of myocardial infarction where absolute coronary flow reserve may be commonly compromised. The role for absolute, relative coronary, and fractional flow reserve are discussed. *Cathet. Cardiovasc. Diagn. 45:174–182, 1998.* © 1998 Wiley-Liss, Inc.

INTRODUCTION

Many clinicians believe that an assessment of coronary blood flow is important to decision making. In stable patients, proceeding with coronary interventions after diagnostic angiography is based on some objective evidence of abnormal coronary blood flow [1]. Several indirect physiologic measurements, such as exercise or pharmacologic stress radionuclide perfusion imaging, left ventricular contractile abnormalities during dobutamine or exercise stress echo, or significant ischemic electrocardiographic changes on routine exercise or ambulatory monitoring are utilized daily for decision making. However, the indirect methods often require additional time and significant expense after catheterization. Some patients may have a suboptimal evaluation or may not even undergo a physiologic evaluation before proceeding with coronary revascularization [2].

Estimates of coronary blood flow responses before and after interventional procedures can be obtained from both intracoronary velocity and pressure, measured with sensor-tipped angioplasty guidewires. Coronary vasodilatory reserve (CVR), the ratio of hyperemic to basal mean velocity, represents the summed result of flow through the coronary artery and myocardial microcirculation and has been used to determine lesion significance [3,4]. A normal CVR identifies both a normal coronary conduit and microvascular response, excluding a coronary lesion from being flow-limiting. To identify co-existent microvascular disease, relative coronary vasodilatory reserve (rCVR, computed as the ratio of coronary flow reserve in the target to coronary flow reserve in a normal reference zone, $CVR_{target}/CVR_{reference}$) has been proposed [4–6]. rCVR has a normal range of 0.8–1.0 [7]. rCVR appears to be a more lesion-specific index than absolute coronary flow reserve (aCVR).

Another approach to assessing coronary blood flow uses the hyperemic post-stenotic pressure in the computation of the fractional flow reserve of the myocardium (FFRmyo) [8–10]. FFRmyo represents the maximal flow across the stenosis compared to the theoretical maximal flow in the same vessel without the stenosis. FFRmyo is computed as the ratio of distal mean coronary pressure and mean aortic pressure during maximal hyperemia and is a specific index to describe the influence of the coronary stenosis on coronary flow to the myocardium.

FFRmyo is independent of microvascular abnormalities, hemodynamics, and rheologic conditions [11].

Since experience in clinical practice is limited for use of these two modalities to assess interventional endpoints in patients after acute myocardial infarction, we present two cases examining coronary hemodynamic results of these 2 modalities in patients undergoing intervention after anterior wall myocardial infarction. The combined measurements highlight areas of agreement and discordance between the two physiologic modalities.

CASE 1

A 44-year-old man presented with an anterior myocardial infarction and ventricular fibrillatory arrest at an outside hospital. Intravenous thrombolysis using reptelase was administered and the patient was transferred for further evaluation. He had been taking aspirin, capoten, lopressor, albuterol, and zocor and continued to smoke cigarettes.

On examination in the laboratory, the blood pressure was 100/60 mm Hg, pulse 70 beats/min. There was no neck vein distention. He had a grade III/VI systolic murmur at the left sternal border radiating to the base of the heart. The remainder of the examination was normal. The electrocardiogram showed Q-waves in leads V_1-V_3 of anterior myocardial infarction in evolution.

Cardiac catheterization was performed from the femoral approach. Left ventriculography demonstrated mild anterolateral hypokinesis with an ejection fraction of 72%. Coronary arteriography found a 50% mid left anterior descending eccentric lesion with TIMI grade 3 flow. There was a 30% mid right coronary artery stenosis. The left circumflex artery was normal.

In view of TIMI grade 3 flow and intermediately severe coronary stenoses, intervention was deferred and the patient was transferred to the Coronary Care Unit for further medical therapy. Eleven days later, after undergoing a negative low-level risk stratification test, the patient complained of having anterior chest pain at home during various activities such as bending over. He denied exertional chest discomfort but had not experienced high activity levels. He continued to smoke cigarettes during this recovery period.

The patient was re-admitted to the Cardiac Catheterization Laboratory for coronary artery lesion assessment and potential intervention. Coronary angiography again revealed a 50–60% mid left anterior descending stenosis (Fig. 1, top). Anterior left ventricular wall motion (by ventriculography) was improved with normal systolic contraction and a global ejection fraction of 65%.

Intracoronary flow velocity reserve measurements were made in the circumflex and left anterior descending coronary arteries in the standard fashion [12]. The circumflex (reference artery) coronary flow reserve was 3.1 (Fig. 1, bottom right). Coronary flow reserve in the (target) left anterior descending artery distal to the intermediate stenosis was 1.9 (Fig. 1, bottom left). rCVR (CVR_{target}/$CVR_{reference}$) was 0.61.

Translesional pressure was obtained with a 2.2F tracking catheter. The resting pressure gradient of 10 mm Hg increased during maximal hyperemia to 30 mm Hg (Fig. 2). The calculated FFRmyo ($pressure_{distal}$/$pressure_{aorta}$ at maximal hyperemia) was 58/80 = 0.73 (normal value $\geq$0.75) [9] (Fig. 2, right). Because of the borderline flow and pressure values and suggestive ischemic symptoms, angioplasty and stent placement were performed. After balloon dilatation with 3.5-mm balloons, there was no change in the coronary hemodynamics nor flow velocity data. A 3.5 x 15 mm J&J stent was positioned and dilated with a high-pressure inflation. The final percent diameter stenosis was <10%. It was noted during the procedure that severe, somewhat atypical chest pain persisted despite having an open artery with no electrocardiographic changes. Intravascular ultrasound revealed a well expanded stent and large lumen (Fig. 3, bottom left). Final flow velocity measurements demonstrated that coronary flow reserve in the target vessel increased to 2.1. rCVR increased to 0.68 (Fig. 3, right). The FFRmyo also remained unchanged at 55/78 = 0.71 (Fig. 4).

The patient was discharged home and recurrent atypical chest pain occurred. A low-level stress test was negative. Medical therapy was increased, but due to persistent complaints during the cardiac rehabilitation activities, the patient underwent a repeat cardiac catheterization 1 month after discharge. The left anterior descending stent site was widely patent. There was a stenotic diagonal branch (<1.5 mm diameter) adjacent to the stent. There were minimal diffuse luminal irregularities of the circumflex and right coronary artery. Ergonovine challenge was negative without evidence of focal coronary vasospasm, angina, or electrocardiographic changes. The patient was discharged on analgesics and anti-ischemic therapy. He has been well for 4 months.

CASE 2

A 67-year-old man with hypertension and diabetes was admitted for severe substernal chest pain. Non-Q-wave myocardial infarction was identified with a peak CK of 2745 and MB fraction of 181 units. Electrocardiogram showed non-specific ST-T wave changes. Initial medical

Pre PTCA

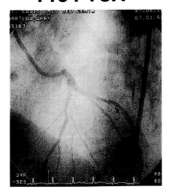

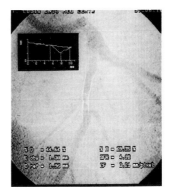

LAD

CFX Reference

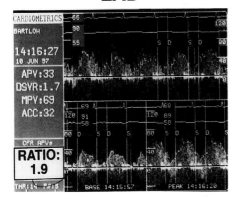

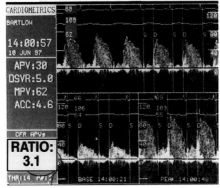

Fig. 1. Top: Coronary cineangiograms before angioplasty demonstrating a 45% QCA diameter stenosis in the left anterior descending (LAD) artery. Bottom left: Coronary flow reserve in the target LAD artery was 1.9. Bottom right: Coronary flow reserve in the reference circumflex (CFX) artery was 3.1. The relative coronary vasodilatory reserve ratio was 0.61. The velocity panels are split into top and bottom with lower panels divided into base (left) and hyperemic (right) flow. The spectral signals are shown on a scale 0–120 cm/sec. The electrocardiogram and aortic pressure are displayed above the velocity spectra. APV = average peak velocity; DSVR = diastolic/systolic velocity ratio; MPV = maximal peak velocity; ACC = acceleration; ratio = coronary vasodilatory reserve.

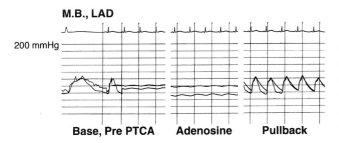

Fig. 2. Distal coronary and aortic pressures before angioplasty at baseline, during adenosine, and during catheter pullback demonstrating a small diastolic pressure gradient. The fractional flow reserve of the myocardium (FFRmyo) computed from values measured at peak adenosine response was 58/80 = 0.71. Scale = 0–200 mm Hg.

therapy with aspirin, heparin, beta-blockers, and topical nitrates was successful in relieving pain. Because of the non-Q-wave myocardial infarction with multiple cardiac risk factors, the patient was transferred for diagnostic cardiac catheterization and potential revascularization.

On physical examination, the blood pressure was 136/84 mm Hg with a pulse of 80/min. There were no neck vein distention nor carotid bruits. The lungs were clear. The heart sounds were normal. There was a systolic ejection murmur heard along the left sternaλ border. The pulses were 2+ throughout. There was no peripheral edema. The electrocardiogram showed normal sinus rhythm, first degree AV block, right bundle branch block, left anterior hemiblock, and small anterior precordial Q waves.

At catheterization, left ventriculography demonstrated severe anterolateral hypokinesis and apical and inferoapical akinesis with an ejection fraction of 26%. There was no mitral regurgitation. Coronary arteriography demonstrated single-vessel coronary artery disease with a 90% stenosis in the mid left anterior descending coronary artery (Fig. 5, left). The circumflex artery was dominant and normal as was the right coronary artery. Coronary angioplasty was then performed after evaluation of CVR and FFRmyo as described in case 1. Coronary flow

Post Stent

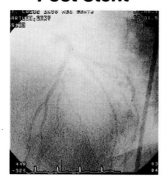

Post PTCA

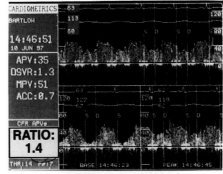

Post Stent

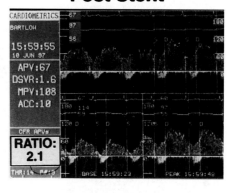

Fig. 3. Top left: Coronary angiogram after stent placement. Right: Coronary flow velocity reserve after angioplasty was 1.4 and after stent placement increased to 2.1, improving (but not normalizing) relative coronary vasodilatory flow reserve to 0.67. The velocity panels are split into top and bottom with lower panels divided into base (left) and hyperemic (right) flow. The spectral signals are shown on a scale of 0–120 cm/sec. The electrocardiogram and aortic pressure are displayed above the velocity spectra. APV = average peak velocity; DSVR = diastolic/systolic velocity ratio; MPV = maximal peak velocity; ACC = acceleration; ratio = coronary vasodilatory reserve. Bottom left: Intravascular ultrasound imaging in the reference and post-stent region with a fully expanded stent.

M.B., Post Stent

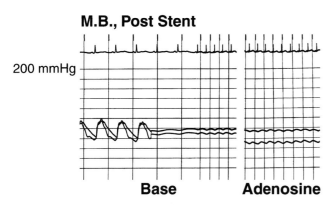

Fig. 4. Post-stent coronary hemodynamics are similar to the pre-angioplasty hemodynamics with fractional flow reserve (FFR) of 55/78 mm Hg = 0.73.

reserve was again measured with a 0.014" Doppler-tipped angioplasty guidewire, but FFRmyo was now measured with a pressure guidewire (Wavewire Endosonics, Sacremento, CA). Coronary flow reserve in the normal reference circumflex artery was 1.4 and in the post-stenotic segment of the left anterior descending artery 1.3 (rCVR = 0.90) (Fig. 6). Translesional coronary pressure and FFRmyo were then measured (Fig. 7). The resting translesional pressure gradient across the left anterior descending artery was approximately 60 mm Hg, distal absolute coronary pressure was 48 mm Hg, and aortic pressure was 114 mm Hg. FFRmyo at rest, without maximal hyperemia, was computed as <0.5. A 3.0-mm Surpass perfusion balloon was advanced over the pressure guidewire. The Doppler wire was also placed in the distal vessel. During balloon inflation, a reduction in the translesional gradient to 40 mm Hg was observed with preserved distal flow (Fig. 8). Absolute distal coronary pressure increased from 48 to 68 mm Hg (Fig. 7, bottom left). On balloon deflation, the resting gradient further decreased to 20 mm Hg (Fig. 7, bottom middle) with absolute increase in distal coronary pressure to 80 mm Hg. On removal of the balloon from the artery, the resting gradient was 8 mm Hg. The final angiographic result was satisfactory with a <10% residual from balloon angioplasty (Fig. 5, right). Post-angioplasty FFRmyo, measured during maximal hyperemia, had a maximal hyper-

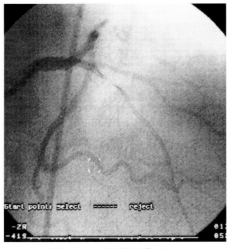
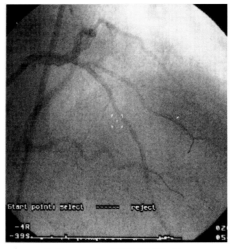

Pre PTCA   ## Post PTCA

Fig. 5. Cineangiographic frames of the left anterior descending (LAD) coronary artery demonstrating 90% stenosis before angioplasty (left) and <10% residual stenosis after angioplasty (right).

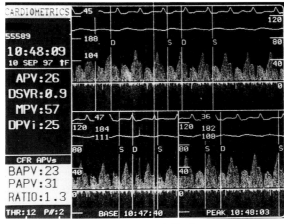
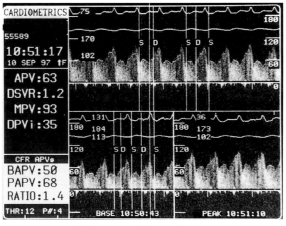

Pre PTCA   ## Post PTCA

Fig. 6. Coronary flow reserve and velocity data measured before angioplasty (left) and after angioplasty (right). The velocity format as in Figure 1. Coronary flow reserve before angioplasty was 1.3 and after angioplasty was 1.4. Note that the basal average peak velocity (BAPV) increased from 23 to 50 cm/sec and peak average peak velocity (PAPV) increased from 31 to 68 cm/sec. (velocity scales 0-120, 0-180 cm/sec).

emic gradient of 10 mm Hg with a value 118/122 or 0.97. Final coronary flow velocity reserve remained similar at 1.4 (Fig. 6, right), but both basal and peak hyperemic flow doubled in this individual. The patient was discharged after an uncomplicated hospital course.

DISCUSSION

Coronary blood flow assessment for ischemia in the post-infarct patient is important but can be problematic. The finding of an intermediately severe coronary stenosis often prompts the cardiologist to proceed with intervention on the target vessel despite having relatively little or no objective evidence of ischemia. The intermediate coronary stenosis in patient 1 was likely not solely responsible for the persistent chest pain syndrome. Coronary hemodynamics were at the borderline of normal and changed minimally after eliminating the target stenosis. The symptoms persisted even after complete elimination of the major coronary narrowing.

In these cases, the hemodynamic significance of a given stenosis was determined by both the pressure and flow methods. The pressure-flow relationship may be influenced by factors other than the stenosis alone, such

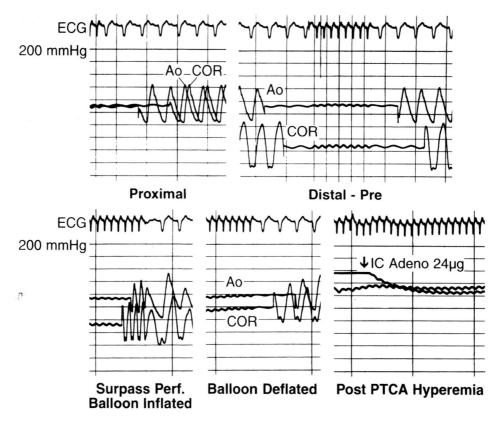

Fig. 7. Top left: Aortic (Ao) and distal coronary (cor) pressures measured with a pressure guidewire in the proximal region of the left anterior descending (LAD) coronary artery. Top right: Translesional pressure gradient before angioplasty (pre). Bottom left: Pressure gradient measured during Surpass perfusion balloon inflation. Bottom middle: Pressure gradient during balloon deflation with balloon across the stenosis. Bottom right: Final result shows post-angioplasty hyperemic gradient with a fractional flow reserve of 0.9. Note the resting gradient is <10 mm Hg. Pressure scale 0–200 mm Hg.

as basal myocardial oxygen demands and microcirculatory abnormalities [4]. The limitations of using coronary lumenography (angiography or intravascular ultrasound imaging) to precisely gauge lesion severity have been acknowledged. Physiologic measurements often provide complementary information to facilitate decisions [13–16]. Distal coronary pressure and a translesional gradient can be measured by use of a guidewire with a pressure transducer at the tip. Similarly, coronary flow velocity reserve can be measured distal to a stenosis. Previous studies have shown that proximal CVR may be normal even with severe lesions since lower pre-lesional branch resistance may direct flow away or around the target coronary stenosis [16–18].

Role of rCVR

In patient 1, the reference CVR was >3.0, suggesting that global microvascular abnormalities were not present [19]. After stent placement, target CVR increased to 2.1, still substantially less than the $CVR_{reference}$ ($aCVR_{reference}$ = 3.1, rCVR = 0.68) indicating that regional flow was limited. Given the minimal pressure loss and near normal FFR, the epicardial conduit at the site of assessment was

likely not a major contributor to reduced flow. The impaired CVR_{target} was likely not due to epicardial obstruction but, in part, the result of the prior myocardial infarction. Since CVR is generally reproducible among vessels [19] and usually unchanged within a 10% variation in heart rate or blood pressure [20], rCVR should theoretically be a more reliable indicator of impaired microvascular function, especially relevant to patients with diabetes mellitus, left ventricular hypertrophy, myocardial infarction, or syndrome X [21]. In contrast, the $CVR_{reference}$ in case 2 was abnormal at 1.4 with CVR_{target} 1.3. The normal rCVR was accompanied by a markedly abnormal FFRmyo. It can be speculated that the degree of $CVR_{reference}$ abnormality was due to 3 factors: prior or contiguous myocardial infarction, hypertension, and diabetes mellitus, all combining to blunt $CVR_{reference}$. In this case, in a patient with an abnormal microcirculation and co-existent atherosclerotic obstruction, the difference between CVR_{target} and $CVR_{reference}$ is reduced and may result in a falsely normal rCVR. When a target vessel supplies a territory of recent or remote myocardial infarction, it might be expected that both aCVR and

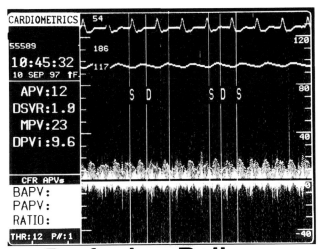

Perfusion Balloon (Surpass) Inflated

Fig. 8. Coronary flow velocity measured during Surpass balloon inflation, demonstrating degree of flow achievable with the inflated balloon at the same pressure gradient as on Figure 7. (Velocity format as in Figure 1.)

rCVR may remain abnormal (or borderline) despite a satisfactory conduit enlargement as evidenced by quantitative coronary angiography, intravascular ultrasound, and FFRmyo.

Because aCVR addresses functional flow through both the conduit and microvascular circulations, the pressure-derived FFRmyo may be more useful for assessing lesions in regions of myocardial infarction. FFRmyo is a stenosis-specific index, independent of hemodynamics, microcirculatory abnormalities, and loading conditions [22,23].

Physiologic Endpoints of Intervention

Use of coronary flow reserve and FFRmyo has been suggested as complementary endpoints for interventional procedures in patients undergoing elective angioplasty. In the DEBATE multicenter trial [24] an aCVR >2.5 and final percent diameter stenosis <35% by quantitative coronary angiography, achieved in 44/224 patients, was associated with low rates (≤16%) of major adverse cardiac events and target lesion revascularization. However, these data were confined to patients with single-vessel coronary artery disease, positive stress testing, and normal left ventricular function. Bech et al. [25] reported FFRmyo >0.9 after elective balloon angioplasty was associated with <15% restenosis rates at 6 months, 1 year, and 2 years follow-up compared to restenosis rates >25% with FFRmyo <0.9.

For patients with target lesions in regions of myocardial infarction, the absence of a significant hyperemic gradient (i.e., normal FFRmyo) and borderline normal aCVR (despite an abnormal rCVR) suggest that a conservative approach and treatment for increased coronary vasomotor tone with nitrates and calcium channel blockers may be worthwhile until provokable or spontaneous ischemia appears. Hemodynamics unchanged by stent placement suggest that the coronary narrowing was likely not the sole source of abnormal coronary flow. One could speculate that perhaps a more diffuse or unsuspected proximal coronary segment may be contributory. For the clinician, it is difficult to resist interventional treatment for non-specific symptoms in patients with intermediately severe lesions when the consequences of potential lesion progression or re-infarction loom in the future.

CVR and Stenting

After balloon angioplasty, CVR normalizes in ≤50% of patients. After stenting in the same patients, CVR can increase >2.0 in ≥80% of cases [26]. The increase in coronary flow reserve appears principally due to the increased coronary lumen, a feature not appreciated by angiography. This mechanism was examined in 42 patients from our laboratory [26]. After angioplasty, CVR increased from 1.7 ± 0.79 to 1.89 ± 0.56 and after stent placement to 2.49 ± 0.68, a value similar to that in a normal adjacent reference vessel. When examined by intravascular ultrasound, vessel cross-sectional area was significantly larger after stenting compared to angioplasty (5.1 ± 2.0 mm² after angioplasty vs. 8.4 ± 2.1 mm² after stent; $P < 0.05$). Linear regression demonstrated target artery lumen cross-sectional area was related to post-procedural coronary vasodilatory reserve (r = 0.47; $P < 0.005$). A persistently impaired CVR after stenting may be due to one or more factors, including obscured conduit obstruction, microvascular abnormalities, or microembolis and a no-reflow phenomenon. In those cases where stenting improved but did not normalize the rCVR, the final CVR_{target} was consistent with a persistently abnormal target vessel microcirculation in the recovering myocardial infarction territory. In case 2, no intravascular ultrasound evidence of lumen obstruction after stenting was present to account for the low CVR_{target}.

It is also interesting to note that although angioplasty may eliminate a significant pressure gradient, CVR may remain unchanged. In case 2, there was a parallel doubling of basal and hyperemic flow with no further augmentation of CVR_{target}. This disparity between pressure and flow suggests an association with conduit enlargement supplying an infarcted and non-functional microcirculation. The clinical significance of this response remains to be studied.

rCVR and FFRmyo

Both rCVR and FFRmyo should be independent of the microcirculatory response and changing hemodynamics.

A strong correlation between rCVR and FFRmyo has been reported [27], suggesting that these two methods are assessing similar flow responses. Their combined use appears complementary. Technical problems in accurately acquiring flow velocity signals may occur in ≤15% of arteries examined in the course of coronary angioplasty. Pressure wire artifacts may also be rarely observed. Borderline or ambiguous data, acquired by either pressure or flow velocity alone, can be theoretically clarified using the complementary technique.

For the most accurate results, FFRmyo should be measured with pressure guidewires, which are commercially unavailable in the United States at this time [11]. The cross-sectional area of a 2.2F pressure catheter will add to the lesion cross-sectional area, artifactually increasing resting and hyperemic pressure gradient and, thus, underestimating the true FFRmyo. In case 1, a pressure guidewire would likely have been associated with an even higher (more normal) FFRmyo before intervention.

Translesional hemodynamics may be influenced by vasomotor changes [28]. For lesion assessment, coronary vasomotor tone is minimized by pre-treatment with intracoronary nitroglycerin. Although safely deferring angioplasty in most stable patients with intermediate stenoses with normal translesional hemodynamics has been reported [29], such an approach has not been validated for patients with unstable lesions or recent myocardial infarction. Nonetheless, careful consideration by lesion assessment and judicious use of angioplasty may avoid inadvertent acceleration of luminal renarrowing in some patients with angiographically intermediate but physiologically mild stenoses.

Clinical Implications

These cases highlight the use and limitations of aCVR, rCVR, and FFRmyo after coronary stenting in patients with recent myocardial infarction. For lesion assessment in regions without myocardial infarction, straightforward intracoronary physiologic criteria in patients have been derived from ischemic testing correlations [30–32] and can support clinical decisions with objective data. For lesion assessment in regions of myocardial infarction, a normal aCVR excludes a significant lesion. However, when an abnormal or borderline aCVR is identified, confirmation of lesion significance with rCVR and/or FFRmyo may be useful.

ACKNOWLEDGMENTS

The authors thank the J.G. Mudd Cardiac Catheterization Laboratory team for technical support and Donna Sander for manuscript preparation.

REFERENCES

1. Ryan TJ, Faxon DP, Gunnar RM, Kennedy JW, King SB, Loop FD, Peterson KL, Reeves TJ, Williams DO, Winters WL: Guidelines for percutaneous transluminal coronary angioplasty. J Am Coll Cardiol 12:529–545, 1988.
2. Topol EJ, Ellis SG, Cosgrove DM, Bates ER, Muller DWM, Schork NJ, Schork MA, Loop FD: Analysis of coronary angioplasty practice in the United States with an insurance-claims data base. Circulation 87:1489–1497, 1993.
3. Geschwind H, Kern MJ (eds): "Guidebook to Endovascular Coronary Diagnostic Techniques." Armonk, NY: Futura Publishing, 1997.
4. Gould KL, Kirkeeide RL, Buchi M: Coronary flow reserve as a physiologic measure of stenosis severity. J Am Coll Cardiol 15:459–474, 1990.
5. Gould KL: Noninvasive assessment of coronary stenoses by myocardial perfusion imaging during pharmacologic coronary vasodilation. I. Physiologic basis and experimental validation. Am J Cardiol 41:267–272, 1978.
6. Strauss HW, Harrison K, Langan JK, Lebowitz E, Pitt B: Thallium-201 for myocardial imaging: Relation of thallium-201 to regional myocardial perfusion. Circulation 51:641–645, 1975.
7. Kern MJ, Donohue TJ, Bach RG, Aguirre FV, Caracciolo EA, Wolford TL: Assessment of intermediate coronary stenosis by relative coronary flow velocity reserve [abstr]. J Am Coll Cardiol 29:21A, 1997.
8. Pijls NHJ, Van Gelder B, Van der Voort P, Peels K, Bracke FALE, Bonnier NJRM, El Gamal MIH: Fractional flow reserve: A useful index to evaluate the influence of an epicardial coronary stenosis on myocardial blood flow. Circulation 92:3183–3193, 1995.
9. Pijls NHJ, de Bruyne B, Peels K, Van der Voort P, Bonnier HJRM, Bartunek J, Koolen JJ: Measurement of myocardial fractional flow reserve to assess the functional severity of coronary artery stenosis. N Engl J Med 334:1703–1708, 1996.
10. de Bruyne B, Paulus WJ, Pijls NHJ: Rationale and application of coronary transstenotic pressure gradient measurements. Cathet Cardiovasc Diagn 33:250–261, 1994.
11. de Bruyne B, Pijls NHJ, Paulus WJ, Vantrimpont PJ, Sys SU, Heyndrickx GR: Trans-stenotic coronary pressure gradient measurements in humans: In vitro and in vivo evaluation of a new pressure monitoring angioplasty guidewire. J Am Coll Cardiol 22:119–126, 1993.
12. Kern MJ, Aguirre FV, Bach RG, Caracciolo EA, Donohue TJ: Translesional pressure-flow velocity assessment in patients. Cathet Cardiovasc Diagn 31:49–60, 1994.
13. White CW, Wright CB, Doty DB, Hiratza LF, Eastham CL, Harrison DG, Marcus ML: Does visual interpretation of the coronary arteriogram predict the physiologic importance of a coronary stenosis? N Engl J Med 310:819–824, 1984.
14. DeFeyter PJ, Serruys PW, Davies MJ, Richardson P, Lubsen J, Oliver MF: Quantitative coronary angiography to measure progression and regression of coronary atherosclerosis: Value, limitations, and implications for clinical trials. Circulation 84:412–423, 1991.
15. Harrison DG, White CW, Hiratzka LF, Doty DB, Varnes DH, Eastham CL, Marcus ML: The value of lesion cross-sectional area determined by quantitative coronary angiography in assessing the physiologic significance of proximal left anterior descending coronary arterial stenosis. Circulation 69:1111–1119, 1984.
16. Donohue TJ, Kern MJ, Aguirre FV, Bach RG, Wolford T, Bell CA, Segal J: Assessing the hemodynamic significance of coronary artery stenoses: Analysis of translesional pressure-flow velocity relationships in patients. J Am Coll Cardiol 22:449–458, 1993.

17. Ofili EO, Kern MJ, Labovitz AJ, St. Vrain JA, Segal J, Aguirre F, Castello R: Analysis of coronary blood flow velocity dynamics in angiographically normal and stenosed arteries before and after endolumen enlargement by angioplasty. J Am Coll Cardiol 21:308–316, 1993.

18. Geschwind HJ, Dupouy P, Dubois-Randé K. Zelinsky R: Restoration of coronary blood flow in severely narrowed and chronically occluded coronary arteries before and after angioplasty: Implications regarding restenosis. Am Heart J 127:252–262, 1994.

19. Kern MJ, Bach RG, Mechem CJ, Caracciolo EA, Aguirre FV, Miller LW, Donohue TJ: Variations in normal coronary vasodilatory reserve stratified by artery, gender, heart transplantation and coronary artery disease. J Am Coll Cardiol 28:1154–1160, 1996.

20. McGinn AL, White CW, Wilson RF: Interstudy variability of coronary flow reserve: Influence of heart rate, arterial pressure, and ventricular preload. Circulation 81:1319–1330, 1990.

21. Strauer B: The significance of coronary reserve in clinical heart disease. J Am Coll Cardiol 15:775–783, 1990.

22. Pijls NHJ, van Son AM, Kirkeeide RL, de Bruyne B, Gould DL: Experimental basis of determining maximum coronary, myocardial, and collateral blood flow by pressure measurements for assessing functional stenosis severity before and after percutaneous transluminal coronary angioplasty. Circulation 87:1354–1367, 1993.

23. De Bruyne B, Bartunek J, Sys SU, Pijls NHJ, Heyndrickx GR, Wijns W: Simultaneous coronary pressure and flow velocity measurements in humans: Feasibility, reproducibility, and hemodynamic dependence of coronary flow velocity reserve, hyperemic flow versus pressure slope index, and fractional flow reserve. Circulation 94:1842–1849, 1996.

24. Serruys PW, Di Mario C, Piek J, Schroeder E, Vrints C, Probst P, de Bruyne B, Hanet C, Fleck E, Haude M, Verna E, Voudris V, Geschwind H, Emanuelsson H, Muhlberger V, Danzi G, Peels HO, Ford AJ Jr, Boersma E for the DEBATE study group: Prognostic value of intracoronary flow velocity and diameter stenosis in assessing the short- and long-term outcomes of coronary balloon angioplasty: The DEBATE Study (Doppler Endpoints Balloon Angioplasty Trial Europe). Circulation 96:3369–3377, 1997.

25. Bech GJW, De Bruyne B, Bonnier HJRM, Wijns W, Heyndrickx G, Michels HR, Koolen JJ, Pijls NHJ: Prognostic value of pressure-derived fractional flow reserve to predict restenosis after regular balloon angioplasty [abstr]. Am J Cardiol 80(7A):56S, 1997.

26. Kern MJ, Dupouy P, Drury JH, Aguirre FV, Aptecar E, Bach RG, Caracciolo EA, Donohue TJ, Dubois-Rande J, Geschwind HJ, Mechem CJ, Kane G, Teiger E, Wolford TL: Role of coronary artery lumen enlargement in improving coronary blood flow after balloon angioplasty and stenting: A combined intravascular ultrasound Doppler flow and imaging study. J Am Coll Cardiol 29:1520–1527, 1997.

27. Baumgart D, Haude M, Liu F, Ge J, Gorge G, Eick B, Dagres N, Shah V, Erbel R: Fractional velocity reserve: A new index for stenosis severity assessment with good correlation to fractional flow reserve [abstr]. J Am Coll Cardiol 29:126A, 1997.

28. Gould KL: Dynamic coronary stenosis. Am J Cardiol 45:286–292, 1980.

29. Kern MJ, Donohue TJ, Aguirre FV, Bach RG, Caracciolo EA, Wolford T, Mechem CJ, Flynn MS, Chaitman B: Clinical outcome of deferring angioplasty in patients with normal translesional pressure-flow velocity measurements. J Am Coll Cardiol 25:178–187, 1995.

30. Miller DD, Donohue TJ, Younis LT, Bach RG, Aguirre FV, Wittry MD, Goodgold HM, Chaitman BR, Kern MJ: Correlation of pharmacologic 99mtc-sestamibi myocardial perfusion imaging with poststenotic coronary flow reserve in patients with angiographically intermediate coronary artery stenoses. Circulation 89:2150–2160, 1994.

31. Joye JD, Schulman DS, Lasorda D, Farah T, Donohue BC, Reichek N: Intracoronary Doppler guide wire versus stress single-photon emission computed tomographic thallium-201 imaging in assessment of intermediate coronary stenoses. J Am Coll Cardiol 24:940–947, 1994.

32. Heller LI, Cates C, Popma J, Deckelbaum LI, Joye JD, Dahlberg ST, Villegas BJ, Arnold A, Kipperman R, Grinstead WC, Balcom S, Ma Y, Cleman M, Steingart RM, Leppo J for the FACTS study group: Intracoronary Doppler assessment of moderate coronary artery disease: Comparison with 201Tl imaging and coronary angiography. Circulation 96:484–490, 1997.

PART VII: UNUSUAL HEMODYNAMICS

A variety of unusual hemodynamic situations arises in the catheterization laboratory related to left and right ventricular pressures, right ventricular infarction, nitroglycerin, pulsus alternans, and extra-cardiac generation of hemodynamic data. We have detailed many of these special conditions in the chapters under this section and have added a more detailed discussion of the presumed straight forward measurement of left ventricular end-diastolic pressure, detailing the pitfalls and artifacts of this important hemodynamic pressure wave form.

Morton J. Kern, MD

Chapter 34

The LVEDP

Morton J. Kern, MD, and Thomas Christopher, MD

INTRODUCTION

The end-diastolic filling pressure (EDP) is often indicative of the hemodynamic health of the ventricle. The left ventricular pressure is available for examination in nearly every catheterization. In some patients undergoing diagnostic angiography, it was thought that right-heart catheterization would add important data, especially regarding the left ventricular filling and pulmonary artery pressures. Right-heart catheterization and measurement of the pulmonary capillary wedge pressure in most patients with coronary artery disease have been replaced by examining the LVEDP before contrast ventriculography. However, at times even this straightforward-appearing pressure wave can be misinterpreted. Although it is well-known and taught that the LVEDP is measured after the "A" wave at the onset of left ventricular isovolemic contraction coincident with the "R" wave, the identification of the true LVEDP may be difficult.

Examine the left ventricular pressure tracing in Figure 1 (provided by Dr. G. Alfred Dodds III, Medical College of Ohio, Toledo, Ohio). The LVEDP was recorded in a 43-year-old woman with exertional chest pain and multiple risk factors for coronary artery disease. The tracing demonstrates several different inflection points of the "A" wave. Note the changing LVEDP of 20 mm Hg (beat 2) with an LVEDP of 42 mm Hg (beats 3–5). On beats 8 and 9, the LVEDP is again at or below 20 mm Hg. What is the true LVEDP and why is this value changing? A multiple-holed catheter (pigtail) may move across the aortic valve and cause the LVEDP to be artifactually higher. With minor differences in positioning over the respiratory cycle, it appears that the pigtail catheter is moving slightly out of the ventricle with one or two of the side holes at the aortic valve. This artifact can be detected

by the pressure waveform and identification of the lowest left ventricular pressure at the initiation of diastole. Note in beat 2 that the minimal diastolic pressure is 10 mm Hg and that in beats 3 and 4 the minimal diastolic pressure is higher, occurring at middiastole, and not at the initiation of the diastolic period. Also, the initial downstroke of left ventricular pressure is delayed further, suggesting aortic pressure contamination which can sometimes occur when side holes of the catheter have moved out of the left ventricle. Thus, stability of the catheter and acquisition of a reliable pressure wave are required for accurate interpretation of the LVEDP.

LVEDP: CLUES TO UNSUSPECTED CONDITIONS

In the routine examination of the left ventricular pressure tracing above, the diastolic waveform, when examined carefully, provided a clue to the error of an abnormally high LVEDP. Myocardial relaxation abnormalities may be suggested by observing the trend of pressure during diastasis. Consider the left ventricular pressure measured in a 42-year-old patient with atypical chest pain syndrome and hypertension (Fig. 2). Nitroglycerin was given prior to left ventriculography. Note the low LVEDP with a continuing decline of pressure over the middiastolic period, with the pressure nadir occurring 50% through the diastolic period. This waveform pattern suggests impaired myocardial relaxation. This patient was found to have severe left ventricular hypertrophy, and an examination of an unsuspected obstructive cardiomyopathy was then performed. No provokable intraventricular pressure gradient was demonstrated. In a similar case in another patient without hypertension, the LVEDP

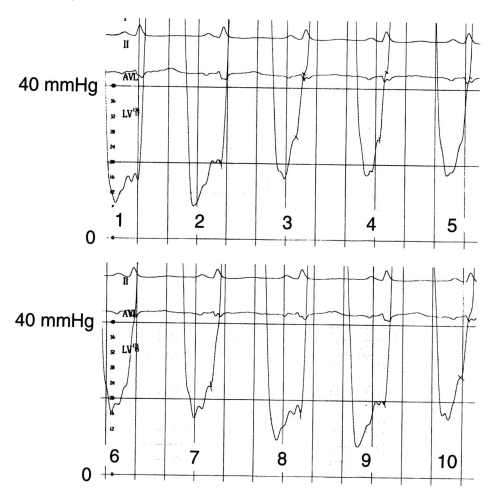

Fig. 1. Left ventricular pressure (0–40 mm Hg scale). Electrocardiogram (leads II and AVL) are shown at the top of the tracings.

waveform was abnormal, with impairment of left ventricular relaxation as described in the previous patient (Fig. 3). A Valsalva maneuver with induction of premature ventricular contractions was performed and demonstrated several beats in which an intraventricular gradient could be produced (Fig. 3, bottom). The diagnosis of hypertrophic myopathy with a nonobstructive classification at rest and provokable interventricular gradient during Valsalva and premature ventricular contractions was made, and beta blockers were recommended. Had the abnormal left ventricular pressure waveform not been appreciated, this diagnosis would not have been entertained or treated.

Insights into the diagnosis of left ventricular dysfunction may be appreciated by examination of simultaneously displayed left and right ventricular pressure waveforms. Abnormalities of ventricular contraction and relaxation, ventricular conduction abnormalities, and restrictive/constrictive pathophysiologic states are often evident. A collection of simultaneously measured left and

right ventricular pressures (Fig. 4) denotes hemodynamic clues to different common clinical problems. What can one deduce from this collection of waveforms?

In Figure 4, top left, the LVEDP is normal at 8–10 mm Hg and the right ventricular pressure is also normal. Although the diastolic period is relatively flat for the first beat, there is normal filling by the third beat. The electrocardiographic rhythm does not demonstrate "P" waves, thus explaining the absence of the "A" wave on the LVEDP. This hemodynamic tracing does not demonstrate any significant pathology, with the exception of a junctional rhythm and relatively low-normal filling pressures which could be mistaken for constrictive physiology (beat 1 only).

Examine Figure 4, top middle, in which the LVEDP is 16 mm Hg. There is a premature atrial contraction (beat 1) which has near-normal filling without apparent influence on right ventricular hemodynamic pressure. Left ventricular relaxation is impaired. The patient has eleva-

T.B.

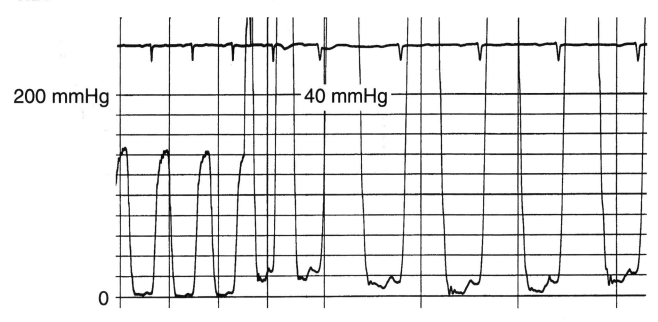

Fig. 2. Left ventricular pressure (0–200 mm Hg and 0–40 mm Hg scales), demonstrating abnormal left ventricular diastolic pressure waveform.

tion of right ventricular pressures and pulmonary hypertension. He is being evaluated for congestive heart failure and chronic mitral regurgitation.

Example 3 (Fig. 4, top right, scale 0–100 mm Hg) was obtained in a patient who has exacerbation of known severe congestive heart failure. Note the LVEDP of approximately 35 mm Hg, varying from 30–40 mm Hg over the 4 beats demonstrated. The extreme elevation of both the minimal diastolic and LVEDP and the high right ventricular systolic and end-diastolic pressures indicates the critical decompensation. In addition, the upslope of contraction is delayed, consistent with severe global left ventricular dysfunction (ejection fraction <20%). Deterioration of ischemic cardiomyopathy was confirmed by ventriculography.

Abnormalities of cardiac rhythm can produce marked distortions in the timing relationship between left ventricular and right ventricular pressures. Note the left and right ventricular end-diastolic pressures in a patient with an abnormal rhythm (Fig. 4, lower left). The LVEDP is 32 mm Hg. Right ventricular end-diastolic pressure is above 22 mm Hg. There is an endocardial pacemaker rhythm which delays and skews the relaxation period of left ventricle pressure, resulting in overlapping of the left ventricular pressure downslope on that of the right ventricular pressure. The unusual alignment of diastolic pressures in this case would provide an additional clue to conduction abnormalities, if these were not evident

already from the coincident electrocardiographic tracings. The high filling pressures were due to nonischemic cardiomyopathy.

Similar findings can be observed in a patient with a left-bundle branch block (Fig. 4, bottom right) in which the LVEDP is 28 mm Hg with a rapid upslope greatly exceeding that of the right ventricular pressure upslope. The compliance of the left ventricle (estimated from slope of diastolic filling pressure) can be compared to the rather slow filling rate (higher compliance) of the right ventricle. This patient had hypertensive congestive heart failure with mild pulmonary hypertension.

DISCUSSION

The interpretation of the LVEDP waveform has contributed to our understanding of ventricular contraction and relaxation. The pressure wave is a reflection of the compliance of the left ventricle and thus indirectly represents the clinical conditions which affect ventricular performance. Early clinical studies of hypertrophic cardiomyopathy emphasized the intraventricular gradient, and recent echocardiographic information has documented the fact that hypertrophic myopathies have abnormal diastolic function with prolonged left ventricular isovolumetric relaxation phases with impaired diastolic filling. The earliest report of improved diastolic function and systolic performance in patients with hypertrophic myopa-

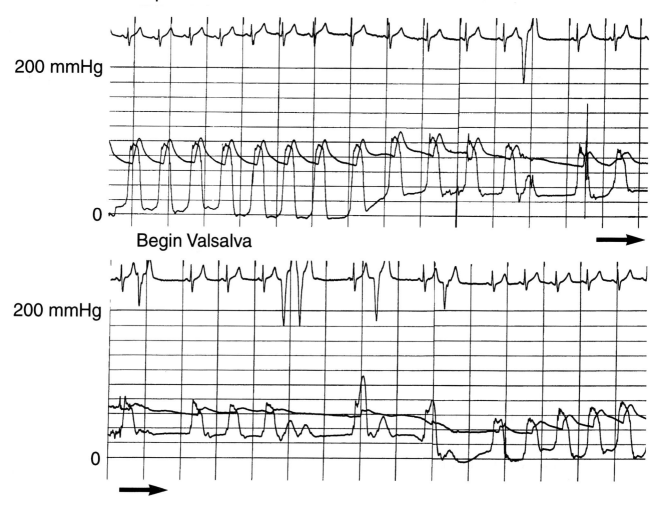

Fig. 3.   Left ventricular and aortic pressures obtained before (top) and during (bottom) Valsalva maneuver with stimulation of ventricular premature contractions (PVC). Note the intraventricular gradient during peak Valsalva with PVCs (bottom middle).

thy after calcium blocker was by Lorell et al. [5] and indicated that nonobstructive hypertrophic cardiomyopathy was responsive to calcium channel blockers to produce substantial hemodynamic and clinical improvement, with amelioration of the abnormal left ventricular diastolic pressure curve. The patients reviewed in Figure 2 and some of the patients in Figure 4 have the abnormal left ventricular relaxation phase present.

The LVEDP immediately precedes the beginning of isometric ventricular contraction in the left ventricular pressure pulse. This point, also known as the "Z" point, is situated on the downslope of the left ventricular "A" wave and marks the crossing over of the left atrial and left ventricular pressures. The LVEDP is normally <12 mm Hg and may be elevated when the left ventricle experiences excessive diastolic volume overload in conditions of mitral or aortic valvular regurgitation or high-volume

shunting (left-to-right) at or distal to the ventricular septum. Impairment of myocardial contractility alters the diastolic pressure-volume relationship and shifts the end-diastolic pressure point upward. Conditions of concentric hypertrophy due to hypertension or valvular stenosis, restrictive or infiltrative cardiomyopathy, or other diseases of the ventricular muscle produce a stiffer chamber and thus alter the pressure-volume curve, elevating the LVEDP.

Left ventricular function has always been associated with changes in the LVEDP in relationship to the existing stroke work for that particular pressure. The curvilinear relationship between stroke work and LVEDP has commonly been called the left ventricular function curve and is a measure of the performance of ventricular activity. The ventricular function curves are shifted upward by positive inotropic interventions and downward by those

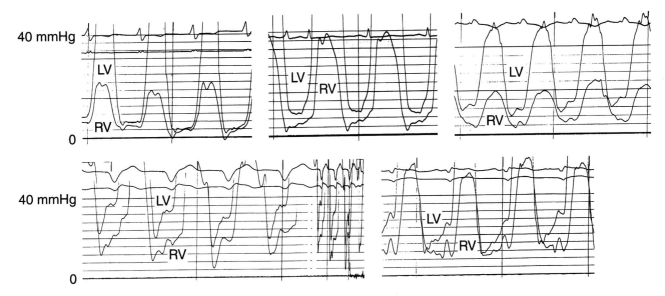

Fig. 4. Simultaneously-recorded left ventricular (LV) and right ventricular (RV) pressures obtained with fluid-filled catheters in a series of patients with cardiovascular abnormalities. Top left, patient with low fitting pressures. Top middle and right, 2 patients with high end diastolic pressures. Bottom left and right, 2 patients with conduction abnormalities. Scale is 0–40 mm Hg except at top right.

impairing inotropic activity. Afterload also may significantly influence the elevation or decline of the ventricular function curve. The compliance of the left ventricle is probably the major determinant of the LVEDP. Compliance is defined as the change in volume divided by the change in ventricular pressure. Both ventricular volume and pressure must be measured simultaneously to compute the compliance value. The slope of the compliance curve is called stiffness, which is the inverse of compliance. Compliance tends to decrease in chronic conditions involving myocardial hypertrophy, restrictive cardiomyopathy, or other infiltrative processes. In patients with cardiac disease, the LVEDP may alter with the provocation of myocardial ischemia. Parker et al. [6] reported their findings on LVEDP changes at rest, during rapid atrial pacing, and on immediate termination of pacing in control patients and patients with coronary artery disease with and without angina. In contrast to normal individuals, left ventricular pressure was elevated in patients with pacing-induced myocardial ischemia, whereas patients without pacing-induced ischemia had a smaller change in LVEDP. The compliance shift due to ischemia was able to alter the reported LVEDP.

CONCLUSIONS

Information about ventricular function, especially diastolic function, can be gleaned from careful examination of the LVEDP waveform. Artifacts of pressure wave-

forms should be identified to avoid confusion with true pathophysiologic responses.

ACKNOWLEDGMENTS

The author thanks the J.G. Mudd Cardiac Catheterization Laboratory for technical support, and Donna Sander for manuscript preparation.

REFERENCES

1. Goodwin JF: Hypertrophic cardiomyopathy: A disease in search of its own identity. Am J Cardiol 45:177–180, 1980.
2. Sanderson JE, Gibson DG, Brown DJ, Goodwin JF: Left ventricular filling in hypertrophic cardiomyopathy: An angiographic study. Br Heart J 39:661–670, 1977.
3. St. John Sutton MG, Tajik AJ, Gibson DG, Brown DJ, Seward JB, Guiliani ER: Echocardiographic assessment of left ventricular filling and septal and posterior wall dynamics in idiopathic hypertrophic subaortic stenosis. Circulation 57:512–520, 1978.
4. Hanrath P, Mathey DG, Siegert R, Bleifeld W: Left ventricular relaxation and filling pattern in different forms of left ventricular hypertrophy: An echocardiographic study. Am J Cardiol 45:15–23, 1980.
5. Lorell BH, Paulus WJ, Grossman W, Wynne J, Cohn PF, Braunwald E: Improved diastolic function and systolic performance in hypertrophic cardiomyopathy after nifedipine. N Engl J Med 303:801–803, 1985.
6. Parker JO, Ledwich JR, West RO, Case RB: Reversible cardiac failure during angina pectoris: Hemodynamic effects of atrial pacing in coronary artery disease. Circulation 39:745–757, 1969.

Chapter 35

Simultaneous Left and Right Ventricular Pressure Measurements

Morton J. Kern, MD, Thomas J. Donohue, MD, Richard G. Bach, MD, and Frank V. Aguirre, MD

INTRODUCTION

The physiology of ventricular pressure generation is more complicated than simple ventricular contraction and ejection [1–5]. Ventricular interaction coupled with septal contractile mechanisms plays a major role in the appearance of individual ventricular pressure waveforms. Moreover, differences in compliance between the two ventricles and timing of activation (conduction) produce interesting hemodynamic records which are reflections of the myocardial diseases effecting one side more than the other. In many cardiac catheterization laboratories simultaneous measurements of right and left ventricular pressures are only performed to evaluate uncommon explanations for cardiac dysfunctions, such as constrictive pericardial disease or restrictive cardiomyopathies. Rarely do cardiologists review simultaneous right and left ventricular pressures during routine hemodynamic studies. As part of the training program in our laboratory, a comparison of simultaneous right and left ventricular pressures during combined complete hemodynamic studies is routinely performed. In this hemodynamic rounds we will review several common and uncommon examples of simultaneous right and left ventricle pressures. The waveforms of constrictive and restrictive physiology have been described in previous rounds [6]. The characteristic configuration and significance of the diastolic ventricular pressure tracings in such patients can be reviewed separately.

NOTES ON HEMODYNAMIC TECHNIQUE

Simultaneous right and left ventricular pressures are easily measured during pullback of the balloon-tipped catheter from the pulmonary artery to the right ventricle while a ventriculography (pigtail) catheter remains within the left ventricle. Standard fluid-filled transducers and tubing provide satisfactory pressure waves which are recorded at fast (50–100 mm/sec) paper speed. Although fluid-filled systems provide clinically useful hemodynamic tracings, high fidelity micromanometer-tipped catheters are needed to identify small pressure differences or contraction/relaxation (dP/dt) data used for research studies.

RIGHT AND LEFT VENTRICULAR PRESSURES IN A PATIENT WITH HYPERTENSION

A 65-year-old man with hypertension had routine diagnostic study for dyspnea and atypical chest pain. Cardiac catheterization was performed from the femoral approach as described earlier [7]. Right heart hemodynamics revealed a mean right atrial pressure of 8mmHg, right ventricular pressure of 65/12mmHg, mean pulmonary capillary wedge pressure of 20mmHg, pulmonary artery pressure of 65/22mmHg. Left ventricular pressure was 162/26mmHg. Cardiac output and oxygen saturations were within normal limits. The simultaneous right and left ventricular pressure tracings are shown on Figure 1. In assessing the ventricular pressures, examine 4 features; 1) the A waves, 2) rates of systolic pressure rise, 3) position of the right ventricular pressure within the left ventricular tracing, and 4) the rate of diastolic pressure decline and mid diastolic upslopes. Recall that these pressures were obtained immediately prior to left ventriculography which demonstrated global hypokinesis

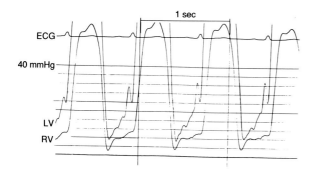

Fig. 1.   Simultaneous right (RV) and left ventricular (LV) pressures in a patient with hypertension.

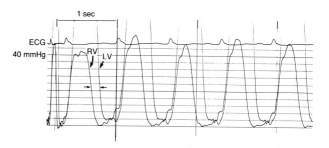

Fig. 2.   Simultaneous right (RV) and left ventricular (LV) pressures in a patient with an intraventricular conduction defect.

and moderate mitral regurgitation. Mild, non-critical coronary artery narrowings were also present. The left ventricular compliance is reflected by both height of the A wave and the diastolic upslope. Note both findings are lower in the right compared to the left ventricle. The left ventricular diastolic pressure has a steep upsloping diastolic filling period. The A wave is also pronounced. The right ventricular pressure tracing is contained (that is, the upstroke and downstroke) equally within the left ventricular pressure waveform. This normal pattern is seen with patients who have normal electrocardiographic conduction and generally normal biventricular function. Despite pulmonary hypertension, the normal diastolic pressure upslope and diminutive A wave suggest that right ventricular compliance is nearly normal.

EFFECTS OF CONDUCTION ON RIGHT AND LEFT VENTRICULAR PRESSURES

Examine the tracings in a 77-yr-old woman with prior history of myocardial infarction (Fig. 2). Normal left heart hemodynamic values and cardiac output were reported. Right heart catheterization revealed mild pulmonary stenosis. Note the shift of the right ventricular upstroke which occurred earlier (40–80msec) under the left ventricular pressure upstroke. The entire right ventricular curve is shifted with an earlier pressure decline shown by the wider spaced tracings during the isovolumetric relaxation period (2 arrows). This shift is attributed to a delay in intraventricular conduction and pressure generation. The QRS complex is consistent with left bundle branch block [8,9]. The review of the A waves, diastolic upstroke and rates of pressure rises reveal normal values with low right and left ventricular end diastolic pressures. Of special interest are the similar observations of Dr. Wiggers over half a century ago using first generation electromechanical pressure manometers [9]. Dr. Wiggers also examined the effects of premature systoles and the subsequent temporary alteration of simultaneous

left and right ventricular pressures [9] (Fig. 3). The precedence of the left over right ventricular contraction force (systole) was noted in a premature beat and that an alteration of systolic pressures of the subsequent beats affected both ventricles (Fig. 3). Similar findings have been observed more recently with high fidelity micromanometer-tipped transducers to identify the precise timing and force of contraction and differences in contractile function between the two ventricles [8].

Compare the positioning of the right ventricular pressure in Figure 2 to the middle beat (arrow) of Figure 4. Right and left ventricular pressures were obtained during a routine catheterization. The electrocardiogram was normal, but the downstroke of the right ventricular pressure overlies that of the left ventricle on several beats (arrows). Why? This pattern was only intermittently present and was a catheter tip artifact. When the tip of the catheter is occluded by the septal wall, the pressure pattern falls directly with left ventricular pressure. The subsequent beats have a normal spacing of the right ventricle pressure upstroke within the left ventricular pressure tracing and its normal spacing during early diastolic relaxation. These tracings are otherwise remarkable for findings of poor left ventricular compliance (large A wave, high minimum diastolic pressure and diastolic upstroke) and the strikingly low right ventricular filling pattern (negative overshoot in early diastole, small A wave, flat diastolic slope).

Another example of conduction delay on the pressure waveforms was found in a 63-yr-old woman with recent chest pain and electrocardiographic findings of acute myocardial infarction. Intermittent hypotension and Wenckebach arrhythmia were noted during the procedure. In the catheterization laboratory, mean right atrial pressure was 25mmHg and mean pulmonary capillary wedge pressure was 22mmHg. The simultaneous right and left ventricular pressures are shown on Figure 5.

An interventricular conduction delay (with ST segment elevation) is associated with a displaced right ventricular pressure downstroke later in the cycle toward the left ventricular pressure diastole on beats #1, 2, 4 and 5.

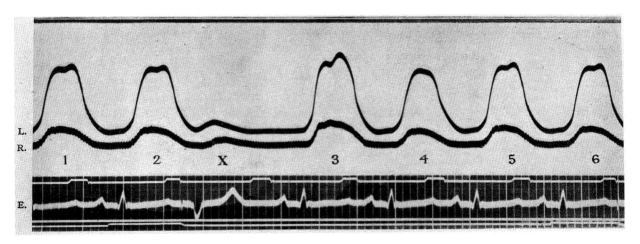

Fig. 3. Original hemodynamic recordings by Dr. Wiggers of simultaneous right and left ventricular pressures in a dog. The effect of a premature systole and subsequent temporary alternation on left and right ventricular pressure curves. Observe precedence of left over right ventricular contraction in premature beat. The alternation affects both ventricles. L = left ventricle; R = right ventricle; E = electrocardiogram, lead II. 1 and 2, normal beats; X, premature ventricular systole of left ventricle; 3–4 and 5–6, alternans couples. With permission from Wiggers CJ (ed). The pressure pulses under certain abnormal types of ventricular contraction. In "The Pressure Pulses in the Cardiovascular System." London: Longmans, Green and Co., 1928, pp 166–181.

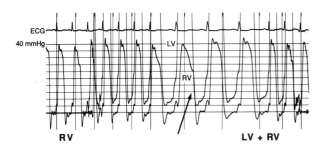

Fig. 4. Simultaneous right (RV) and left ventricular (LV) pressures in a patient without an intraventricular conduction defect. Why is pressure overlapping at the arrow?

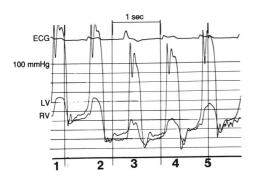

Fig. 5. Simultaneous right (RV) and left ventricular (LV) pressures in a patient with intraventricular conduction defect.

The interventricular conduction delay of a right bundle branch block pattern has normal early septal excitation-contraction of the left ventricle with 40–100msec delay in right ventricular excitation. From these tracings, why does beat #3 have an early right ventricular upstroke? What is the clinical diagnosis? An acute inferior myocardial infarction with right ventricular involvement is responsible for elevation and near equilibration of diastolic pressures, especially evident on beat #5. The compliance of the ventricles is obscured by the constrictive/restrictive dip and plateau patterns. Right and left ventricular filling pressures in this patient are elevated due to recent infarction. When examining patients with abnormal right ventricular pressures, the concordance (matching) of diastolic waveforms should be placed in the clinical context. Low but matched diastolic pressures may separate after rapid volume administration indicating normal function, whereas in restrictive myopathy, the diastolic concordance may persist [4]. Beat #3 is a fusion beat with normalized conduction (note the P and T waves). The right ventricular pressure on this beat is different with the upstroke and downstroke occurring earlier inside the left ventricular pressure.

PACEMAKER PRESSURE RESPONSES

Ventricular pacemaker activation and left bundle branch block may also produce unusual patterns of right and left ventricular pressure waves. Simultaneous right and left ventricular pressures were obtained in an elderly patient with congestive heart failure and a permanent pacemaker undergoing right and left heart catheterization (Fig. 6). The compliance of both ventricles was thought to be similar with absent A waves (due to ventricular pacing) and normal diastolic upslopes. A delayed rate of pressure rise and delayed relaxation of the right ventric-

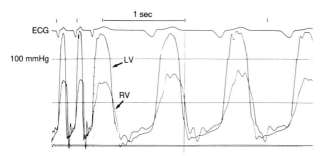

Fig. 6. Simultaneous right (RV) and left ventricular (LV) pressures in a patient with a permanent pacemaker.

ular pressure waveform can be seen with the later part of the right ventricular pressure (arrow) falling outside the left ventricular pressure curve. This abnormal pattern can be attributed, in part, to the pacemaker rhythm. In addition, the slow upstroke reflects abnormal right ventricular systolic function. Note the right ventricular pressure is 72/20mmHg. A delay of the right ventricular pressure rise could be caused by damping within the right ventricular catheter, but the resonant frequency of the pressure responses seems to be within normal range (consider the sinusoidal variations during the peak systolic and early diastolic periods). This unusual timing relationship of right and left ventricular pressures is a result of left bundle branch block and pacemaker in a patient with ventricular dysfunction. In patients with left bundle branch block (Fig. 7), maximal right ventricular contraction (dP/dt) usually preceeds left ventricular maximal contraction suggesting the abnormal ventricular activation of the pacemaker has an important action on right and left ventricular function.

First degree conduction abnormalities can also be reflected in the hemodynamic pressure tracings of both ventricles. The atrial contraction is easily discernable on simultaneous right and left ventricular pressures in a patient with first degree block (Fig. 8). The atrial pressure wave of beat #2 shows up as a positive deflection in the left ventricular pressure, but as a small negative deflection in the right ventricular pressure wave. The right ventricular pressure in this patient is normally located within the left ventricular pressure outline. The explanation for a negative P wave is unknown. Compare the A waves in this patient to those in Figure 9 with a pacemaker rhythm. The right and left ventricular pressures show striking A waves (beat #1) when P waves occur in normal sequence to ventricular activation. The ventricular pressures also show the contribution of atrial filling by augmented systolic pressure. On beat #2, no A waves are seen and differences in diastolic filling slopes are indicative of compliance differences between the two ventricles. As P wave activity occurs again, first on the

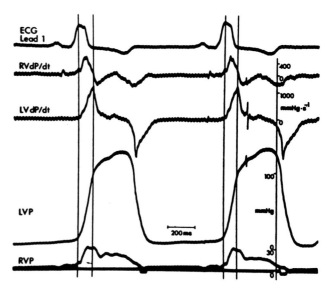

Fig. 7. Simultaneous right and left ventricular pressures and dP/dt recorded from a subject with left bundle branch block. The small right ventricular dP/dt peak precedes the onset of the rise of left ventricular dP/dt which is delayed. A secondary rapid rise of right ventricular dP/dt occurs after the onset of left ventricular dP/dt and is followed by an unusually slow decline. This pattern reflects the contractile function and interaction between the ventricular chambers. With permission from Feneley MP, Gavaghan TP, Baron DW, Branson JA, Roy PR, Morgan JJ. Contribution of left ventricular contraction to the generation of right ventricular systolic pressure in the human heart. Circulation 71:473–480, 1985.

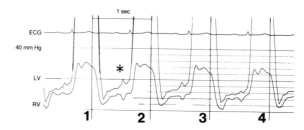

Fig. 8. Simultaneous right (RV) and left ventricular (LV) pressures in a patient with first degree atrioventricular block.

T wave (beat #4) and then after the T wave (beat #5), the atrial contribution to ventricular pressures can be easily appreciated. The effect of pacing on the timing of right and left ventricular pressure patterns in this patient was minimal.

VENTRICULAR PRESSURES IN A PATIENT WITH MITRAL STENOSIS

Mitral or pulmonary valvular lesions may be associated with markedly different ventricular chamber compliance. Differences in ventricular pressures may become apparent during cardiac arrhythmias with varying

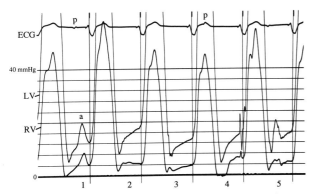

Fig. 9. Simultaneous right (RV) and left ventricular (LV) pressures in a patient with a pacemaker rhythm.

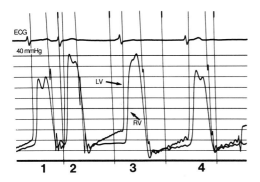

Fig. 10. Simultaneous right (RV) and left ventricular (LV) pressures in a patient with mitral stenosis.

SUMMARY

In addition to demonstrating constrictive and restrictive cardiac physiology, simultaneous right and left ventricular pressure measurements can be helpful to identify various aspects of myocardial dysfunction. Intracardiac conduction defects will displace the right ventricular pressure under the left ventricular pressure upstroke and identify differences in the timing of ventricular contraction. Right ventricular dysfunction will also produce abnormal right ventricular pressure waveforms which may overlap left ventricular pressure and contribute to abnormalities in right atrial and ventricular pressure waveforms.

ACKNOWLEDGMENT

The authors wish to thank the J.G. Mudd Cardiac Catheterization Laboratory Team and Donna Sander for manuscript preparation.

REFERENCES

1. Holt JP, Rhode EA, Kines H. Pericardial and ventricular pressure. Circ Res 8:1171–1181, 1960.
2. Glantz SA, Parmley WW. Factors which affect the diastolic pressure-volume curve. Circ Res 42:171–180, 1978.
3. Goldstein JA, Harada A, Yagi Y, Barzilai B, Cox JL. Hemodynamic importance of systolic ventricular interaction, augmented right atrial contractility and atrioventricular synchrony in acute right ventricular dysfunction. J Am Coll Cardiol 16:181–189, 1990.
4. Hoit BD, Dalton N, Bhargava V, Shabetai R. Pericardial influences on right and left ventricular filling dynamics. Cir Res 68:197–208, 1991.
5. Janicki JS, Weber KT. The pericardium and ventricular interaction, distensibility, and function. Am J Physiol 238 (Heart Circ Physiol 7):H494–H503, 1980.
6. Kern MJ, Aguirre FV. Hemodynamic rounds: Interpretation of cardiac pathophysiology from pressure waveform analysis: Pericardial compressive hemodynamics, Part I, II and III. Cathet Cardiovasc Diagn 25:336–342; 26:34–40; 26:152–158, 1992.
7. Kern MJ (ed), Deligonul U, Gudipati C. Hemodynamic and ECG data. In "The Cardiac Catheterization Handbook. St. Louis: Mosby Year Book, Inc., 1991, pp 98–201.
8. Feneley MP, Gavaghan TP, Baron DW, Branson JA, Roy PR, Morgan JJ. Contribution of left ventricular contraction to the generation of right ventricular systolic pressure in the human heart. Circulation 71:473–480, 1985.
9. Wiggers CJ (ed). The pressure pulses under certain abnormal types of ventricular contraction. In "The Pressure Pulses in the Cardiovascular System." London: Longmans, Green and Co., 1928, pp 166–181.
10. Thompson CR, Kingma I, MacDonald RPR, Belenkie I, Tyberg JV, Smith ER. Transseptal pressure gradient and diastolic ventricular septal motion in patients with mitral stenosis. Circulation 76:974–980, 1987.

RR cycles. Consider the hemodynamic tracings obtained in a 42-yr-old woman with mitral stenosis. Simultaneous right and left heart pressures (Fig. 10) demonstrate hemodynamic findings typical for atrial fibrillation. Diastolic filling rates (slopes) differ between ventricles during long pauses (beat #3). The left ventricular diastolic pressure has no A wave and a more rapid upstroke compared to the right ventricular pressure tracing which shows a long plateau before ventricular ejection. On beat #3, filling of the right ventricle appears completed by early diastole, whereas filling of the left ventricle continues throughout the cycle because of high left atrial pressure. This pattern also reflects differences in chamber compliance, as well as the influence of long RR cycle length (10). The flat right ventricular diastolic filling period of beat #3 is effected by respiratory activity on subsequent beats.

Chapter 36

Hemodynamic Manifestations of Ischemic Right Heart Dysfunction

Sharon G. Cresci, MD, and James A. Goldstein, MD

Acute right coronary artery (RCA) occlusions proximal to the right ventricular (RV) branches compromise RV free wall (RVFW) perfusion, resulting in RV dysfunction in nearly 50% of patients with transmural infero-posterior myocardial infarctions [1–3]. A spectrum of hemodynamic perturbations is manifest in approximately 50% of patients with ischemic RV involvement. In its most severe form, the clinical syndrome of predominant RV infarction (RVI) develops, characterized by right heart failure with clear lung fields and hypotension [1–5]. Hemodynamic evaluation in such patients typically reveals disproportionate elevation of right sided filling pressures, equalization of right and left sided diastolic pressures and low cardiac output despite intact left ventricular (LV) function [1–5].

Though for many years the right ventricle was considered functionally unimportant in the maintenance of the circulation, the hemodynamic contributions of intact RV function are now well documented [6–8]. Under normal conditions, RV systolic pressure is generated by shortening and thickening of the RVFW along its longitudinal and horizontal axes, resulting in a peristaltic wave of contraction from apex to outflow tract toward the septum. Furthermore, the septum is an integral architectural and mechanical component of the RV chamber and even under physiologic conditions, LV-septal contraction contributes to RV performance through systolic ventricular interactions mediated by the septum [6].

The mechanical importance of intact RVFW contraction is emphasized by the deleterious hemodynamic effects of RVFW dysfunction. Acute ischemia leads to RVFW dyskinesis and depressed global RV performance [7–11]. RV systolic dysfunction, manifest in the RV waveform by a slow upstroke, diminished peak pressure and delayed relaxation, reduces transpulmonary flow and results in diminished LV preload and decreased cardiac output despite preserved LV contractility [7–11]. RVFW ischemia also causes severe RV diastolic dysfunction [7–12]. Depressed RV systolic performance results in gross RV enlargement and ischemia both impairs

RV relaxation and renders the right ventricle intrinsically stiff. At the beginning of diastole, the right ventricle is dilated and its filling pressure elevated, thereby imparting increased resistance to early filling. There is progressively increased impedance to inflow as the right ventricle fills and ascends a steep noncompliant diastolic pressure-volume curve [9–11]. This progressive pandiastolic resistance to RV filling is manifest in the RV waveform as a rapid rise in diastolic pressure to an elevated plateau and in the right atrial (RA) waveform by elevated mean RA pressure and a blunted y descent [9–11].

RV diastolic dysfunction adversely affects LV diastolic properties [7–12]. Acute RV dilatation and elevated RV diastolic pressure shifts the interventricular septum toward the volume deprived left ventricle, thereby impairing LV compliance and further limiting LV filling. Abrupt RV dilatation within the non-compliant pericardium leads to elevated intrapericardial pressure [7,8,10,11]. The resultant pericardial constraint further impairs both RV and LV compliance and filling both directly and by intensifying the adverse effects of diastolic ventricular interactions [7–11]. Furthermore, as both ventricles fill and compete for space within the crowded pericardium, the effects of pericardial constraint contribute to the pattern of progressive pandiastolic impedance to RV filling, reflected hemodynamically by a blunted RA y descent, RV "dip and plateau" pattern and elevated, equalized diastolic filling pressures [7–11].

DETERMINANTS OF RV PERFORMANCE WITH ACUTE RV DYSFUNCTION:

Under conditions of acute RVFW dysfunction, RV performance is dependent on LV septal contractile contributions transmitted via systolic ventricular interactions mediated by the septum through both paradoxical septal motion and primary septal contributions [9–11]. In early isovolumic systole, unopposed LV-septal pressure generation creates a left-to-right transseptal pressure gradient, resulting in early systolic septal bulging into the RV cavity. This paradoxical motion not only contributes to early generation of RV systolic pressure, but also helps stretch the dyskinetic RVFW, a prerequisite to providing a stable buttress upon which later LV-septal thickening and shortening can generate peak RV pressure and effective pulmonary flow [9–11]. These interactions result in a bifid RV systolic pressure waveform, with the initial peak correlating with early paradoxical septal bulging and the later peak with maximal LV-septal shortening and peak systolic pressure generation.

The status of RA function is also an important determinant of hemodynamic performance under conditions of acute RV dysfunction [9–11,13]. Atrial function can be viewed as a tripartite process comprised of: 1) *Diastolic reserve (capacitance) properties* related to venous return and atrial compliance [14–20]; 2) *conductance function,* determined by tricuspid valve resistance and RV diastolic properties; and 3) *active transport,* related to atrial contraction [19,20]. The principles governing the mechanical behavior of atrial myocardium are similar to those operating in ventricular muscle. Thus, the strength of atrial contraction, reflected in the upstroke and peak amplitude of the RA a wave, is determined by the intrinsic atrial inotropic state, modulated by extrinsic neurohumoral stimuli, and influenced by atrial preload (maximal atrial volume) and afterload (imposed by the tricuspid valve and right ventricle) [16–20].

Evaluation of the RA waveform provides insight into the status of RA function [9–11,13–20]. Interpretation of the RA waveform may be facilitated by timing waveform components not only to the ECG, but also to mechanical correlates from simultaneous RV or pulmonary artery pressures [13]. The RA waveform components include: 1) The *a wave,* a positive deflection immediately following the P wave on the ECG and immediately preceding ventricular systole. The upstroke and amplitude of the a wave reflect the strength of atrial contraction. 2) The *x descent,* a negative deflection following the a wave and coincident with the QRS complex and mechanical ventricular systole. The x descent reflects both atrial relaxation and systolic intrapericardial pressure changes. 3) The *c wave,* a positive wave coinciding with early RV pressure generation and tricuspid valve closure, just following the QRS complex. The c wave likely represents mild early tricuspid valve regurgitation. When present, the c wave separates the x descent into two components, the x portion prior to the c wave reflecting atrial relaxation, and the x′ descent following the c wave representing systolic intrapericardial depressurization. 4) The *v wave,* a positive deflection during ventricular systole, reflecting passive atrial filling or,

when exaggerated, tricuspid regurgitation. 5) the *y descent,* a negative deflection following the v wave during ventricular diastole and just following the T wave but prior to the subsequent P wave. The slope of the y descent is an indicator, in part, of RV compliance.

In the setting of acute RVI, RV systolic and diastolic dysfunction impose increased preload and afterload on the right atrium, resulting in elevated mean RA pressures and a blunted y descent indicative of pandiastolic resistance to RV filling. These loading conditions stimulate both augmented RA contraction, reflected in the RA waveform as a more rapid upstroke and increased peak amplitude of the a wave, as well as enhanced RA relaxation, reflected by a steep x descent [9–11,13]. Experimental animal studies demonstrate that enhanced RA transport is an important compensatory mechanism that optimizes RV filling and performance (Fig. 1) [9–11]. Conversely, ischemic depression of atrial function, manifest as elevated mean RA pressure but depressed a wave and x descent, results in more severe hemodynamic compromise [10,11].

The strength of RA contraction is an important determinant of hemodynamic stability in clinical RVI [13]. Such patients manifest one of two distinct RA waveform patterns that share in common a blunted y descent reflecting pandiastolic resistance to RV filling, but are differentiated by the status of RA contraction and relaxation, as reflected in the morphology of the a wave and x descent [10,13]. Patients with RCA occlusion proximal to the RV branches but distal to the RA branches manifest RVI with enhanced RA contraction/relaxation resulting in an augmented a wave and steep x descent ("W" pattern) in the RA trace (Fig. 2). RCA occlusion proximal to the RA branches result in RA ischemia/infarction and depressed RA function manifest by a depressed a wave and x descent ("M" pattern) (Fig. 3). These findings have prognostic and therapeutic impact [13]. Patients with enhanced RA contraction have higher peak RV pressure, better cardiac output and more favorable therapeutic response to volume infusion and inotropic stimulation relative to those with depressed atrial function. However, when patients with augmented RA contraction lose this compensatory atrial kick due to atrioventricular asynchrony, more severe hemodynamic compromise results. Similarly, ischemic depression of atrial contractility is associated with more severe hemodynamic compromise.

CASE STUDIES

Occlusion of the Mid-RCA: RV ischemic dysfunction with augmented RA function. A 65-year-old man presented with an acute inferior myocardial infarction complicated by second degree atrioventricular block, el-

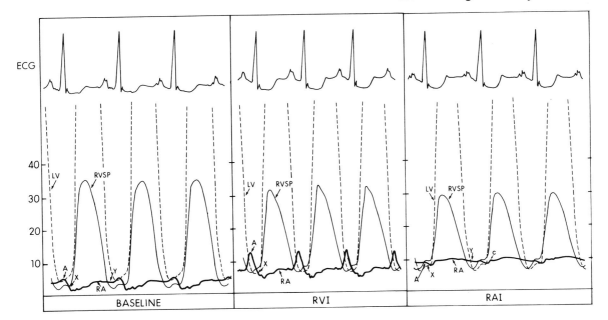

Fig. 1. Sequential superimposed hemodynamic changes. After right ventricular ischemia (RVI), peak right ventricular systolic pressure (RVSP) was depressed and right ventricular relaxation delayed. Mean right atrial (RA) pressure increased and its a wave became markedly augmented (arrow) and dominated the diastolic filling period. There was a prominent right atrial x and a comparatively blunted y descent. Left ventricular (LV) and right ventricular diastolic pressure were elevated and equal-ized. Subsequent right atrial ischemia (RAI) further increased mean right atrial pressure with severe depression of the a wave and blunting of the previously prominent x descent, with associated further reduction in right ventricular systolic pressure. ECG = electrocardiogram. (All pressures are measured in mm Hg.) Reprinted with permission from the Am Coll of Cardiol, J1 Am Coll Cardiol 18:1564–1572, 1985.

evated jugular venous pressure and hypotension. Echocardiography revealed marked RV dilatation, severe RVFW dysfunction, and an inferior LV wall motion abnormality but overall normal LV ejection fraction. Coronary angiography demonstrated RCA occlusion proximal to the RV branches but distal to the RA branches.

Hemodynamic evaluation with a fluid-filled, balloon-tipped catheter (Fig. 4) demonstrated a broadened, depressed RV systolic waveform with a diminished upstroke, decreased and bifid peak pressure and delayed relaxation. These changes reflect depressed RV contractility and the compensatory effects of systolic ventricular interactions. RV filling pressure was elevated early in diastole, with a rapid rise to a plateau indicative of progressive pandiastolic impedance to RV filling. Though mean RA pressure was elevated, the upstroke and peak amplitude of the a wave were increased ("W" pattern), indicating augmented RA contraction. A steep x descent was evident, reflecting enhanced RA relaxation, whereas the y descent was blunted representing pandiastolic resistance to RV filling. Simultaneous superimposed RA and pulmonary capillary wedge pressure (not shown) revealed equalization of diastolic pressures, attributable to the effects of pericardial restraint.

Proximal RCA occlusion: RV and RA ischemic dysfunction. A 72-year-old man presented with an acute inferior myocardial infarction complicated by severe hypotension with predominant right heart failure. Echocardiography revealed severe RVFW dysfunction, RV dilatation and an inferior LV wall motion abnormality with overall normal LV ejection fraction. Coronary angiography demonstrated RCA occlusion proximal to the RA branches, with no evidence of collateral flow.

Hemodynamic evaluation (Fig. 5) demonstrated RV waveform alterations similar to those in case 1 and characteristic of RV systolic dysfunction. The RV upstroke was depressed with its peak pressure diminished and a broad systolic wave with delayed relaxation was evident. RV diastolic pressure was elevated with a "dip and plateau" pattern. As in the prior case, mean RA pressure was markedly elevated and the y descent blunted, reflecting the effects of impedance to RV filling. In contrast, the upstroke and peak amplitude of the a wave were markedly depressed and the x descent diminished ("M" pattern), consistent with ischemic depression of RA contraction and relaxation (figure 4). Gross RA dilatation and akinesis were observed at thoracotomy for emergency revascularization in this patient, indicating the presence of RA ischemia/infarction.

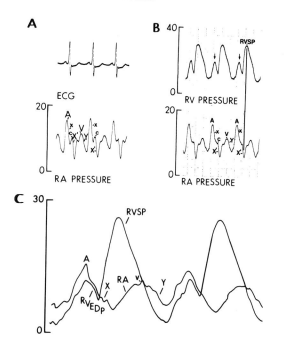

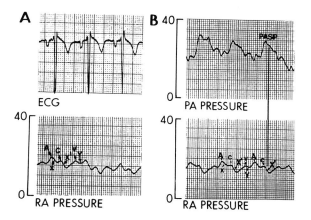

Fig. 3. Tracings of simultaneous right atrial (RA) pressure and electrocardiogram (ECG) (panel A) from a patient with an M pattern demonstrate most prominent negative deflection (x') coincident with T wave suggesting a y descent. However, timing of RA pressure with pulmonary artery systolic pressure (PASP) (panel B) demonstrates that this descent is coincident with peak PASP and therefore a systolic x' descent. Reprinted with permission from Circulation 82:359–368, 1990.

Fig. 2. Hemodynamic recordings from a patient with a W pattern. Peaks of W are formed by prominent a waves, and most prominent right atrial (RA) descent occurs just before T wave of electrocardiogram (ECG) (panel A). Simultaneous RA and right ventricular (RV) pressures (panel B) demonstrate that this prominent descent coincides with peak RV systolic pressure (RVSP) and is therefore an x' systolic descent, followed by a comparatively blunted y descent. Peak RVSP is depressed, RV relaxation is prolonged, and there is a dip and rapid rise in RV diastolic pressure. Prominent RA a waves are reflected in the right ventricle as an augmented end-diastolic pressure (EDP) rise (arrows). These wave form relations are confirmed by simultaneous superimposed RA/RV pressure recordings (panel C). Reprinted with permission from Circulation 82:359–368, 1990.

DIFFERENTIATION OF RVI AND PERICARDIAL CONSTRICTION

The equalized diastolic filling pressures and the RV "dip and plateau" pattern observed in patients with RV infarction may be seen in those with constrictive pericarditis as well. However, careful examination of the RA waveform permits differentiation of these conditions. In constrictive pericarditis, there is rapid unimpeded filling of the right ventricle in the first third of diastole, reflected in the RA waveform as a brisk y descent. However, as RV volume reaches the limits of the constraining pericardial shell in later diastole, an abrupt increase in impedance to RV inflow results in a rapid rise in RV pressure to an elevated level, reflected in the RV waveform as a "dip and plateau" pattern. Though a similar RV morphology may be seen with acute RVI, the pandiastolic impedance to RV inflow results in a blunted RA y descent, which therefore serves to distinguish these conditions.

THERAPEUTIC OPTIONS

Treatment of RV infarction should focus on the general considerations of optimizing oxygen supply-demand which are critical to the management of all patients with acute ischemic heart disease [21]. Patients with acute transmural infero-posterior myocardial infarction should undergo noninvasive testing with right sided chest leads (V3R-V4R) and two dimensional echocardiography to detect the presence of RV involvement. In patients with RV dilatation and RV wall motion abnormalities, careful attention to optimizing preload may prevent or minimize hemodynamic compromise. More specifically, vasodilators and diuretics should be administered with great caution. In patients with the hemodynamic syndrome of predominant RVI, attention should first be given to restoration of physiologic rhythm. Thereafter, volume challenge is indicated for persistent low output. When hypotension and low output persist despite these measures, invasive hemodynamic monitoring is indicated. Parenteral inotropic stimulation, which may act by augmenting LV-septal contractile contributions to RV performance [11], rather than via direct improvement in RVFW contraction is usually effective in stabilizing patients not responsive to more conservative measures. Inotropic therapy should be instituted with dopamine when mean arterial pressure is less than 60 mm Hg in order to optimize perfusion to both left and right circulatory systems. Otherwise, dobutamine is more appropriate as the initial inotropic agent. Intraaortic balloon pumping, by improving coronary perfusion to both left and right circulations, may be beneficial in patients with refractory

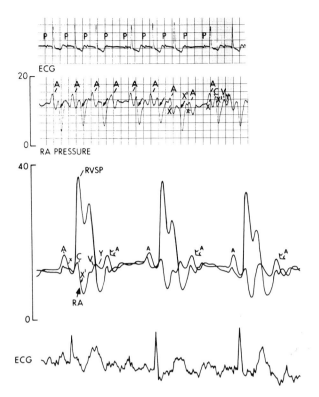

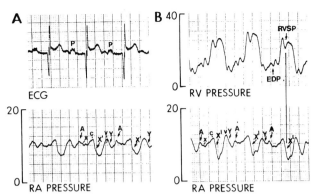

Fig. 5. Tracings of M pattern of right atrial (RA) pressure. When timed by electrocardiogram (panel A), most prominent negative deflection in right atrium is coincident with T wave, suggesting a diastolic y descent. In contrast, its relation to right ventricular (RV) pressure (panel B) demonstrates that this prominent descent coincides with peak RV systolic pressure (RVSP), indicating a systolic x' descent, whereas diastolic y descent is blunted. M pattern comprises a depressed a wave, x descent before a small c wave, a prominent x' descent, a small v wave, and a blunted y descent. Peak RV systolic pressure (RVSP) is depressed and bifid (arrow) with delayed relaxation and an elevated end-diastolic pressure (EDP). Reprinted with permission from Circulation 82:359–368, 1990.

Fig. 4. Hemodynamic recordings from a patient with a W pattern and severe low cardiac output precipitated by 2° atrioventricular block (upper panel). Recording of right atrial (RA) pressure and electrocardiogram (ECG) (upper panel) demonstrates augmented a waves and prominent x' and blunted y descents, confirmed by simultaneous superimposed RA and right ventricular (RV) pressure recordings (lower panel). Presence of both x and x' descents, delineated in conducted beats only (upper panel), demonstrates an additional problem with identification of components of RA pressure waveform. RV systolic pressure (RVSP) morphology is bifid, and a diastolic dip and plateau pattern is evident. Slight variation in timing of simultaneous superimposed RA/RV pressure recordings may be due to differences in maximal frequency response. RVEDP, RV end-diastolic pressure. Reprinted with permission from Circulation 82: 359–368, 1990.

low output. The role of acute RV revascularization, whether with thrombolytic agents, acute angioplasty or urgent coronary bypass surgery, has not been adequately defined. However, recent experimental studies suggest that, by virtue of comparatively more favorable oxygen supply-demand characteristics compared with the left ventricle, the right ventricle may be more resistant to infarction and thereby manifest a more salutary response to reperfusion in general and late reperfusion in particular [22].

CONCLUSIONS

In summary, right heart ischemia results in intrinsic pathophysiologic changes in right heart performance and

elicits compensatory physiologic mechanisms that are reflected in characteristic hemodynamic alterations. Careful evaluation of RV and RA waveforms provides useful information regarding the status of right heart function that may have therapeutic and prognostic implications.

REFERENCES

1. Cohn JN, Guiha NH, Broder MI, Constantinos JL: Right ventricular infarction: Clinical and hemodynamic features. Am J Cardiol 33:209–214, 1974.
2. Lopez-Sendon J, Garcia-Fernandez MA, Coma-Canella I, Yanguela MM, Banuelos F: Segmental right ventricular function after acute myocardial infarction: Two-dimensional echocardiographic study in 63 patients. Am J Cardiol 51:390–396, 1983.
3. Dell'Italia LJ, Starling MR, Crawford MH, Boros BL, Chaudhuri TK, O'Rourke RA, Heyl B, Amon W: Right ventricular infarction: Identification by hemodynamic measurements before and after volume loading and correlation with noninvasive techniques. J Am Coll Cardiol 4:931–939, 1984.
4. Dell'Italia LJ, Starling MR, Blumhardt R, Lasher JC, O'Rourke RA: Comparative effects of volume loading, dobutamine, and nitroprusside in patients with predominant right ventricular infarction. Circulation 72:1327–1335, 1985.
5. Shah PD, Maddahi J, Berman DS, Pichler M, Swan HJC: Scintigraphically detected predominant right ventricular dysfunction in acute myocardial infarction: Clinical and hemodynamic correlates and implications for therapy and prognosis. J Am Coll Cardiol 6:1264–1272, 1985.
6. Meier GD, Bove AA, Santamore WLP, Lynch PR: Contractile function in canine right ventricle. Am J Physiol 239:H794–H804, 1980.
7. Goldstein JA, Vlahakes GJ, Verrier ED, Schiller NB, Tyberg JV,

Ports TA, Parmley WW, Chatterjee K: The role of right ventricular systolic dysfunction and elevated intrapericardial pressure in the genesis of low output in experimental right ventricular infarction. Circulation 65:513–522, 1982.

8. Tani M: Roles of the right ventricular free wall and ventricular septum in right ventricular performance and influence of the parietal pericardium during right ventricular failure in dogs. Am J Cardiol 52:196–202, 1983.

9. Goldstein JA, Harada A, Yagi Y, Barzilai B, Cox JL: Hemodynamic importance of systolic ventricular interaction, augmented right atrial contractility and atrioventricular synchrony in acute right ventricular dysfunction. J Am Coll Cardiol 16:181–189, 1990.

10. Goldstein JA, Tweddell JS, Barzilai B, Yagi Y, Jaffe AS, Cox JL: Right atrial ischemia exacerbates hemodynamic compromise associated with experimental right ventricular dysfunction. J Am Coll Cardiol 18:1564–1572, 1985.

11. Goldstein JA, Tweddell JS, Barzilai B, Yagi Y, Jaffe AS, Cox JL: Importance of left ventricular function and systolic ventricular interaction to right ventricular performance during acute right heart ischemia. J Am Coll Cardiol 19:704–711, 1992.

12. Lorell B, Leinbach RC, Pohost AM, Gold HK, Dinsmore RE, Hutter AM, Pastore JO, Desanctis RW: Right ventricular infarction. Clinical diagnosis and differentiation from cardiac tamponade and pericardial constriction. Am J Cardiol 43:465–471, 1979.

13. Goldstein JA, Barzilai B, Rosamond TL, Eisenberg PR, Jaffe AS: Determinants of hemodynamic compromise with severe right ventricular infarction. Circulation 82:359–368, 1990.

14. Braunwald E, Frahm CJ: Studies on Starling's Law of the heart. Circulation 24:633–642, 1961.

15. Grant C, Bunnell IL, Greene DG: The reservoir function of the left atrium during ventricular systole. Am J Med 37:36–43, 1964.

16. Brawley RK, Oldham N, Vasko JS, Henney RP, Morrow AG: Influence of right atrial pressure pulse on instantaneous vena cava blood flow. Am J Physio 211:347–353, 1966.

17. Kalmanson D, Veyrat C, Chiche P: Atrial versus ventricular contribution in determining systemic venous return. Cardiovasc Res 5:293–302, 1971.

18. Sarnoff SJ, Gilmore JP, Brockman SK, Mitchell JH, Linden RJ: Regulation of ventricular contraction by the carotid sinus: Its effect on atrial and ventricular dynamics. Circ Res 8:1123–1136, 1960.

19. Williams JF, Sonnenblick EH, Braunwald E: Determinants of atrial contractile force on the intact heart. Am J Physiol 209:1061–1068, 1965.

20. Sarnoff SJ, Gilmore JP, Mitchell JH: Influence of atrial contraction and relaxation on closure on mitral valve. Circ Res 11:26–35, 1962.

21. Goldstein JA: Pathophysiology of hemodynamically severe right ventricular infarction. Coronary Artery Disease 1:314–322, 1990.

22. Laster SB, Shelton TJ, Barzilai B, Goldstein JA. Response of the ischemic right ventricle to reperfusion. J Am Coll Cardiol 17(2):164A, 1991.

Commentary

EDITORIAL COMMENTS: HEMODYNAMIC MANIFESTATIONS OF ISCHEMIC RIGHT HEART DYSFUNCTION

Morton J. Kern, MD

Patients with right ventricular infarction often present with striking abnormalities of right heart hemodynamics. The extent and detail of these hemodynamic alterations has been eloquently elucidated by Drs. Cresci and Goldstein in Hemodynamic Manifestations of Ischemic Right Heart Dysfunction. The changes observed in right atrial pressure during different degrees of ischemic right ventricular dysfunction are discussed as new observations and interpretations of the traditional A, C, and V waveforms. Further striking changes can be observed with the addition of right atrial ischemia superimposed on right ventricular ischemia. These findings are unique and rarely described in earlier studies. The elegant investigational work of the authors confirms commonly observed changes in right heart hemodynamics and accurately reflects and furthers clarifies the underlying physiologic mechanisms.

This chapter illustrates the changes in right atrial and ventricular pressures during the progressive ischemia of right coronary occlusion which may be commonly observed in patients. Simultaneous right and left ventricular hemodynamic patterns often demonstrate constrictive/restrictive physiology during acute right ventricular infarction. I have taken the liberty of adding the following clinical example to complete the common findings.

Right atrial and simultaneous right and left ventricular pressures (Fig. 1) were measured in a 43 year old woman with acute inferior myocardial infarction, persistent chest pain and ventricular arrhythmias after receiving intravenous streptokinase. Coronary artery bypass grafting was performed in 1987 with saphenous vein grafts to the left anterior descending and diagonal branch. The right coronary artery had not been bypassed. The systolic pressure was 90mmHg. The electrocardiogram showed ST elevation in the inferior leads, reciprocal ST depression in leads, V_1-V_6. Right-sided electrocardiogram showed ST elevation in lead V_4. Periods of Mobitz's type I AV block were noted. Coronary arteriography revealed total occlusion of the proximal right coronary artery with patent vein grafts to the left system. The initial right atrial pressure (Fig. 1A) demonstrated a mean right atrial

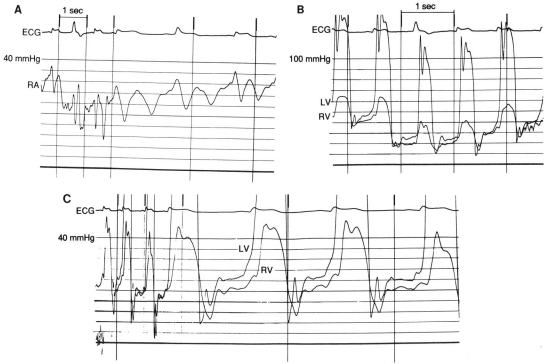

Fig. 1.   A: Right atrial (RA) pressure in a patient with acute inferior myocardial infarction (0-40mmHg scale). B: Simultaneous right (RV) and left ventricular (LV) pressures in the same patient as figure 1 (0-100mmHg scale). C: Simultaneous right (RV) and left ventricular (LV) pressures in the same patient as figure 1 (0-40mmHg scale).

pressure of approximately 28mmHG with nearly equal A and V waves with the M-shaped configuration as described by Drs. Cresci and Goldstein. Right ventricular pressure was also elevated (approximately 50/28mmHg). Prior to coronary angioplasty, the configuration of the right and left ventricular diastolic pressure waveforms were nearly matched with an early diastolic dip and a relatively flat period of diastasis prior to atrial systole (Fig. 1 B and C). Following coronary angioplasty, with resolution of chest pain and restoration of a consistent sinus rhythm, left and right ventricular end-diastolic pressure declined with persistence of the matching of the

diastolic waveforms similar to that of constrictive physiology. These tracings further illustrate the role of pericardial constraint in the patient with significant right ventricular ischemic dysfunction.

Review of the waveforms in this chapter should bring new insight into the hemodynamic mechanisms and consequences of right ventricular ischemia for the clinician.

REFERENCE

1. Cresci SG, Goldstein, J: Hemodynamic manifestations of Ischemic Right Heart Dysfunction. Cathet Cardiovasc Diagn (in press).

Chapter 37

Effects of Nitroglycerin

Morton J. Kern, MD, Frank V. Aguirre, MD, and Thomas C. Hilton, MD

INTRODUCTION

Nitroglycerin is the most commonly used medication in the cardiac catheterization laboratory. The hemodynamic effects of systemic and coronary vasodilation are often striking and, in general, are therapeutic. Nitroglycerin is routinely administered sublingually, intravenously, or intraarterially during coronary and left ventricular angiography. Significant increases in the caliber and flow responses of the coronary arteries as well as reduction of left ventricular filling pressures are well documented [1–3]. However, the varied hemodynamic influences of nitroglycerin reported during myocardial ischemia [3,4] may not be readily apparent from routine responses observed in stable patients. The purpose of this Hemodynamic Rounds is to review the hemodynamic effects of nitroglycerin with particular reference to ventricular unloading and acute ischemia. The case examples illustrate the systemic and coronary influence of this potent, short-lived, and important medication.

NITROGLYCERIN AND VENTRICULAR UNLOADING

A 72-yr-old woman with severe triple vessel coronary artery disease and hypertension had intermittent chest pain preceding the diagnostic coronary angiogram. At the conclusion of coronary angiography, elevated left ventricular pressure was measured through an 8 French pigtail catheter (Fig. 1). Before reviewing the hemodynamic tracings, consider the following issues. What is the upper limit of left ventricular end-diastolic pressure (above which the risk of problems increases) for patients undergoing left ventriculography? Based on the pressure tracing and clinical presentation, would this patient likely have a problem during or following left ventriculography? Finally, is volume unloading necessary for this individual?

Examine the pressure tracings. Left ventricular systolic pressure is 200 mm Hg, with end-diastolic pressure approximately 22 mm Hg (Fig. 1). Prior to contrast ventriculography, sublingual nitroglycerin (0.4 mg) was administered. The effects of nitroglycerin shown at the right side of Figure 1 occurred within 2 min. Nitroglycerin reduced the systolic pressure from 200 mm Hg to 155 mm Hg and end-diastolic pressure to approximately 2 mm Hg.

It should be obvious from this typical hemodynamic tracing that sublingual nitroglycerin produced a marked reduction in left ventricular preload, dropping the left ventricular filling pressure from 22 mm Hg to 2 mm Hg, with corresponding reduction in the left ventricular systolic pressure. This is a characteristic response to sublingual nitroglycerin, especially evident in patients with high left ventricular end-diastolic pressure. The decrease in left ventricular filling pressure with vasodilators such as nitroglycerin (and sodium nitroprusside) is characterized by a downward shift in the left ventricular pressure-volume relationship [5,6]. During rest, nitrates routinely reduce left ventricular systolic pressure between 10 mm Hg and 15 mm Hg [5], while reducing left ventricular end-diastolic volume 25–30% and left ventricular end-systolic volume 30–35%. These effects are also present during ischemia. During the ischemic stress of supine exercise, systemic nitroglycerin also demonstrates significant reduction in end-diastolic pressures and left ventricular end-systolic volume in comparison to intracoronary nitrates [7]. These findings support the systemic effects of preload reduction more than coronary dilation as predominantly responsible for the antiischemic effects of nitroglycerin [2,4].

Patients with elevated left ventricular end-diastolic pressure may have ongoing ischemia that does not become symptomatic until after left ventriculography. High left ventricular end-diastolic pressures (>30 mm Hg) have been associated with the development of accelerated angina and congestive heart failure in the catheterization laboratory in some patients [8,9]. Nigroglycerin should be routinely administered (either sublingual or systemically) for left ventricular end-diastolic pressures >20 mm Hg. Depending on the volume status of the individual, preload reduction with small doses of nitroglycerin can result in a significant decrease in filling pressures, as demonstrated in this patient. Patients with hypertension and high left ventricular end-diastolic pressures, especially those with coronary artery disease and hypertrophy, have an increased potential for subclinical ischemia and generally respond favorably to prophylactic nitroglycerin.

To maintain a satisfactory systemic pressure after ventriculography should a marked vasodilatory effect of radiographic contrast media occur, we infused fluids to increase the left ventricular end-diastolic pressure between 5 mm Hg and 10 mm Hg. It is not routinely necessary to administer volume after nitroglycerin, but the hemodynamic effect of nitroglycerin can be used as an indicator of the volume status to prevent hypotension either following contrast-induced vasodilatation or later in the post-catheterization period in which contrast-induced diuresis may further deplete the marginal volume status of such individuals.

ISCHEMIA AND NITROGLYCERIN

A 61-yr-old woman with unstable angina was admitted to the hospital for cardiac catheterization. In the catheterization laboratory, routine right and left heart hemodynamic measurements were obtained before coronary angiography and ventriculography. During these measurements, the patient complained of her typical chest pain while resting during the midportion of the study. Pulmonary capillary wedge and pulmonary artery pressures were measured during and after spontaneous resolution of angina (Fig. 2A, left). Examine the pressure tracings during spontaneous ischemia. Giant "V" waves seen on the pulmonary capillary wedge tracing are nearly 60 mm Hg. The "V" can also be appreciated on the downslope of the pulmonary artery pressure tracing. The mean pulmonary capillary wedge pressure with chest pain was 35 mm Hg and approximately equal to the pulmonary artery diastolic pressure. While we were preparing to administer nitroglycerin, chest pain resolved. The ischemia-related pressure changes were dramatically improved. Examine the pressure tracings again (Fig. 2A, right). The pressure scale is changed from 100 mm Hg to 40 mm Hg. During myocardial ischemia, the mean pulmonary capillary wedge, V wave, and pulmonary artery pressures were markedly elevated. After sponatneous relief of ischemia, pulmonary artery pressure is 32/16 mm Hg; the pulmonary artery "V" wave cannot be seen and the pulmonary capillary wedge pressure is reduced to approximately 10 mm Hg. A few minutes later ischemia recurred (Fig. 2B, left). Observe the hemodynamics before administration of nitroglycerin and compare these hemodynamics with those of the spontaneous occurrence and resolution of ischemia. The pressure scale has again been changed in Figure 2B to 0–200 mm Hg. Before nitroglycerin (Fig. 2B, left), aortic pressure is 138/64 mm Hg, mean pulmonary capillary wedge pressure 30 mm Hg with V waves to 42 mm Hg; pulmonary artery pressure is 60/20 mm Hg. Note again the distinct change

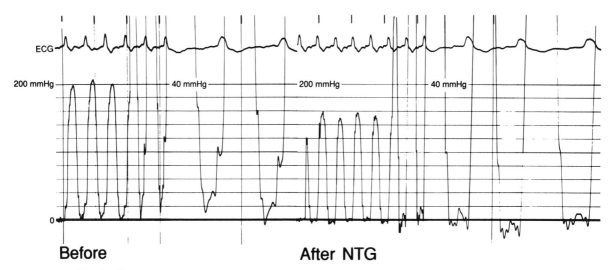

Fig. 1.   Hemodynamic tracings of left ventricular end-diastolic pressure before and after nitroglycerin in patient 1. See text for details.

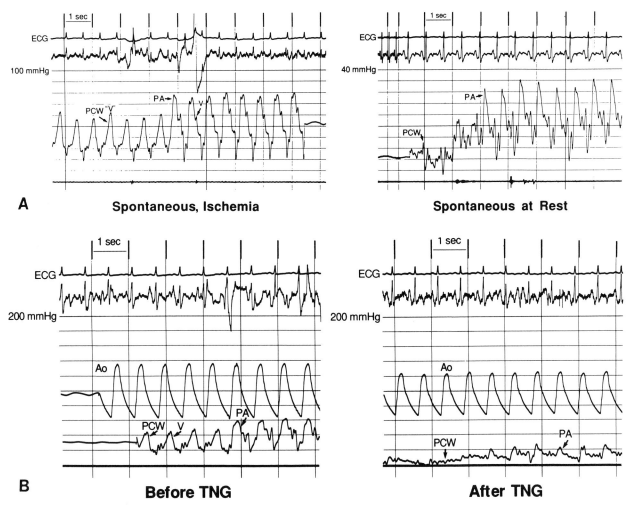

A Spontaneous, Ischemia

Spontaneous at Rest

B Before TNG

After TNG

Fig. 2. A: Hemodynamic tracing of right heart pressure during the spontaneous development of ischemia and its spontaneous resolution prior to the administration of nitroglycerin. PCW, pulmonary capillary wedge pressure; PA, pulmonary artery pressure; V, "V" wave. Note the difference in scale between the left and right panels from 100 mm Hg to 40 mm Hg. B: The arterial and pulmonary artery pressures prior to nitroglycerin (left) during an episode of ischemia and its relief after nitroglycerin (right). Note that the scale on both tracings is 0–200 mm Hg for both pulmonary artery and aortic pressures. Ao, aortic pressure; PA pulmonary artery pressure; PCW, pulmonary capillary wedge pressure.

in waveform between the pulmonary capillary wedge pressure with large V waves and the pulmonary artery pressure during the preischemic period. Nitroglycerin (0.4 mg sublingual) is given and within 3 min aortic pressure falls (122/68 mm Hg), mean pulmonary wedge pressure is now 6–8 mm Hg without V waves, and pulmonary artery pressure is 22/10 mm Hg. Nitroglycerin-induced relief of chest pain was dramatic. The most striking difference between spontaneous and nitroglycerin-induced relief of ischemia is the dramatic preload reduction demonstrated by the greater decline in mean pulmonary capillary wedge and pulmonary artery pressures. Spontaneous resolution of ischemia causes less shift in the pressure-volume relationship of the left ventricle than the nitroglycerin-induced reduction in ischemia.

NITROGLYCERIN AND CORONARY BLOOD FLOW

Does sublingual nitroglycerin improve coronary blood flow to relieve myocardial ischemia in patients with coronary artery disease [10]? A 73-yr-old man with severe angina refractory to calcium channel blockers and topical nitroglycerin was admitted for cardiac catheterization. Coronary angiography revealed severe triple vessel coronary artery disease, with left ventricular ejection fraction of 46% with anterior hypokinesis. After coronary angiography, coronary blood flow responses with calcium channel blockers were measured under an approved research protocol. Coronary sinus thermodilution and high-fidelity dual-micromanometer-tipped left ventricular catheters were positioned for hemodynamic study.

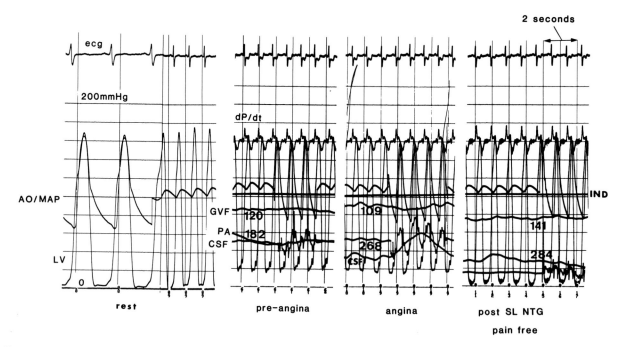

Fig. 3. The effect of sublingual nitroglycerin on total and regional coronary blood flow during spontaneous ischemia. Increasing coronary flow is directed toward the bottom of the figure. Numbers under the coronary sinus and great vein flow signals are the average flow in mililiters/minute averaged over a 5 sec time period. Ao, aortic pressure; CSF, coronary sinus flow; GVF, great vein flow; LV, left ventricular pressure; MAP, mean arterial pressure; PA, pulmonary artery pressure (Reprinted from Kern et al. [10] with permission of the publisher.)

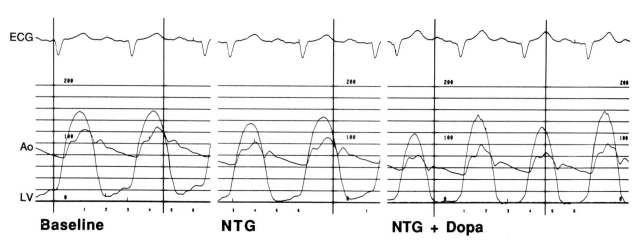

Fig. 4. Simultaneous aortic and left ventricular pressures in a patient with severe aortic stenosis at baseline, after 0.4 mg sublingual nitroglycerin and after sublingual nitroglycerin with low-dose dopamine infusion (5 μg/kg/min). Note the decline in pressures after nitroglycerin and the pulsus alternans after the administration of dopamine. See text for details.

Although unanticipated, hemodynamics measurements were obtained continuously before, during, and after an episode of typical angina. Prior to the onset of chest pain, blood pressure (Fig. 3, left) was 160/70 mm Hg with a left ventricular end-diastolic pressure of 12 mm Hg. While preparing the study medication, asymptomatic ST depression was observed preceding the onset of chest pain (Fig. 3, pre-angina). The observed preanginal

hemodynamic alterations were consistent with a hierarchy of ischemic events later described to occur reproducibly during controlled, transient ischemia produced by angioplasty [11]. Blood pressure was unchanged at approximately 160/78 mm Hg, but left ventricular end-diastolic and minimal diastolic pressures were increased to 30 mm Hg and 20 mm Hg, respectively (Fig. 3, pre-angina). Great cardiac vein flow (an index of anterior left

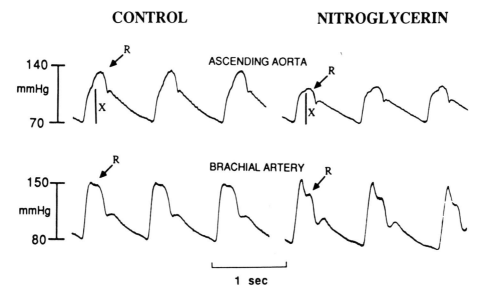

Fig. 5. Pressure waves recorded in the ascending aorta (top) and brachial artery (bottom) under control conditions and after 0.3 mg sublingual nitroglycerin in human adult. The right panel demonstrates the effects of nitroglycerin. (Reproduced from Nichols and O'Rourke [13] with permission of the publisher.)

ventricular blood flow) was 120 ml/minute with coronary sinus (global left ventricular) flow of 182 ml/min. The mean pulmonary artery pressure was also elevated at 30 mm Hg (0–100 mm Hg scale for pulmonary artery). After 1 min of ST segment depression, angina occurred, gradually becoming more severe (Fig. 3, angina). Great cardiac vein flow decreased to 109 ml/min, whereas coronary sinus flow increased to 268 ml/min. Left ventricular end-diastolic, minimal diastolic, and mean pulmonary artery pressure remained elevated as in the preanginal period. Nitroglycerin produced the expected result. Within 2 min after receiving 0.4 mg sublingual nitroglycerin, the angina abated and ST segment changes returned toward normal with marked improvement in great cardiac vein flow, increasing to 141 ml/min. Coronary sinus flow increased to 284 ml/min. Coincident with improved blood flow and reduced clinical ischemia, left ventricular end-diastolic pressure declined to normal values. The mean pulmonary artery pressure also fell to 16 mm Hg.

Peripheral venous dilation decreasing myocardial oxygen consumption through preload reduction has been well established [1,2], but the nitrate-induced increase in coronary blood flow to ischemic myocardium through reversal of coronary vasoconstriction has been a controversial subject [5,6]. Evident from this case, the mechanism relieving ischemia is a sum of the two drug actions of both myocardial oxygen demand reduction and augmentation of coronary flow when coronaries can respond to vasodilation. These detailed hemodynamic observa-

tions in patient 3 demonstrated that coronary blood flow may be significantly, albeit regionally, improved simultaneous with the reduction in the determinants of myocardial oxygen demand in at least some patients with severe coronary artery disease.

NITROGLYCERIN, ANGINA, AND AORTIC STENOSIS

Nitroglycerin may reduce anginal-like chest pain which is unrelated to coronary artery disease. A 74-year-old man with mild aortic stenosis, increasing fatigue, and angina pectoris underwent diagnostic cardiac catheterization. Simultaneous left ventricular and aortic pressures (Fig. 4) demonstrated an aortic gradient of approximately 30 mm Hg with a cardiac output of 4.9 liter/min, resulting in a calculated aortic valve area of approximately 0.9 cm^2. Coronary arteriography was normal. Left ventriculography showed global hypokinesis with an ejection fraction of 32%. To assess the influence of changing loading conditions and cardiac output on aortic valve gradient, sublingual nitroglycerin and dopamine (5 μg/kg/min) were administered and hemodynamics reexamined (Fig. 4). Nitroglycerin reduced left ventricular end-diastolic and minimal diastolic pressures from approximately 28 mm Hg to 18 mm Hg and from 10 mm Hg to 2 mm Hg, respectively. Left ventricular systolic pressure also fell, without increasing the transvalvular pressure gradient. When low-dose dopamine was infused, augmenting contractility and cardiac output, pul-

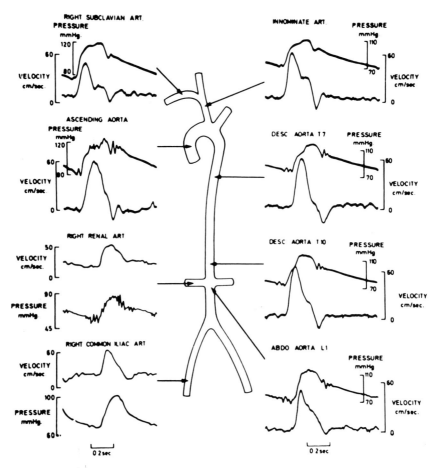

Fig. 6. Pressure and velocity waveforms in different arteries recorded in a patient undergoing diagnostic cardiac catheterization. Signals were obtained with an electromagnetic catheter transducer. (Reproduced from Nichols and O'Rourke [13] with permission of the publisher.)

sus alternans was observed and was augmented over that seen with nitroglycerin. The aortic stenotic gradient showed alternating pressure gradients with the strong and weak beats. The increase in cardiac output to 6.5 liter/min with a mean gradient of 45 mm Hg did not alter the aortic valve area calculations (0.9 cm^2). Note that dopamine and nitroglycerin further decreased left ventricular filling pressures. Nitroglycerin predominantly reduced preload in this patient, but had little effect on the valve area. As a rule, vasodilators should not be employed in patients with significant aortic stenosis. The production of pulsus alternans was unexpected. Pulsus alternans occurs in patients with aortic stenosis and has been attributed to alternations in afterload (wall stress) and contractile state, but not to preload [12]. We speculate that the nitroglycerin in this patient produced a reflex increase in sympathetic tone resulting in pulsus alternans because of the impaired cardiac contractile reserve. However, in the previous studies [12], patients with aortic stenosis and pulsus alternans were given nitroglycerin and did not have this effect based on observ-

able direct or indirect (reflex mediated) changes in contractile state. Whether this is a finding related to reduced preload reserve or not remains under study.

NITROGLYCERIN AND THE AORTIC PRESSURE WAVEFORM

With nitroglycerin, the aortic pressure wave shows a more distinct dicrotic notch and a more prominent secondary reflected wave (Fig. 5). The changing waveform with nitroglycerin has been reviewed in detail by Nichols and O'Rourke [13]. The ascending aortic pressure wave after nitroglycerin is significantly modified, as shown by a drop in the height of the anacrotic notch and augmentation of the dicrotic notch by wave reflections. This reflected wave physiology is more pronounced as one measures pressure further in the peripheral circulation (Fig. 6). The mechanism for nitroglycerin's effect on the pressure waveform is not precisely known. Nitroglycerin, a nonendothelial-dependent vasodilator, decreases arterial stiffness and improves arterial distensibility and

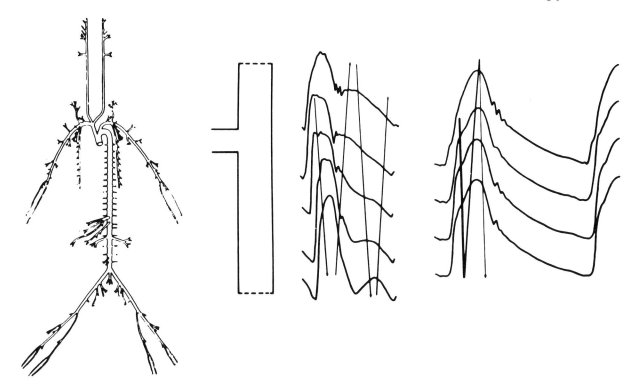

Fig. 7. Graphic explanation of pressure wave amplitude and contour differences between central aortic and peripheral arteries on the basis of wave travel and reflection. The systemic arterial system (left) is similar to an asymmetric T tube, with the short limb representing all arteries in the upper part of the body and the long limb representing descending arota and arteries in the lower part of the body. The ends of the T tube represent resultant terminations of individual arteries in both the upper and lower parts of the body. Pressure waves in different arteries of dogs are displayed second to right and in a patient with arteriosclerosis at far right (at half amplitude). The changes in waveform occur based on the reflection and rereflection of the pulse wave with respect to ventricular ejection. (Reproduced from Nichols and O'Rourke [13] with permission of the publisher.)

thus reduces arterial pressure. Nitrates, in low dosages, dilate arteries without effecting arterioles, whereas calcium channel antagonists and angiotensin converting enzyme (ACE) inhibitors dilate both arteries and arterioles. Nitrates have little effect on the largest arteries, such as the aorta, or on the smallest arteries, the arterioles, but substantial effects on arteries of medium size. Exactly how dilatation improves distensibility in arteries is currently under investigation [13–17]. A suggested mechanism is that arterial smooth muscle is in series with some stiffer collagen components, but in parallel with the elastic lamini [16]. Contraction of smooth muscle tenses the collagen components, whereas dilation transfers stress to the elastic lamellae, thus improving distensibility. The release of endothelial-derived relaxing factor and the common pathway of nitrate activation of guanylate cyclase has also been proposed [17]. Despite these hypotheses, the exact mechanism of nitroglycerin on the vascular responses remains unresolved. These effects may also be due to the greater dilatation of subbranches than of the parent branch with subsequent reduction in the amplitude of the reflected wave returning from the periphery (Fig. 7). This explanation is based on nitroglycerin's effect on the caliber of small peripheral arteries minimizing the contribution of arterial distensibility. Probably both caliber and distensibility are altered with nitroglycerin and contribute to the beneficial effect. With regard to cardiac function, a favorable effect is produced as a result of reduced wave reflection in the impedance modulus at various heart rate frequencies as well as in the peak aortic and left ventricular end-diastolic pressure independent of the influence on coronary vasodilatation and reduction of myocardial ischemia [7,13].

SUMMARY

Nitroglycerin has dependable, short-lived veno- and arterial vasodilatory effects ameliorating ischemia through both preload reduction and coronary vasodilation. Nitroglycerin should be used prior to left ventriculography in patients with elevated left ventricular end-diastolic pressure. The arterial pressure waveform alteration of nitroglycerin can be explained on the basis of changes in arterial distensibility and reflected wave patterns and may vary considerably among individuals with different degrees of atherosclerosis.

ACKNOWLEDGMENTS

The authors thank the J. Gerard Mudd Cardiac Catheterization Team and Donna Sander for manuscript preparation.

REFERENCES

1. McGregor M: The nitrates and myocardial ischemia. Circulation 66:689–692, 1982.
2. Kaski JC, Plaza LR, Meran DO, Araujo L, Chierchia S, Maseri A: An improved coronary supply: Prevailing mechanisms of action of nitrates in chronic stable angina. Am Heart J 110:238–245, 1985.
3. Liu P, Houle S, Burns RS, Kimball B, Warbick-Cerrone A, Johnston L, Gilday D, Weisel RD, McLaughlin PR: Effect of intracoronary nitroglycerin on myocardial blood flow and distribution on pacing-induced angina pectoris. Am J Cardiol 55:1270–1276, 1985.
4. Ganz W, Marcus HR: Failure of intracoronary nitroglycerin to alleviate pacing-induced angina. Circulation 46:880–889, 1972.
5. Kingma I, Smiseth OA, Belenkie I, Knudtson ML, MacDonald RPR, Tyberg JV, Smith ER: A mechanism for the nitroglycerin-induced downward shift of the left ventricular diastolic pressure-diameter relation. Am J Cardiol 57:673–677, 1986.
6. Brodie BR, Grossman W, Mann T, McLaurin LP: Effects of sodium nitroprusside on left ventricular diastolic pressure-volume relations. J Clin Invest 59:59–68, 1977.
7. DeCoster PMN, Chierchia S, Davies GJ, Hackett D, Fragasso G, Maseri A: Combined effects of nitrates on the coronary and peripheral circulation in exercise-induced ischemia. Circulation 81:1881–1886, 1990.
8. Grossman W (ed): Cardiac ventriculography. In: "Cardiac Catheterization and Angiography, 3rd ed. 1986, p 204.
9. Deligonul U, Kern MJ, Serota H, Roth R: Angiographic data. In Kern MJ (ed): "The Cardiac Catheterization Handbook." St. Louis: Mosby Year Book, 1991, p 245.
10. Kern MJ, Eilen SD, O'Rourke R: Coronary vasomotion in angina at rest and effect of sublingual nitroglycerin on coronary blood flow. Am J Cardiol 56:484–485, 1985.
11. Labovitz AJ, Lewen MJ, Kern MJ, Vandormael M, Deligonul U, Kennedy HL: Evaluation of left ventricular systolic and diastolic dysfunction during transient myocrdial ischemia. J Am Coll Cardiol 10:748–755, 1987.
12. Laskey WK, Sutton MSJ, Untereker WJ, Martin JL, Hirshfeld JW Jr, Reichek N: Mechanics of pulsus alternans in aortic valve stenosis. Am J Cardiol 52:809–812, 1983.
13. Nichols WW, O'Rourke MF: "McDonald's Blood Flow in Arteries: Theoretical, Experimental and Clinical Principles, 3rd ed." Philadelphia: Lea & Febiger, 1990, pp 421–432.
14. Cohen MV, Kirk ES: Differential response of large and small coronary arteries to nitroglycerin and angiotensin. Circ Res 33:445–453, 1973.
15. Feldman RL, Pepine CJ, Conti CR: Magnitude of dilation of large and small coronary arteries by nitroglycerin. Circulation 64:324–333, 1981.
16. O'Rourke MF, Avolio AP, Yaginuma T: Arterial dilation as a mechanism for favorable effects of nitroglycerin in man. In: "Proc 6th Int Adalat Symp, Geneva." 1985, p 13.
17. O'Rourke MF, Kelley RP, Avolio AP, Hayward CS: Potential for reversing the ill-effects of angina and of arterial hypertension on central aortic systolic pressure and on left ventricular hydraulic load by arterial dilator agents. Am J Cardiol 63:381–441, 1989.

Chapter 38

Pulsus Alternans

W. Jeffrey Schoen, MD, J. David Talley, MD, and Morton J. Kern, MD

INTRODUCTION

Pulsus alternans, first described by Traube in 1872, is the regular alternation of strong and weak cardiac contractions in the absence of respiratory or cycle length variation [1,2]. It is detected by palpation of a peripheral artery or by sphygmomanometry with a regular alteration of the intensity of the Korofkoff sounds. Total alternans occurs when the left ventricular systolic pressure is less than aortic pressure on alternate beats so that the aortic valve does not open with apparent halving of the pulse rate. Pulsus alternans is usually found in patients with severe myocardial disease due to aortic stenosis, systemic arterial hypertension, cardiomyopathy, or coronary heart disease [3]. It has, however, been described in patients with normal hearts for brief periods during or after supraventricular tachycardia.

Pulsus alternans may also be transiently induced by premature ventricular contractions [4], orthostatic factors [5], rapid atrial pacing [6], inferior vena caval occlusion [7], as well as myocardial ischemia [8]. Intracoronary contrast injection during angiography in a patient with hypertensive cardiomyopathy has also been reported to attenuate pulsus alternans [9].

CASE HISTORY AND HEMODYNAMIC DATA

A 52-yr-old male was admitted with dyspnea. Shortly after admission, the patient had a respiratory and cardiac arrest and was successfully resuscitated. After two weeks of convalescing, palpation of the peripheral pulses revealed reduced amplitude with every other beat. Jugular veins were 5 cm at 30°. Lungs were clear. The apical impulse was enlarged, in the anterior axillary line, 6th intercostal space and associated with a soft S_3 gallop.

Cardiac catheterization showed significant (> 80%) lesions in both the left anterior descending and right coronary arteries. Left ventriculography demonstrated an enlarged chamber with a calculated left ventricular ejection fraction (by area length method) of 16%.

The systolic aortic and left ventricular pressures (Fig. 1) demonstrated a consistent alternating pattern with a reduced pressure every other beat of approximately 20 mmHg. Interestingly, the left ventricular waveform on the "weak" beats is different by its reduced peak and time to peak pressure, as well as a subtle alteration of the rapid phase of relaxation. A similar alteration in peak systolic pressure is also noted on every other beat in the right ventricular and pulmonary artery tracings (Fig. 2). Pulmonary and left ventricular diastolic pressures are significantly elevated, consistent with biventricular dysfunction. The time to peak systolic pressure is also prolonged in the weaker beats of right-sided pressures, consistent with the hypothesized mechanism of alternating diminished contractility. Right ventricular pulsus alternans may occur independently, concordantly or discordantly with left ventricular alternans [10,11]. Atrial alternans has also been described [12].

This patient demonstrated *pulsus alternans* by both clinical and hemodynamic criteria. Physical findings associated with pulsus alternans included alternating intensity of heart sounds and an S_3 gallop. Pulsus alternans may be augmented by maneuvers which decrease venous return, such as head tilting, standing, or administration of nitroglycerin.

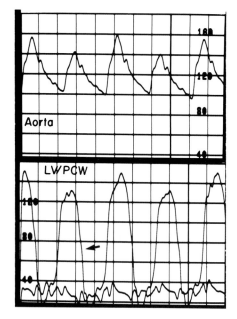

1

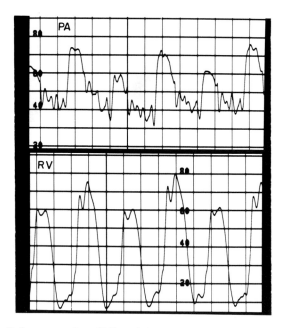

2

Fig. 1. Aortic and left ventricular (LV) pressure tracings demonstrate mechanical alternans with peak systolic pressure reduced to 20 mmHg every other contraction. The left ventricular relaxation pattern of weak beats shows subtle delay and an altered waveform (arrow). Of note, the pulmonary capillary wedge (PCW) tracing does not significantly vary during this recording. See text for details.

Fig. 2. Pulmonary artery (PA) and right ventricular (RV) pressure tracings demonstrate mechanical alternans occurring in a similar fashion to left ventricular hemodynamics of Figure 1.

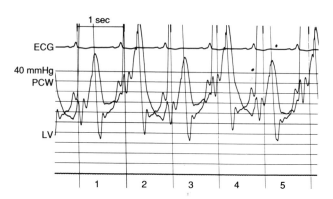

Fig. 3. Left ventricular (LV) and pulmonary capillary wedge (PCW) pressure tracings in a patient with large A and V waves of alternating magnitude. See text for details.

Pulsus alternans must be differentiated from conditions with similar physical examination characteristics. *Pulsus bigeminus* occurs when the cardiac rhythm is bigeminal, with either atrial or ventricular pairing with the premature beats having decreased stroke volume and systolic peak pressure. *Pulsus paradoxus* is the decrease in pulse amplitude during the inspiratory phase of respi-

ration. In this condition, when a patient has a rapid respiratory rate which is equal to half the pulse rate, the physical findings may resemble pulsus alternans, with apparent decrease in pulse amplitude every other beat.

MECHANISMS OF PULSUS ALTERNANS

Weber et al. [13] induced pulsus alternans in the canine heart when anaerobic metabolism was reached by increasing the filling volume, heart rate, and contractility and by decreasing coronary perfusion. When the aerobic limit of the myocardium was exceeded, myocardial performance declined with resultant pulsus alternans [13]. Pulsus alternans is thought to be primarily due to decreased myocardial contractility on alternate beats, with relatively less effect produced by changes in preload, afterload, or diastolic relaxation [4,6,14]. Decreased contractility is attributed to deletion of the number of myocardial cells contracting on alternate beats. This reduction in the contractile cell population is thought to be caused by intracellular calcium cycling involving the sarcoplasmic reticulum leading to localized electrical mechanical dissociation [15]. Another postulated mechanism for the alternations in pulse pressure evolved from Frank Starling's mechanism due to alterations in diastolic volume [5,16]. However, measured diastolic volumes in patient studies [7] suggest the earlier mechanism may play a predominant role.

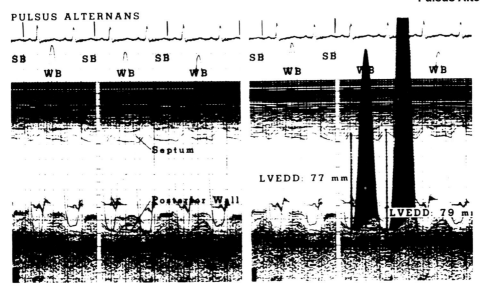

Fig. 4. Simultaneous echocardiography and pressure measurements during induction of pulsus alternans. Left ventricular pressure and M-mode echocardiography (on left panel) are unretouched, with septal posterior wall and weak beats (WB) and strong beats (SB) shown accentuated in black (on right panel). A small but statistically significant difference in left ventricular end-diastolic dimension occurs between strong and weak beats. With permission from reference #7.

A 62-yr-old patient with congestive failure underwent cardiac catheterization for mitral regurgitation and continuing left ventricular dysfunction. Right and left heart hemodynamics were obtained in a routine fashion. Examine the hemodynamic tracings of the simultaneous left ventricular and pulmonary capillary wedge pressures (Fig. 3). Note the differences in the height of the V and A waves during sinus rhythm on the odd numbered beats. The alternation of V waves was consistent with the pulsus alternans produced in the systemic pressure. The left atrial filling curve (compliance) was appropriately influenced with a greater degree of mitral regurgitation (larger V wave) for greater systolic ejection (regurgitant pressure).

The theory of pressure generation and alternation of contractility on the beat-to-beat basis with unimpaired diastolic parameters was reported by Bashore et al. [7]. Pulsus alternans was induced by preload reduction with balloon occlusion of the inferior vena cava, performed during measurements of left ventricular function. Reduction in preload in 11 patients with non-ischemic cardiomyopathy produced sustained pulsus alternans in 5. The strong beats demonstrated systolic characteristics similar to baseline values despite a decline in both left ventricular end-diastolic diameter and left ventricular end-diastolic pressure (Fig. 4). The weak beats demonstrated reduction in peak systolic pressure, fractional shortening, and peak positive dP/dt. Diastolic parameters were not different between baseline beats and the strong beats. Left ventricular end-diastolic wall stress differed somewhat between baseline beats compared with weak, but not strong beats. Significant differences in peak systolic pressure, positive dP/dt and fractional shortening were present between strong and weak beats (Fig. 5), but no difference in any measured diastolic parameter were observed. These data were consistent with an augmentation and deletion of intrinsic contractile forces in association with an alternation in preload on a beat-to-beat basis during pulsus alternans.

Of the many associations of pulsus alternans, myocardial ischemia appears to contribute to both the alternation and attenuation of the pressure waveforms. Pulsus alternans observed prior to coronary angiography in a patient with severe cardiomyopathy was significantly attenuated during contrast injection [9]. Pulsus alternans may also disappear after administration of digitalis [17] and during continued deterioration of left ventricular function [18]. Both the new appearance of pulsus alternans and the disappearance of pulsus alternans should alert the clinician to possible deteriorating myocardial function.

ACKNOWLEDGMENT

The authors thank Donna Sander for manuscript preparation.

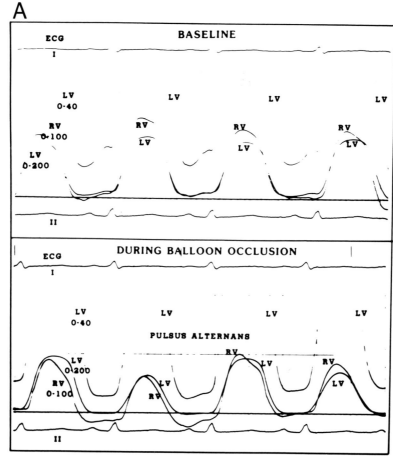

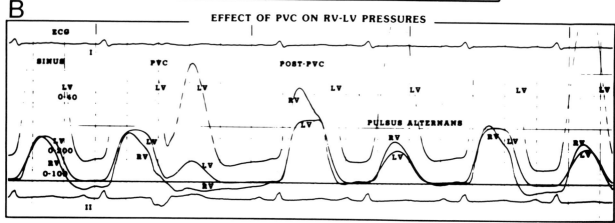

Fig. 5. A: Concordant right ventricular (RV) and left ventricular (LV) pulsus alternans. Subtle baseline concordant right and left ventricular alternans is dramatically accentuated during inferior vena caval balloon occlusion. B: Induction of right ventricular (RV) and left ventricular (LV) pulsus alternans following prema-ture ventricular contractions (PVC) following beat #2. The mild baseline pulsus alternans shown is accentuated following the post-extra systolic accentuation of the pressure. The concordance of right and left ventricular pulsus alternans is again demonstrated. With permission from reference #7.

REFERENCES

1. Traube L: Ein fall von pulsus bigeminus nebst bemerkungen über die leberschwellungen bei klappen fehlern und über acute leber-atrophie. Ber Klin Wochenschr 185–188;221–224, 1872.

2. Laskey WK, St. John Sutton M, Unterecker WJ, Martin JL, Hirschfield JW: Mechanics of pulsus alternans in aortic valve stenosis. Am J Cardiol 52:809–812, 1983.

3. Braunwald E (ed): "Heart Disease: A Textbook of Cardiovascular Medicine." Philadelphia: McGraw-Hill, 1988, p 481.

4. Hess OM, Surber EP, Ritter M, Krayenbuehl HP: Pulsus alternans: Its influence on systolic and diastolic function in aortic valve disease. J Am Coll Cardiol 4:1–7, 1984.

5. Lewis BS, Lweis N, Gotsman MS: Effect of postural changes on pulsus alternans. An echocardiographic study. Chest 75:634–636, 1979.

6. McGaughey MD, Maughan WL, Sunagawa K, Sagawa K: Alternating contractility in pulsus alternans studied in the isolated canine heart. Circulation 71:357–362, 1985.

7. Bashore TM, Walker S, VanFossen D, Schaffer PB, Fontana ME, Unverferth DV: Pulsus alternans induced by inferior vena caval occlusion in man. Cathet Cardiovasc Diagn 14:24–32, 1988.

8. Elbaum DM, Banka VS: Pulsus alternans during spontaneous angina pectoris. Am J Cardiol 58:1099–1100, 1986.

9. Ring ME, Kern MJ, Genovely H, Serota H, Vandormael M: Attenuation of pulsus alternans during coronary angiography. Cathet Cardiovasc Diagn 20:193–195, 1990.

10. Hada Y, Wolfe C, Craige E: Pulsus alternans by biventricular systolic time intervals. Circulation 65:617–626, 1982.

11. Desser KB, Benchimol A: Phasic left ventricular blood velocity alternans in man. Am J Cardiol 36:309–314, 1975.

12. Verheugt FWA, Scheck H, Meltzer RS, Roelandt J: Alternating atrial electro-mechanical dissociation as contributing factor for pulsus alternans. Br Heart J 48:459–461, 1982.

13. Weber KT, Janicki JS, Sundram B: Myocardial energetics: Experimental and clinical studies to address its determinants and aerobic limit. Basic Res Cardiol 84:237–246, 1989.

14. Miller WP, Liedtke AJ, Nellis SH: End systolic pressure diameter relationships during pulsus alternans in intact pig hearts. Am J Physiol 250:H606–H611, 1985.

15. Lab MJ, Lee JA: Changes in intracellular calcium during mechanical alternans in isolated ferret ventricular muscle. Circ Res 66:585–595, 1990.

16. Gleason WL, Braunwald E: Studies on Starling's Law of the Heart. VI. Relationship between left ventricular end-diastolic volume and stroke volume in man with observations on the mechanism of pulsus alternans. Circulation 25:841–847, 1962.

17. Windle JD: Clinical observations on the effects of digitalis in heart disease with pulsus alternans. Q J Med 10:274, 1917.

18. Ryan JM, Schieve JF, Hull HB, Osner BM: The influence of advanced congestive heart failure on pulsus alternans. Circulation 12:60–63, 1955.

Chapter 39

Extra Hearts—Section I

Morton J. Kern, MD, Ubeydullah Deligonul, MD, and Leslie Miller, MD

INTRODUCTION

This "hemodynamic rounds" will delve into the curiosities of pressure waveforms from patients with transplanted hearts. Some of these types of patients may never be seen in smaller clinical centers or even in some major centers. Heart transplant hemodynamics can be confusing, but are also interesting as very unusual and rare findings. Nonetheless, the principles applied to interpreting hemodynamics in native hearts are even more important when examined in the context of a transplanted heart. For special interest, we have selected several of our more unusual tracings. If one reviews the hemodynamic tracings prior to reading the text explanation, the curiosities of pressure delivery in functioning and nonfunctioning "extra" hearts will be even more educational.

CASE PRESENTATIONS AND DISCUSSION
"Extra" Arterial Pressure

A 43-yr-old man with a history of mitral valve replacement for mitral stenosis developed coronary artery disease and class IV left ventricular failure due to ischemic cardiomyopathy which was refractory to medical therapy. Because of long standing pulmonary hypertension, a surgical procedure was performed (to be discussed below). Retrograde left and right heart catheterization was performed. Measurement of aortic pressure was obtained through an 8 French femoral side arm sheath. Simultaneous left ventricular pressure was measured with a 7 F pigtail catheter. The hemodynamic tracings are shown in

Figures 1 and 2. Examine the arterial pressure wave (Fig. 1). The electrocardiogram has an irregularly irregular rhythm. An aortic gradient is observed in Figure 1, beats #1, #2 and #3. Explain the waveform configuration and pressure generation of beats #4, #5 and #6 on this figure? Before moving to Figure 2, when can aortic pressure "normally" exceed left ventricular pressure?

Figure 2 is a continuous tracing from Figure 1 of the patient described above showing deterioration of left ventricular pressure despite maintained aortic pressure. The catheter position is unchanged and aortic pressure continues around 120/70 mm Hg. What is causing the change in left ventricular pressure?

Consider another patient: a 37-yr-old man having had the same procedure as the preceding patient. The "surgical" treatment for refractory idiopathic congestive heart failure was successful. The arterial pressure and electrocardiogram are shown in Figure 3 and demonstrate a highly irregular arterial pulse pattern with a more regular electrocardiogram. Explain the systolic arterial pressure wave in the absence of apparent high grade atrial or ventricular ectopy.

This puzzling sequence of tracings represents unusual examples of pressure generation occurring from 1 or 2 ventricles in patients after *heterotopic heart* transplant (Fig. 4). Heterotopic heart transplantation has a long experimental history and was the technique used by Christian Barnard and his colleagues in South Africa performing the first clinical heart transplantation in 1967. Although 95% of all heart transplantations done in 1990 have been orthotopic replacements, heterotopic heart transplantation is indicated in patients with pulmo-

295

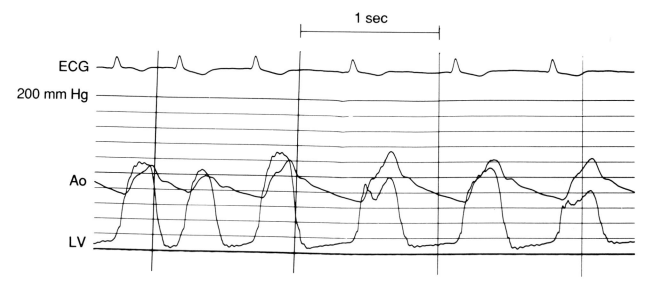

Fig. 1.   Simultaneous aortic (Ao) and left ventricular (LV) pressures (200 mm Hg scale). See text for details.

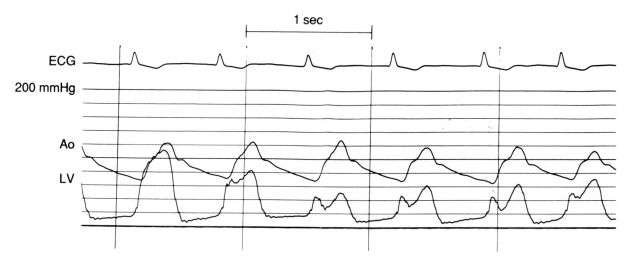

Fig. 2.   Simultaneous aortic (Ao) and left ventricular (LV) pressures (200 mm Hg scale). See text for details.

nary hypertension who need left ventricular assistance. Orthotopic replacement of a "new" donor heart, unaccustomed to high pulmonary artery pressures would result in severe, potentially fatal right ventricular failure after transplantation. The vascular communications of heterotopic transplantation are varied [1]. One common method used in the patient examples is as follows: the aorta of the accessory (donor) heart is attached end-to-side directly to the aorta of the native heart and the donor pulmonary artery by graft to the native pulmonary artery. A communication between both left atria is created (large "atrial" septal defect) to allow filling of the donor left ventricle. The donor right ventricle is filled by right atrial

flow from the native heart. Since the function of the native left ventricle is generally very poor and, at times, insufficient to influence systemic pressure, the arterial pulse depends principally on the Frank-Starling mechanism of filling of the donor heart. However, the electrocardiographic complex which is most prominent may not be that of the native heart, often accounting for the disparity between electrocardiographic rhythm and pressure waves.

There are several advantages of heterotopic over orthotopic heart transplantation. The donor heart acts as a built-in left ventricular assist device and maintains the systemic circulation. Heterotopic heart transplantation

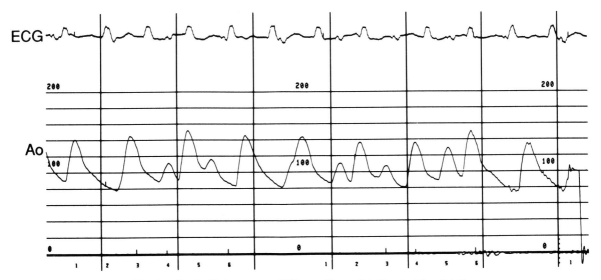

Fig. 3.   Aortic (Ao) pressure (200 mm Hg scale). See text for details.

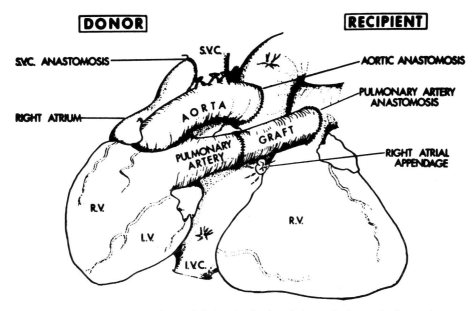

Fig. 4. Graphic representation of heterotopic heart transplant surgical anastomoses. SVC = superior vena cava; IVC = inferior vena cava; RV = right ventricle; LV = left ventricle.

allows for possible recovery of recipient heart failure after viral myocarditis and can be performed in the presence of very high pulmonary vascular resistance as hypertrophied native right ventricle continues to support the pulmonary circulation. However, the transplanted heterotopic heart patient also carries severe risk of systemic emboli from thrombus in the poorly contracting recipient left ventricle and requires long term anticoagulation. Moreover, the native ventricle may be subject to continuing angina related to ischemic cardiomyopathy. The

risk of infection in the recipient heart is also a continuing problem.

Customary hemodynamic waveforms may be significantly affected by the dysrhythmic activity of the recipient heart, occasionally requiring high doses of antiarrhythmic agents. Abnormal hemodynamic patterns of donor left ventricular pressure may indicate early transplant rejection. Failing function of the heterotopic transplant often appears as a significant decline in the magnitude and slowed and diminished pattern of the

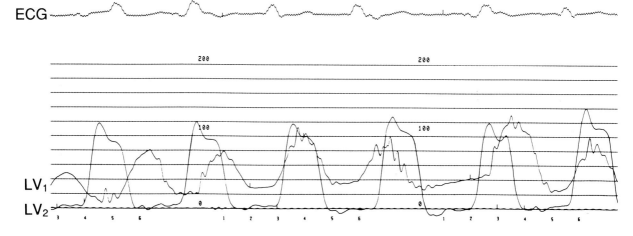

Fig. 5. Simultaneous left ventricular (LV₁, LV₂) pressures (200 mm Hg scale). LV₁ = native left ventricle; LV₂ = donor left ventricle. See text for details.

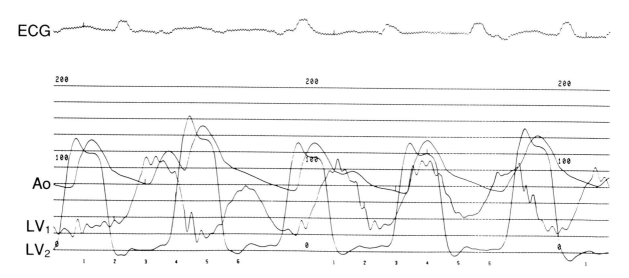

Fig. 6. Simultaneous aortic (Ao) and left ventricular (LV₁, LV₂) pressures (200 mm Hg scale). LV₁ = native left ventricle; LV₂ = donor left ventricle. See text for details.

peripheral pressure wave. The ratio of the arterial pulse of each of the 2 contracting ventricles is thought to be an indicator of impending cardiac rejection [1].

In many patients, the donor heart functions as a pressure "assist" pump. The donor heart influences the systemic pressure in 2 ways: 1) co-pulsation, in time with the native heart, or 2) counterpulsation, pumping in the native heart's diastole. These coincident or counterpoint beats are evidenced by the changing waveform of aortic pressure and occasionally by the 2 different QRS complexes inscribed on the electrocardiographic tracing above the pressure waves. The timing of the 2 left ventricular pressures and influence on aortic pressure can be seen in Figures 5 and 6, which were taken from patient #2, whose arterial pressure was provided in Figure 3. The subtle small waves in the electrocardiogram mistakenly appearing as P waves are the electrocardiographic complexes of the donor heart with the largest complexes being the native heart. This rhythm is more complicated because a VPC in the donor heart may not be detected electrocardiographically and confuse the pressure wave interpretation. However, in patients with reduced native left ventricular function insufficient to exceed systemic pressure, the magnitude of arterial pressure is dependent on donor heart R-R interval and Frank-Starling filling-force relationship.

The intrinsic cardiac rhythm for many patients may be atrial fibrillation with the donor heart in a sinus rhythm.

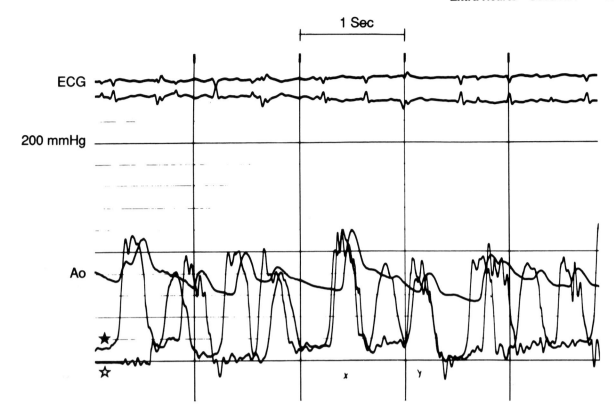

Fig. 7. Simultaneous aortic (Ao) and left ventricular (LV) pressures (200 mm Hg scale). Black star represents left ventricular pressures of the donor heart. Open star represents left ventricular pressure of the native heart. See text for details.

In Figures 1 and 2, there was coincident timing of the native and donor left ventricular pressures, explaining why native left ventricular pressures could fall under the higher aortic pressure wave. Synchrony of the two hearts was maintained for long periods of times, giving the impression that native left ventricular pressure was sufficient to generate adequate pressure in the systemic circulation. Most of the native left ventricular beats in Figure 2 were clearly insufficient to generate arterial pressure. The false gradient (aortic higher than left ventricular pressure) demonstrated in beat #1 (Fig. 1) is a result of pressure being satisfactory in the native heart with reduced output of the donor heart. The highest aortic pressure (beat #4, Fig. 1 and beat #3, Fig. 6) occur with co-pulsation of the ventricles. The lowest arterial pressure waves (beat #2, Fig. 1 and beat #3, Fig. 6) occur during dysynchrony of ventricular contraction may be evident. The timing cycle of the co-pulsation and counterpulsation beats is particularly evident in Figure 7. To determine which electrocardiographic signal and which waveform originates from the donor versus native heart, drop a vertical line from the QRS and identify the corresponding pressure upstroke. Usually the weaker pressure is the native heart.

Co-Pulsation and Counterpulsation

A 42-yr-old man with pulmonary hypertension, class IV refractory congestive heart failure received a heterotopic heart transplant 6 weeks prior to evaluation (Fig. 7). The electrocardiogram demonstrates 2 QRS complexes, representing the donor and native hearts. The donor left ventricular pressure (identified with the dark star) and the recipient's native left ventricular pressure (identified with the open star) show their influence on the aortic pulse pressures. Compare the synchrony of the 2 hearts on beats labelled X and Y. The size of the aortic pulse waves depend on the co-pulsation or counterpulsation (i.e., synchrony) of native and donor left ventricular pressure augmentation. Synchrony of 2 left ventricular pressures produces a large aortic pulse (X beat). The next beat barely generates a small arterial pulse wave with only the native left ventricular pressure. The following beat (Y beat) has both left ventricular pressures, but the native left ventricle is not filled adequately preceding the "premature" contraction.

Although considered artifact by the unsuspecting, the electrocardiographic rhythm consistently demonstrates the 2 different QRS complexes, 1 for each ventricle, and

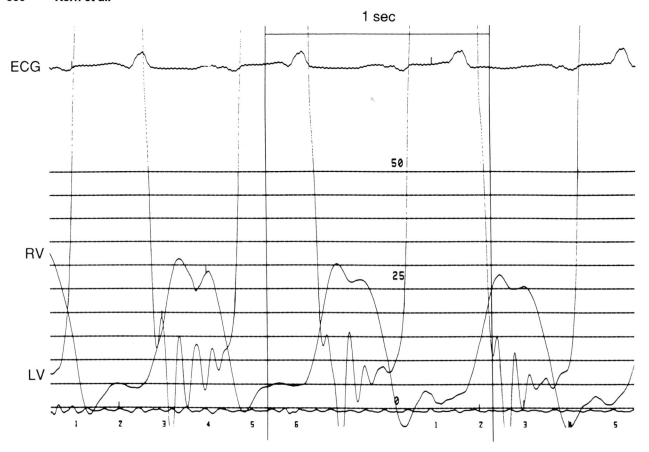

Fig. 8. Simultaneous right ventricular (RV) and left ventricular (LV) pressures (50 mm Hg scale). Notice small abnormal QRS complex of the native left ventricle.

corresponds to arterial pressure wave pattern. The hemodynamic responses of the 2 ventricles over time become clinically important when considering early allograft rejection.

As one might expect, right ventricular pressure in the donor heart is normal and is independent of native left ventricular contraction (Fig. 8). In this example, the native QRS on the electrocardiogram is small and nearly unrecognizable relative to the large donor QRS complexes coupled to right ventricular pressure.

"Extra" Atrial Pressure

Atrial activity, at times, becomes dysynchronus from ventricular contraction in certain *orthotopic* and *heterotopic* transplant patients. A 52-yr-old man had received *orthotopic* transplant 1 year prior to study. Left ventricular and aortic pressures measured simultaneously show elevated systemic pressures (180/100 mm Hg), no aortic-left ventricular gradient and only mild elevation of left ventricular-end diastolic pressure (Fig. 9A). However, the diastolic left ventricular pressure waveform is consistently, but irregularly, deformed by "notches" in mid

to late diastole (Fig. 9B). Although uncommon, atrial contraction stimulated from the remaining native atrial tissue can produce this pressure artifact. The 'A' wave may occur at variable times in the diastolic or systolic periods and appear separate from electrocardiographic atrial activity of the donor heart (Figs. 9B, 9C).

Consider the right heart pressure tracings in a 53-yr-old man 6 months after orthotopic transplantation (Figs. 10, 11). Dysynchronous atrial activity is also evident. Residual native atrial activity is more easily discerned on the electrocardiogram in this patient (than Fig. 9) and shown by the 'P¹' wave relative to the "normal" 'P' wave. The sinus (p) beats have their normal 'A' and 'V' waves, but when the ectopic atrial beat (p¹) appears, the right atrial waveform becomes distorted (see beats A¹). Also note the diastolic right ventricular pressure notch (astrisk, Fig. 11). The dysynchronous atrial contraction superimposed on right ventricular systole may be appreciated on beat #2. Although hemodynamically interesting, atrial dysynchrony does not present a serious clinical problem.

Applying the traditional hemodynamic principles to

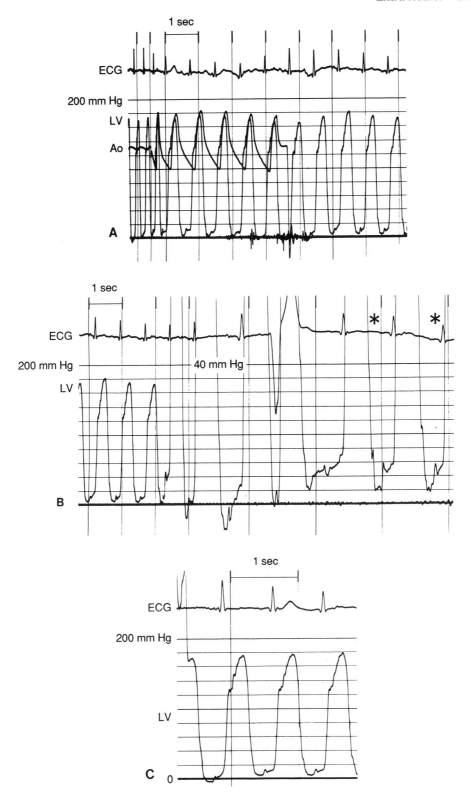

Fig. 9A. Simultaneous aortic (Ao) and left ventricular (LV) pressures (200 mm Hg scale). See text for details.

Fig. 9B. Simultaneous aortic (Ao) and left ventricular (LV) pressures (both 200 mm Hg and 40 mm Hg scale). See text for details.

Fig. 9C. Left ventricular pressure (0–200 mm Hg scale). See text for details.

302   Kern et al.

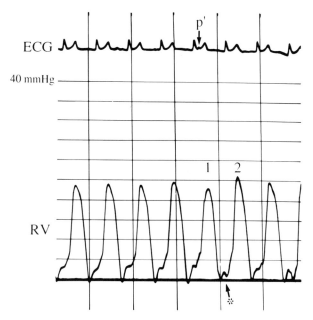

Fig. 10. Right ventricular (RV) pressure in a patient with cardiac transplantation (40 mm Hg scale). See text for details.

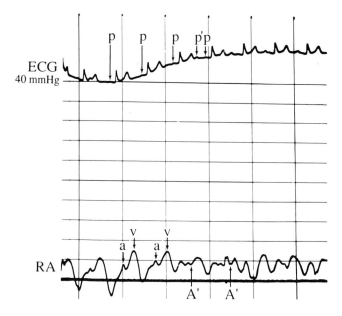

Fig. 11. Right atrial (RA) pressure in a patient with cardiac transplantation (40 mm Hg scale). See text for details.

the cardiac cycle with its attendant electrical-mechanical events is complicated in patients with "extra" hearts. When *non-physiologic* events are present, investigate all possible sources of artifact, along the fluid path to the transducer, catheter malposition, and congenital or *"acquired"* anatomic anomalies.

REFERENCES

1. Melvin KR, Pollick C, Hunt SA, McDougall R, Goris ML, Oyer P, Popp RL, Stinson EB. Cardiovascular physiology in a case of heterotopic cardiac transplantation. Am J Cardiol 49:1301–1307, 1982.
2. Novitzky D, Cooper DKC. Surgical techniques of orthotopic and heterotopic heart transplantation. In Cooper DKC, Lanza RP (ed.): "Heart Transplantation: The Present Status of Orthotopic and Heterotopic Heart Transplantation." MTP Press Limited, 1984, pp 103–127.
3. Cooper DKC. Advantages and disadvantages of heterotopic transplantation. In Cooper DKC, Lanza RP (ed.): "Heart Transplantation: The Present Status of Orthotopic and Heterotopic Heart Transplantation." MTP Press Limited, 1984, pp 305–320.

Chapter 40

Extra Hearts—Section II

Morton J. Kern, MD, and Ubeydullah Deligonul, MD

INTRODUCTION

This "hemodynamic rounds" will examine the pressure waves generated by a mechanical assist device as an "extra heart." Cardiac assist devices function in 2 principal ways: either partially supporting or completely supporting systemic pressure. Current partial support devices include only intra-aortic balloon pumps. Complete support devices generate flow through centripetal, roller-type, clam-shell, or other unique pump designs and are used as left, right or biventricular support devices [1–4]. The total artificial heart is only one of several types of these complete support devices. Pressure waves generated by these devices depend on the contribution of both mechanical and intrinsic myocardial pulsatile activity.

CASE PRESENTATION AND DISCUSSION
Myocardial Ischemia and the Extra Heart

A 52-yr-old man with severe coronary artery disease underwent coronary artery bypass graft surgery after a complicated myocardial infarction in 1985. Because of progressive ischemia and atherosclerosis in the saphenous vein grafts, a second coronary artery bypass surgery, complicated by a cardiac arrest, was performed. Successful resuscitation was accomplished with the institution of a left ventricular cardiac assist device. He was fully active with a normal exercise capacity in the hospital. Unusual serum antibodies precluded earlier donor heart matching. The patient did well for 9 mo after device implantation, while awaiting cardiac transplanta-

tion. Despite a well-functioning assist device, angina pectoris with decreasing exercise tolerance became incapacitating. A cardiac catheterization and exercise hemodynamic study was performed. Aortic and left ventricular pressures were simultaneously measured from an 8 French femoral sheath and 7 F pigtail catheter in the left ventricle (Fig. 1). Explain the arterial pressure without a corresponding left ventricular pressure. The waveform of aortic pressure indicates an "extra heart" must be performing the work to generate a systemic pulse. Note the electrocardiogram does not correlate to the aortic pressure, but does precede each left ventricular pressure wave. Left ventricular pressure rarely exceeds minimal aortic pressure. Why are alternate left ventricular pressures higher? Which mechanical mechanisms trigger the assist device? The "extra heart" in this patient was a clam-shell type pump [4]. The Novacor® and other similar pulsatile ventricular support devices function by employing volume triggers, producing a pressure pulse when the "new" left ventricle is passively filled to a pre-determined volume. "Heart rate" is then driven by filling pressures (and volume) related to systemic muscular activity. When examining simultaneous left and right ventricular pressures (Fig. 2), a majority of beats demonstrate relatively small differences in the ventricular pressures without features of myocardial restrictive physiology.

The variation of the left ventricular pressure is related to the rate of emptying through the apex conduit to the pump. As one might expect, left ventriculography is unusual, showing the volume of contrast passing through the left ventricle and exiting from the apex conduit into

303

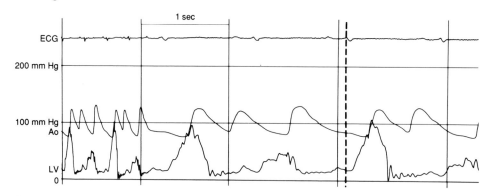

Fig. 1. Aortic (Ao) and left ventricular (LV) pressure in a patient with an extra heart. The timing of the QRS corresponds to the left ventricular pressure (dotted line). Aortic pressure is generated in a pulsatile manner unrelated to left ventricular pressure. See text for details.

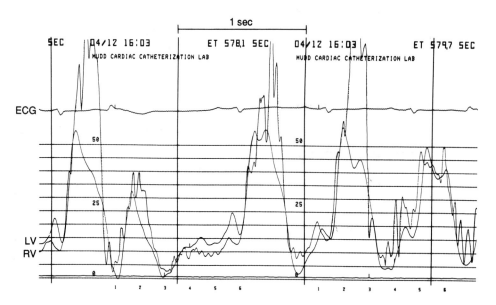

Fig. 2. Simultaneous left ventricular (LV) and right ventricular (RV) pressures in the patient above (0–50 mm Hg full scale). Note the correspondence of pressures of the left and right ventricles in most beats. There is no evidence of restrictive physiology. See text for details.

the assist device (Fig. 3A). With each pump, the stroke volume is moved to the ascending aorta through the abdominally implanted conduit from the clam-shell pump (Figs. 3B,C). Reduced left ventricular pressure occurs when the timing of pump filling exceeds the timing of the native left ventricular ejection, and thereby results in the alteration of left ventricular pressures.

To assess the etiology of cardiac dysfunction, coronary angiography was performed and showed total occlusion of the left anterior descending, right coronary and circumflex arteries. The single saphenous vein graft to the right coronary artery had a 50% ostial narrowing with mid graft 90% lesion. Contrast opacification of the posterior descending artery and faint circumflex collaterals were noted. An exercise hemodynamic study was also performed. Aortic and left ventricular pressures,

coronary sinus thermodilution blood flow (catheter inserted through the left antecubital vein), continuous pulmonary artery oxygen saturation, and pressures were measured during weighted leg raising for 6 min (Fig. 4, Table I). Exercise increased the assisted heart rate (103 to 113 bpm), mean arterial pressure (99 to 128 mm Hg), aortic diastolic pressure (88 to 115 mm Hg), left ventricular end diastolic pressure (18 to 25 mm Hg), and pulmonary artery pressures (45/15 to 75/28 mm Hg). Cardiac output (by thermodilution and confirmed by the console values) rose minimally (5.2 to 6.5L/min) with marked decline in pulmonary artery oxygen saturation (78 to 40%) and accompanying symptomatic fatigue and mild angina. Coronary blood flow (great cardiac vein) increased (43 to 56ml/min) with only modest lactate generation. Consider the hemodynamic results of exercise in

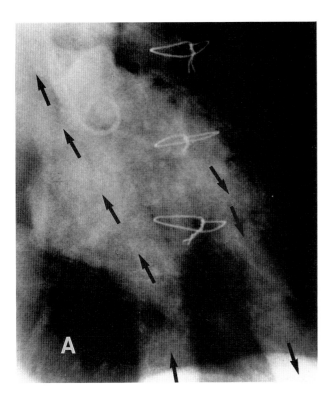

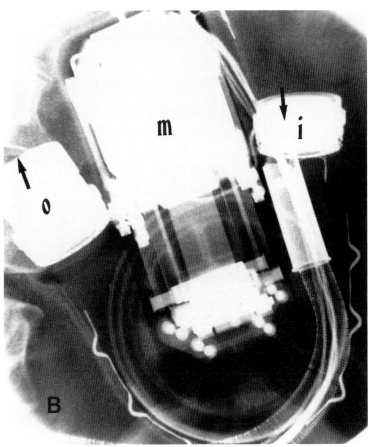

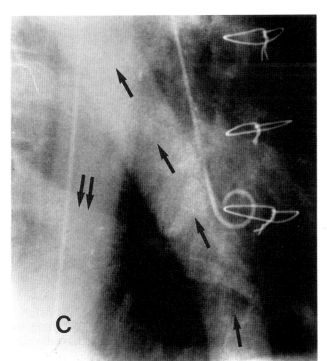

this patient with a left ventricular assist device with regard to exercise responses in normal subjects. Exercise normally increases heart rate > 25%, decreases aortic diastolic pressure due to decreased systemic vascular resistance, minimally changes right ventricular and pulmonary artery pressures, and markedly increases cardiac output and coronary blood flow at least 4-fold. In our patient, the blunted heart rate and the increase in diastolic aortic and mean systemic pressures indicate failure to lower systemic vascular resistance appropriately. The decline in pulmonary artery oxygen saturation is a markedly exaggerated response compared to a normal subject.

Fig. 3. (A) Ventriculogram after injection of contrast into the mid ventricle. Contrast empties through the apex of the heart (3 black down arrows). (B) It enters the input port of the Novacor® pump (I with the down arrow), exits through the output port (0 with the up arrow) and returns to the aorta via conduit (Figure 3A, 5 upward arrows) to the aorta. (C) Late phase of the left ventriculogram with the pump to aortic conduit filling (4 arrows) and the descending aorta filled with (2 black down arrows). The aortic valve does not open.

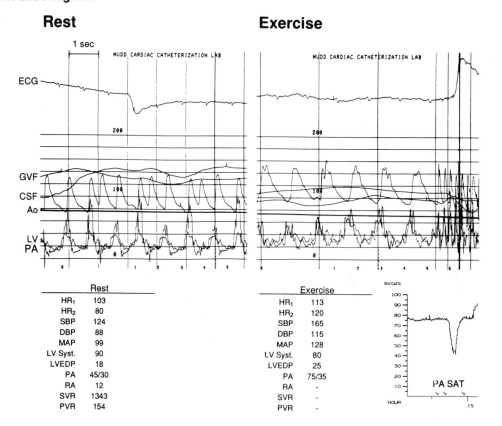

Fig. 4. Hemodynamics at rest and during exercise, measuring great cardiac vein flow (GVF), coronary sinus flow (CSF), aortic pressure (Ao), left ventricular pressure (LV) and pulmonary artery pressure (PA). The higher coronary blood flow is toward the bottom of the tracing. In the lower right corner is a continuous signal of pulmonary artery oxygen saturation showing a decline at peak exercise from 78 to approximately 40%.

TABLE I. Hemodynamic Data*

	HR_{native}	HR_{pump}	BP	MAP	LVP	PA	RA
Rest	80	103	124/80	99	65/18	38/15	12
Exercise	120	113	150/98	128	65/25	65/25	—

| | CO_{Td} | CO_{pump} | SVR | PVR | Oxygen saturations (%) | | |
					Ao	PA	CS
Rest	5.18	6.46	1343	154	94	75	36
Exercise	5.90	6.47	—	—	97	42	41

| | Lactate (mEq/L) | | | GVF (ml/min) | MVO_2 (mL/dL) |
	Art	CS	Diff		
Rest	1.3	1.1	0.2	43	273
Exercise	6.0	4.3	2.3	96	406

*HR = heart rate (bpm); BP = blood pressure (mm Hg); MAP = mean arterial pressure (mm Hg); LVP = left ventricular pressure (mm Hg); PA = pulmonary artery pressure (mm Hg); RA = right atrial pressure (mm Hg); CO_{TD} = thermodilution cardiac output (L/min); CO_{pump} = assist device pump output (L/min); SVR = systemic vascular resistance (dynes.sec.cm^{-5}); PVR = pulmonary vascular resistance (dynes.sec.cm^{-5}); CS = coronary sinus; GVF = great cardiac vein flow; Diff = aorta-CS difference.

The increase in pulmonary artery pressures also required explanation with a left ventricular pump which is presumed to be substituting for native left ventricular work. The limited capacity of the assist pump to empty the native left ventricle results in increased left ventricular end diastolic pressure and also pulmonary pressures. As one might anticipate, limited coronary blood flow through this severely diseased heart might be due to arterial conduit blockage, as well as attenuated oxygen demand, with myocardial muscle performance supplemented by mechanical support. Despite mechanical ventricular assistance, myocardial oxygen demand was increased and signs of ischemia occurred.

Can one explain the increase in left ventricular end diastolic pressure and MVO_2 in a left ventricle that supposedly is *not* doing its normal share of pressure work? We speculate that the marked increase in pulmonary pressures reflects ischemia from the inferior left ventricular and right ventricular functioning zones. Right ventricular ischemia in the unassisted right ventricle might well be the cause of progressive dyspnea with compromised function of the remaining active myocardium of the inferior and lateral walls. Progression of coronary artery disease in the right coronary artery bypass graft (the only remaining arterial blood suppy) was evident. Limited blood flow to the inferior left ventricular distribution most likely affected the pressure responses to exercise.

Unfortunately, a complete answer to the questions raised cannot be provided from the hemodynamic data alone. Several issues regarding alteration of left and right ventricular chamber dimensions, mitral and tricuspid regurgitation, and left ventricular ischemic dysfunction require combined echocardiographic imaging. This unusual hemodynamic case is illustrative of both the insights and limitations of hemodynamic data interpretation. In situations where complex questions of physiology are anticipated, optimal results would be obtained with combined echocardiographic and hemodynamic techniques, a subject to be addressed in a future "rounds."

REFERENCES

1. Pennington DG, Samuels LD, Williams G, Palmer D, Swartz MT, Codd JE, Merjavy JP, Lagunoff D, Joist H. Experience with the Pierce-Donachy ventricular assist device in postcardiotomy patients with cardiogenic shock. World J Surg 9:37–46, 1985.
2. Davis PK, Pae WE, Miller CA, Parascandola SA. Myocardial oxygen consumption: Comparison between left atrial pulsatile synchronous and asynchronous bypass. Trans Am Soc Artif Intern Organs 35:461–463, 1989.
3. Moulopoulos SD, Topaz S, Kolff WJ. Diastolic balloon pumping (with carbon dioxide) in the aorta. A mechanical assistance to the failing circulation. Am Heart J 63:669, 1962.
4. DeBakey ME. Left ventricular bypass pumps for cardiac assistance. Am J Cardiol 27:3–11, 1971.

Chapter 41

Extra Hearts—Section III

Morton J. Kern, MD, and Ubeydullah Deligonul, MD

INTRODUCTION

Previously, we have described the hemodynamics in a patient with a pulsatile left ventricular clam-shell type assist device. The systemic pressure was generated by the clam-shell pumping with decompression of left ventricular filling and pressure. This type of pump is generally associated with reduced myocardial oxygen demand and is, at times, considered to "rest" the heart [1,2].

Recently, portable cardiopulmonary bypass has emerged as an emergency "extra heart" to support circulatory collapse after acute myocardial infarction, cardiac arrest in the catheterization laboratory during diagnostic or therapeutic intervention [3,4]. This hemodynamic rounds will address several issues related to the hemodynamics occurring during portable cardiac bypass.

CASE PRESENTATION AND DISCUSSION
A Blood Pressure With a Closed Aortic Valve

A 34-yr-old woman had severe crushing chest pain with electrocardiographic evidence of extensive anterior and lateral myocardial infarctions. Because of a history of uncontrolled hypertension, thrombolytic therapy was not administered. Twelve hours after admission to a community hospital, hypotension and ventricular tachyarrhythmias occurred. Emergency helicopter transport was performed. On arrival in the intensive care unit, the patient had cardiac arrest. Initial resuscitative efforts were successful with subsequent intubation and placement of femoral arterial and venous sheaths. Intravenous infusions of dopamine, lidocaine, and bretylium were

required to maintain a systolic blood pressure of 80 mm Hg and stable sinus tachycardia. One hour after initial resuscitation and stabilization, hypotension and ventricular arrhythmias recurred. Because of failure to maintain a systolic pressure of 60 mm Hg, emergency portable cardiopulmonary bypass was instituted inserting an 18 French arterial cannulation into the right femoral artery and a 20 French cannulae into the inferior vena cava (Fig. 1). Systemic blood flow using a centripetal pump system was maintained at 4.0L/min, generating a mean blood pressure of 85 mm Hg. The patient was transferred to the cardiac catheterization laboratory for diagnostic study and possible angioplasty.

The electrocardiogram at the time of catheterization, while on cardiopulmonary bypass, showed new right bundle branch block, left axis deviation, and low anterior R wave voltage (Fig. 2). Coronary angiography showed a normal and co-dominant right coronary artery, 90% left main stenosis, and 100% occlusion of both the left anterior descending and circumflex arteries (Fig. 3). Left ventricular function was assessed before the cardiovascular surgeon would consider emergency coronary artery bypass grafting. Examine the hemodynamic pressure tracings measured through an 8 French pigtail catheter in the left ventricle (Fig. 4). Left ventricular pressure is 58/20 mm Hg (left side, panel A, beats 1–4) and is abnormal in both rate of pressure development and pattern of left ventricular relaxation as indicated by the sharp downslope across diastole. Continuous pressure recording during left ventricular-aortic catheter pullback is shown at the right side of the tracing after beat 4. The pressure scale is changed to 0–200 mm Hg. The phasic character of left ventricular pressure quickly changes to a

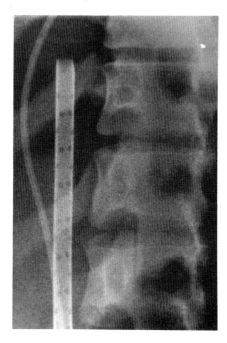

Fig. 1. Angiogram of inferior vena cava showing the long 20 F venous cannula of the cardiopulmonary bypass circuit located just beneath the inferior right atrial entrance. A pulmonary artery balloon flotation catheter can be seen traversing the inferior vena cava. The catheter was inserted from the left femoral vein.

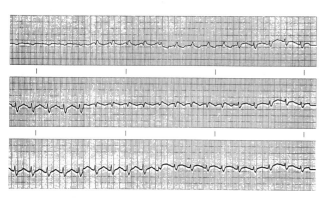

Fig. 2. The electrocardiogram during portable cardiopulmonary bypass. Sinus tachycardia with left axis deviation, poor R wave progression and diffuse low voltage across the anterior leads was different from the previous tracing with marked ST elevation over leads V$_1$–V$_4$.

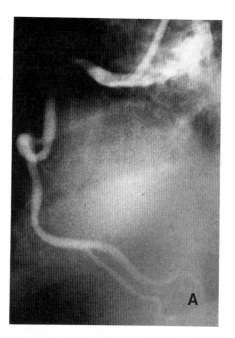

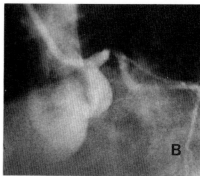

Fig. 3. A: Normal right coronary artery in the LAO projection. B: Subtotal occlusion of the left coronary artery with only an obtuse marginal branch evident. Neither the left anterior descending nor the circumflex artery were visualized. The aortic valve did not open during contrast injection.

mean pressure of the cardiopulmonary bypass circuit when the catheter is pulled across the aortic valve.

From the difference in left ventricular-aortic pressure, it is obvious the aortic valve cannot open. To demonstrate the pressure at which the aortic valve did open, the flow rate of the cardiopulmonary bypass pump was turned down while continuously recording aortic pressure (Fig. 4, panel B). Note the phasic arterial pressure

waves do not appear until the mean aortic pressure falls below 60 mm Hg. These phasic waves reflect the left ventricular pressure opening the aortic valve. During cardiopulmonary bypass, the left ventricle is contracting against a closed aortic valve with no means of left ventricular decompression. Mitral regurgitation was not evident hemodynamically. Left ventricular strain and wall stress is certainly elevated, as is myocardial oxygen demand [5]. However, aortic pressure is maintained sufficient to perfuse the cerebral, renal and coronary circulations.

The critical nature of cardiopulmonary bypass augmented coronary perfusion was also demonstrated shortly after turning down the cardiopulmonary bypass system, reducing the mean blood pressure to < 60 mm Hg. The aortic and right atrial pressures were recorded

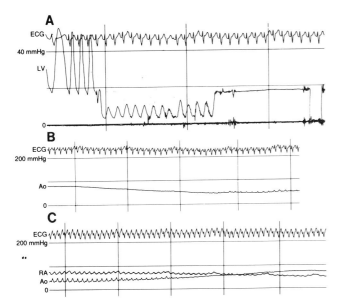

A

ECG

40 mmHg

LV

0

B

ECG

200 mmHg

Ao

0

C

ECG

200 mmHg

RA
Ao

0

Fig. 4. Hemodynamics obtained with a 7 F pigtail catheter in the left ventricle. Panel A shows left ventricular pressure on a 0–40 mm Hg scale (beats 1–4, left side) and 0–200 mm Hg scale (beats 5 and on toward the right). Left ventricular pressure demonstrated a slow increase in pressure generation and abnormal pressure decline during diastole. After beat 17, the catheter was pulled into the aorta and the mean systemic pressure of the portable cardiopulmonary bypass can be observed. Panel B shows the alteration of pressure waveform during reduction of cardiopulmonary bypass flow volume to reduce systemic pressure below that of left ventricular pressure. The far right of the tracing shows phasic beats of aortic valve opening. Panel C shows the right atrial pressure (RA) and aortic pressure (Ao) during very low cardiopulmonary bypass flow rate. As flow rate is increased, the aortic pressure increases to a mean of 85 mm Hg and right atrial pressure falls from 16 to 10 mm Hg. See text for details.

during cardiopulmonary bypass flow at a low level, generating a mean pressure of < 40 mm Hg (Fig. 4, panel C, left side). Aortic pressure is 55/40 mm Hg and right atrial pressure is 16 mm Hg (0–40 mm Hg scale). The rhythm degenerated into a wide complex tachyarrhythmia (compare to panel B). With increasing cardiopulmonary bypass flow and restoration of an adequate systemic pressure, the phasic aortic pressure is obliterated and the right atrial pressure falls as inferior vena caval blood is returned to the cardiopulmonary bypass circuit. With maintanence of coronary perfusion pressure, the rhythm was converted into a sinus tachycardia.

Because of the critical need to assess myocardial function > 18 hr after near total occlusion of the left coronary artery, a 15 cc contrast injection (low osmolar media, 15 cc/second) into the left ventricle. The contraction pattern and regions of potential viability were measured using a digital angiographic technique. It is important to reduce the cardiopulmonary bypass flow to permit

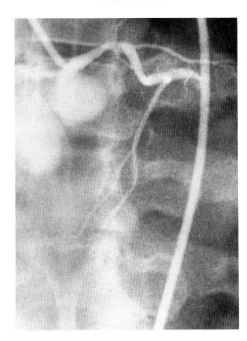

Fig. 5. The left coronary artery after coronary angioplasty of the left main and proximal circumflex coronary lesions. The left anterior descending artery could not be recanalized.

aortic valve opening during ventriculography for a realistic assessment of left ventricular contraction. A severely reduced ejection fraction would not be surprising when viewing the left ventricle trying to eject blood through a closed aortic valve. In this patient, the left ventricular ejection fraction was < 10% with global hypokinesis and inferior, as well as anterior akinesis. A decision for emergency coronary angioplasty was made after consultation with the cardiothoracic surgeon. Incomplete revascularization of the left main and circumflex arteries was achieved (Fig. 5). The occluded left anterior descending artery could not be reopened. The patient expired 36 hr later because of acidosis, hypoxia, and renal failure.

''Extra hearts'' of the cardiopulmonary bypass variety without ventricular decompression can maintain systemic perfusion, but do so at the cost of increased myocardial work. Systemic pressure support facilitates emergency resuscitation and should be employed briefly until revascularization can be performed. The hemodynamic waveforms in this patient illustrate the paradox of systemic perfusion with increased myocardial ischemia. Without restoration of coronary perfusion, myocardial salvage, and ultimately survival, is highly unlikely.

REFERENCES

1. Smalling RW, Cassidy DB, Merhige M, et al. Improved hemodynamic and left ventricular unloading during acute ischemia using

the left ventricular assist device compared to intra-aortic balloon counterpulsation (abstr). J Am Coll Cardiol 13:160A, 1989.

2. Shani J, Hollander G, Nathan I, et al. Percutaneous left atrial-femoral artery bypass with a pulsatile pump: Initial experience in cardiogenic shock (abstr). J Am Coll Cardiol 13:53A, 1989.

3. Vogel RA, Shawl F, Tommaso C, O'Neill W, Overlie P, O'Toole J, Vandormael M, Topol E, Tabari KK, Vogel J, Smith S Jr, Freedman R, White C, George B, Teirstein P. Initial report of the National Registry of Elective Cardiopulmonary Bypass Supported Coronary Angioplasty. J Am Coll Cardiol 15:23–29, 1990.

4. Shawl FA, Domanski MJ, Wish MH, Davis M. Percutaneous cardiopulmonary bypass support in the catheterization laboratory: Technique and complications. Am Heart J 120:195–203, 1990.

5. Stack RK, Pavlides GS, Justeson G, Schreiber TL, O'Neill WW. Hemodynamic and metabolic effects of cardiopulmonary support during PTCA (abstr). J Am Coll Cardiol 15:250A, 1990.

Chapter 42

Adult Congenital Anomalies

Morton J. Kern, MD, Frank V. Aguirre, MD, Thomas J. Donohue, MD, and Richard G. Bach, MD

INTRODUCTION

The most common adult congenital heart lesions are ventricular septal defects, atrial septal defects, and corrected complex lesions in childhood, such as Tetralogy of Fallot [1,2]. Adult congenital cardiac abnormalities produce unusual hemodynamic tracings, often characteristic of the resultant valvular or myopathic dysfunction. A variety of right atrial pressure waveforms have been previously presented [3] reflecting tricuspid valve lesions and right ventricular dysfunction. An unusual example of one adult congenital cardiac condition can be diagnosed by simultaneous electrocardiography and right heart hemodynamics. In conjunction with this case, we discuss ventricular septal defects. Oxygen saturation data with selected green dye curves are presented to illustrate several important aspects of intracardiac shunts.

ATRIAL PRESSURE WITH A VENTRICULAR ELECTROGRAM

A 29-year-old white male with a history of congenital heart disease, which included a diagnosis of an ostium secundum type atrial septal defect, was evaluated for palpitations. Physical examination revealed a blood pressure of 118/78mmHg with a heart rate of 73/minute and regular rhythm. There was a loud split S_1 and fixed splitting of S_2. There was a grade II/VI systolic ejection murmur at the left sternal border. The remainder of the examination was unremarkable. Electrophysiologic study demonstrated retrograde accessory pathways on programmed stimulation. Two-dimensional and transesophageal echocardiograms demonstrated an abnormality of the tricuspid valve and right atrium and confirmed an ostium secundum atrial septal defect with abnormal septal motion consistent with right ventricular volume overload. There was moderate tricuspid regurgitation. Using the Doppler technique, the pulmonary to systemic blood flow ratio was estimated at 1.4:1. The 12-lead electrocardiogram demonstrated right atrial and ventricular enlargement with right bundle branch block (Fig. 1).

Right and left heart cardiac catheterization was performed using a 6 French arterial sheath and an 8 French venous sheath. A 7 French balloon-tipped catheter was advanced to the right atrium. Per routine, right atrial oxygen saturations and pressures were obtained. The catheter was advanced into the right ventricle and then to the pulmonary capillary wedge position with balloon deflation to record pulmonary artery pressure. Simultaneous left and right heart hemodynamics were obtained (see Table I). An oxygen saturation run was performed during right heart catheter pullback (Table II). Immediately after pullback, the atrial septal defect was crossed with the balloon-tipped catheter and pulmonary venous saturations were obtained. A minimal oxygen step-up was detected in the right heart chambers. Systemic cardiac output was 3.1L/min (index of 1.6L/min/m²). Pulmonary flow was 3.4L/min (index of 1.7L/min/m²), resulting in a calculated Qp/Qs ratio of 1.1:1. Systemic and pulmonary vascular resistances were 2,194 dynes. sec.cm⁻⁵ and 141 dynes.sec.cm⁻⁵, respectively.

Left ventriculography showed normal contraction with an ejection fraction of 62%. Moderate (2+) tricuspid regurgitation was observed on the right ventriculogram with slight right-to-left contrast shunting when injecting into the right atrial chamber.

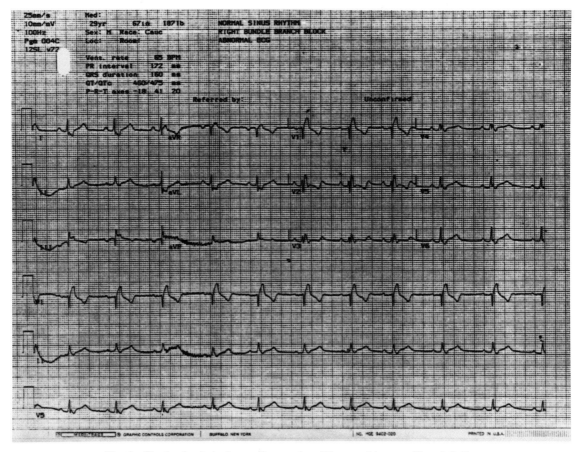

Fig. 1. Twelve-lead electrocardiogram in a 29-year-old man with palpitations.

TABLE I. Hemodynamic Data in Patient #1

Right atrial mean (a,v) (mmHg)	4 (6,5)
Right ventricular (mmHg)	23/5
Pulmonary artery (mmHg)	23/11
Pulmonary capillary wedge mean (a,v) (mmHg)	8 (8,6)
Left ventricular (mmHg)	105/10
Aortic (mmHg)	105/70
Cardiac output/Cardiac index (L/min, L/min^2)	3.1/1.6
Systemic vascular resistance (dynes.sec.cm^{-5})	2195
Pulmonary vascular resistance (dynes.sec.cm^{-5})	141
Qp/Qs	1.1:1

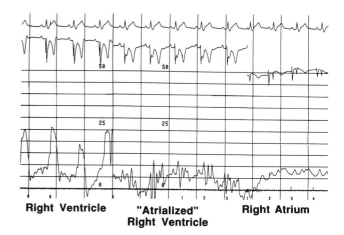

Right Ventricle   "Atrialized"   Right Atrium
Right Ventricle

Fig. 2. Right heart catheter pullback in patient #1. The lower electrocardiographic tracing is an intracavitary electrogram. See text for details.

Because of a characteristic echocardiogram, a simultaneous intracavitary electrogram and hemodynamic recording were obtained with a Zucker (pacing end-hole, woven Dacron, USCI, Inc.) catheter during right ventricular catheter pullback (Fig. 2). Examine the hemodynamic tracing and observe the right ventricular pressure as it changes to right atrial pressure at a time when the intracavitary electrogram continues to reflect contact with right ventricular myocardium. On further pullback, the right ventricular electrogram then converts into a normal right atrial electrogram with minor alteration of the pressure wave. The transition to atrial pressure with a

simultaneous ventricular electrogram is the classic hemodynamic finding of Ebstein's anomaly and, although rarely seen, serves to illustrate the use of hemodynamics in documenting the histologic atrialization of the right ventricle with pressure becoming "atrialized" during ventricular electrocardiographic activity.

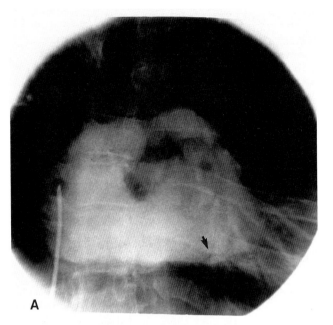 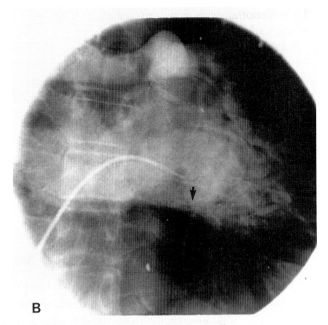

Fig. 3. A. Right ventriculogram in a 29-year-old man in Figure 1. The right ventricle is small. The tricuspid valve (arrow) is markedly displaced downward into the right ventricular cavity. B: Right atrial angiogram emphasizing the size of the right atrium and location of the tricuspid valve.

Ebstein's anomaly occurs in fewer than 1% of patients with congenital heart disease [5]. Although no family or genetic transmission of the syndrome is described, congenital cardiac anomalies in infants of mothers taking lithium have been reported. Ebstein's anomaly is characterized by a downward displacement of the tricuspid valve into the right ventricle. Anomalous attachments of the tricuspid leaflets are a result of dysplastic formation. The displaced tricuspid valve involves both the right atrium and right ventricle. The tricuspid valve takes a funnel-like form leading into the right ventricle with the septal and inferior cusps adherent to the right ventricular wall at a variable distance from the AV junction (Fig. 3). The anterior leaflet of the tricuspid valve is large and dysplastic, often with rudimentary septal and inferior leaflets connecting to the body of the right ventricle. The tricuspid valve is also variably regurgitant. The inflow region of the right ventricle is generally hypoplastic with a fibrotic and poorly contractile ventricular wall. The atrialized portion of the right ventricle may be thin-walled, dilated, or thick and fibrotic with variations in the size and degree of tricuspid leaflet displacement.

As demonstrated in this patient, a patent foramen ovale or atrial septal defect is present in more than 75% of patients with Ebstein's anomaly [4,6]. Left-sided Ebstein's anomaly has been reported in corrected transposition of the great vessels [8].

The clinical presentation of Ebstein's anomaly usually involves symptoms of dyspnea, fatigue and occasionally cyanosis, usually occurring during exertion. Dyspnea and fatigue may occur in the absence of cyanosis. Chest pain resembling angina has also been reported [5]. As the patient progresses through childhood and adolescence, right heart failure increasingly becomes the predominant cause of death. As occurred in our patient, atrial tachyarrhythmias are present in approximately 25% of patients with 15% of patients dying suddenly. Approximately 10% of these patients have accessory pathways. Nearly 25% of patients may die before the age of 10 and 87% die before the age of 25 with few adults surviving > 50 years [7–9]. Increasing heart size, cyanosis, and paradoxical embolization or other complications of right-to-left shunting are more prevalent with increasing age. Infectious endocarditis is uncommon unless other cardiac lesions are also present.

Typical findings during cardiac catheterization usually involve elevation of right atrial pressure. As shown, the magnitude of right atrial A and V waves depend on the compliance of the right atrium, amount of interatrial shunting, and right ventricular end diastolic pressure. The typical atrialized hemodynamics with the right ventricular electrocardiographic complex alone does not unequivocally identify Ebstein's anomaly. However, false positives are rare. The catheter in the location of the atrialized right ventricle usually induces ventricular extra systoles despite recording atrial pressure. Also, the catheter position in Ebstein's anomaly is left of the spine in the posterior/anterior projection, confirming the unusual location of pressure with the electrogram.

Cardiac catheterization in patients with Ebstein's anomaly may be associated with increased risks relative to other cardiac anomalies since catheterization-related serious arrhythmias have been reported in as high as 28% of patients. Death in 5% of such patients has been noted [7–9]. Nonetheless, we believe patients who have Ebstein's anomaly requiring electrophysiologic testing should have complete catheterization to identify the extent and degree of hemodynamic abnormalities and intracardiac shunting.

INTRACARDIAC SHUNTS

Intracardiac shunts may be the most common congenital anomalies encountered in adults and can be detected by 5 methods: oximetry, indocyanine green dye dilution curves, angiography, radionuclide angiographic techniques [10], and inhaled hydrogen arrival time [11]. Measurement of the arrival time of inhaled hydrogen gas using a platinum-tipped catheter in the venous circulation [11] permits detection and localization of left-to-right shunting. However, actual quantitation of a shunt necessitates serial oximetry or indicator dilution techniques. The oximetry findings of the intracardiac shunt in the first patient example were clincially insignificant. Sophisticated techniques for shunt detection often relegate oximetric and hemodynamic confirmation to a secondary role. However, standard oxygen saturation sampling has clinical importance in modern catheterization laboratories because of acute presentations of patients with complications of ischemic heart disease, postseptostomy assessment after mitral valvuloplasty, and unsuspected atrial or ventricular septal defects. Oxygen saturations should be collected in duplicate (1–3 cc heparinized syringes), if possible, and from the sites shown on Table II.

For left-to-right shunts, oxygen saturation data are generally clinically satisfactory with good correlation to hemodynamic findings. A brief simplified formula for rapid computation of left-to-right atrial septal defects can be obtained by computing the arterial (art) minus mixed venous oxygen (MVO_2) saturation over the pulmonary vein (PV) minus pulmonary artery (PA) oxygen saturation, providing a quick Qp/Qs ratio [(Art − MVO_2)/(PV − PA)]. Well-known limitations of the oximetric technique include a low sensitivity. Oximetry may fail to detect shunts smaller than a 20% shunt fraction. The Fick principle to calculate blood flow presumes a steady state during the diagnostic run and must also assume that complete mixing is achieved instantly during sampling of blood at representative locations. A high systemic flow tends to equalize arteriovenous difference across the

TABLE II. Oxygen Saturation Data in Patient #1

Site	Saturation (%)
Inferior vena cava (low)	85
Inferior vena cava (right atrial)	70
Right atrial (low)	71
Right atrial (mid)	67
Right atrial (high)	68
Superior vena cava (right atrial)	63
Superior vena cava (high)	64
Right ventricular (tricuspid valve)	71
Right ventricular (apex)	70
Right ventricular (outflow)	73
Pulmonary artery (right)	73
Pulmonary artery (main)	73
Left atrial (pulmonary vein)	96
Left ventricular	96

heart. Elevated systemic blood flow thus produces mixed venous oxygen saturation that is higher than normal and intrachamber variability also higher than normal. When systemic blood flow is reduced, the mixed venous oxygen saturation is lower. A larger step-up must be detected before significant right-to-left shunting is diagnosed. More sensitive techniques such as green dye or inhaled hydrogen arrival time may be needed to exclude right-to-left shunting. For right-to-left shunts, the localization technique is more difficult. Saturation data demonstrating a "step-down" on the left heart is not always diagnostic since desaturation of arterial blood has several contributing explanations.

The quantitation of a shunt depends on accurate measurement of blood flow through the right and left heart using indicator dilution (thermodilution or green dye) and Fick or angiographic cardiac output techniques. Advantages and limitations of these methods have been described in detail elsewhere [10,12,13].

Consider the case of a 39-year-old woman with progressive dyspnea. Long-standing pulmonary hypertension was present with a clinical and echocardiographic examination revealing a ventricular septal defect. She had been away from follow-up medical care for several years and now presents with markedly increasing dyspnea. Aortic pressure was 95/72 mmHg. Right heart pressures revealed pulmonary hypertension (Fig. 4) with pulmonary artery pressure of 100/50 mmHg, right ventricular pressure of 100/10 mmHg and mean right atrial pressure approximately 15 mmHg with prominent A and V waves. Mean pulmonary capillary wedge pressure was also elevated to approximately 25 mmHg with striking A and V waves (Fig. 4C). The elevation of mean pulmonary capillary wedge pressure was thought to be a predominant cause of dyspnea. Oxygen saturations on the right heart did not demonstrate a stepup with right atrial, right ventricular, and pulmonary artery saturations nearly

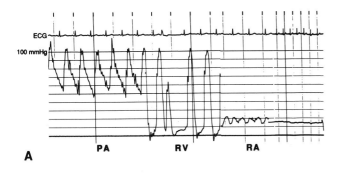

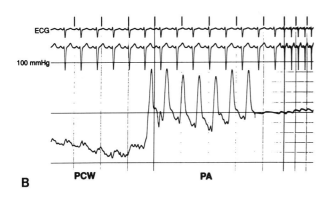

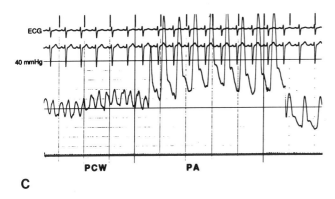

Fig. 4. A. Right atrial (RA), right ventricular (RV), and pulmonary artery (PA) pressures (0–100 mmHg scale) in a patient with arterial desaturation. B: Pulmonary artery (PA) and pulmonary capillary wedge (PCW) pressure in the patient in A (0–100 mmHg scale). C: Pulmonary artery (PA) and pulmonary capillary wedge (PCW) pressure in the patient in A (0–40 mmHg scale).

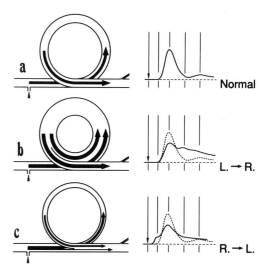

Fig. 5. Diagram of intracardiac shunting. A: Normal circuit through the lungs (upward circle). The dye curve on the right shows normal tracing when injecting into the pulmonary artery and sampling in the systemic artery. B: Left-to-right shunting (L→R) shows additional flow through the pulmonary circuit (larger upward circle) with dye dilution curve showing flattened peak with later recirculation hump as the dye recirculates through the lungs and out to the systemic circulation a second time. C: Right-to-left shunt (R→L) showing addition of flow to systemic circulation with relatively reduced pulmonary flow (smaller upward circle). Dye dilution curve shows early shoulder with flattened peak and attenuated late downstroke. Areas beneath curves are used for quantitation. See ref. #12.

the same at 52%. Arterial oxygen saturation was 88%. Because of the documented ventricular septal defect by noninvasive methods, green dye curves to confirm and localize the shunt were obtained.

An injection of a small bolus of green dye with sampling of arterial blood from the femoral artery normally produces a brisk upstroke with a uniform curve. Recirculation causes characteristic deflections of dye early on the curve for right-to-left shunts or late on the curve for left-to-right shunts (Fig. 5). In our patient, when injecting into the pulmonary artery and sampling in the aorta, the dye passes through the pulmonary circuit and left heart with no evidence of recirculation of left-to-right shunting (Fig. 6). However, on injection of green dye into the right ventricle, an early recirculation deflection can be seen with a less prominent but similar rise in the major bolus of green dye as it passes through the left heart (Fig. 7). On futher pullback into the right atrium, the pattern of green dye traversing from right to left is duplicated with a slightly later appearance of the recirculation deflection and similar pattern of green dye bolus travel through the right heart, indicating the shunt to be at the ventricular level. Dye circulation curves have been used to quantitate flow by computing the area beneath the curve [13].

Ventricular septal defects may be divided into the membranous, muscular, canal type, and supra cristal types. The location has prognostic importance in the presence of associated lesions. Membranous septal type defects occur in 25% of cases and are located inferior to the crista supraventricularis. Fibrous tissue proliferation after infancy may close these defects. Rare septal aneu-

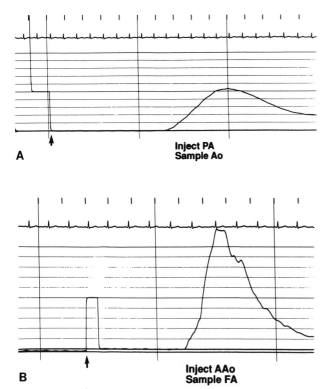

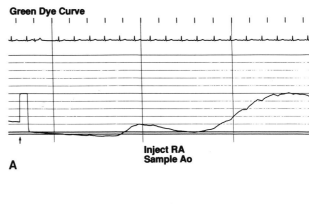

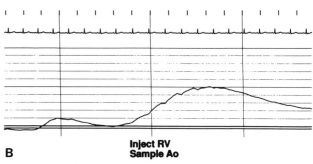

Fig. 6. A: Green dye curve injection site is the pulmonary artery (PA) and sampling in the aorta (Ao). Injection occurs at arrow. B: Green dye curve when injecting into the proximal aorta (AAo) and sampling in the femoral artery (FA).

Fig. 7. A: Green dye curve injection site is the right atrium (RA) and sampling in the aorta (Ao). See text for details. B: Green dye curve injection site is the right ventricle (RV) and sampling in the aorta (Ao). See text for details.

rysms in this region have been reported to protrude into the right ventricle, sometimes becoming large and obstructive [14].

Muscular septal defects comprise 10% of ventricular septal defects and may be single or multiple, located in the supra crista area. Atrioventricular canal type defects (also approximately 10% of ventricular septal defects) occur largely in patients with Down's syndrome and are commonly associated with abnormalities of the AV valves. Supra crystal infra-aortic ventricular septal defects are the least common entity comprising < 5% of patients (in infancy). These defects are located beneath the aortic annulus, above and anterior to the crista supraventricularis, and are generally hemodynamically insignificant, unless the aortic valve becomes regurgitant.

A stepup in the oxygen content of 4–6 volumes percent at the ventricular level identifies ventricular septal defect with left-to-right shunting [10]. Ventriculography performed in the left anterior oblique view with the septum en face may also visualize the defect with contrast opacification of the right ventricle during left ventriculography. Green dye curves are extremely sensitive to detecting very small shunts. A comparison of oximetry and indicator dilution techniques for the assessment of

left-to-right intracardiac shunting in adults demonstrates a close correlation by both techniques. Hillis et al. [15] note that shunt volume by oximetry exceeded shunt volume by indocyanine green technique by 20% in a majority of adult patients. In infants indicator dilution technique yielded larger shunt values than did the oximetric technique.

The early appearance of an indicator in the systemic circulation on Figure 7 identifies a right-to-left shunt [16]. There is an early hump in the dye curve prior to the primary peak. The indocyanine green technique can detect right-to-left shunts as small as 2.5% of the systemic cardiac output [15]. Serial injection sites are used to detect shunts at the level of the atrium, ventricle, and pulmonary artery. Moving the injection site more distally further localizes the shunt by noting when the early appearance of the "hump" on the primary curve is no longer evident. Right-to-left shunting across an atrial septal defect or patent foramen ovale would be best detected by injection into the inferior vena cava because of preferential streaming of the blood [17]. The Valsalva maneuver often will accentuate shunt through a patent foramen ovale because of the hemodynamics of right atrial pressure increasing more than left atrial pressure during phase II.

SUMMARY

Congenital anomalies are unusual in adults, but characteristic hemodynamic data faciliate precise diagnoses. A complete evaluation, including assessment for intracardiac shunts, is usually indicated in patients prior to major surgical procedures or electrophysiologic interventions.

ACKNOWLEDGMENTS

The authors thank the J.G. Mudd Cardiac Catheterization Laboratory Team and Donna Sander for manuscript preparation.

REFERENCES

1. Mitchell SC, Korones SB, Berendes HW: Congenital heart disease in 56,109 births: Incidence and natural history. Circulation 43:323, 1971.
2. Liberthson RR: Congenital heart disease in the child, adolescent and adult patients. In Johnson RA, Haber E, Austin GE (ed): "The Practice of Cardiology." Boston: Little Brown, 1980, pp 755–887.
3. Kern MJ, Deligonul U: Hemodynamic rounds: interpretation of cardiac pathophysiology from pressure waveform analysis. II. The tricuspid valve. Cathet Cardiovasc Diagn 21:278–286, 1990.
4. Lev M, Liberthson RR, Joseph RH, et al: The pathologic anatomy of Ebstein's disease. Arch Pathol 90:334, 1970.
5. Vacca JB, Bussmann DW, Mudd JG: Ebstein's anomaly: Complete review of 108 cases. Am J Cardiol 2:210, 1958.
6. Nora JJ, Nora AH, Toews WH: Lithium, Ebstein's anomaly and other congenital heart defects. Lancet 2:594, 1974.
7. Watson H: Natural history of Ebstein's anomaly of tricuspid valve in childhood and adolescence. An international cooperative study of 505 cases. Br Heart J 36:417, 1974.
8. Marcelletti C, McGoon DC, Mair DC: The natural history of truncus arteriosus. Circulation 54:108, 1976.
9. Braunwald E, Gorlin R: Cooperative study on cardiac catheterization. Total population studied, procedures employed and incidence of complication. Circulation 37(suppl III):III-8, 1968.
10. Dalen JE, Grossman W (ed): Shunt detection and measurement. In "Cardiac Catheterization and Angiography," 2nd ed. Philadelphia: Lea & Febiger, 1980, pp 131–143.
11. Hugenholtz PG, Schwark T, Monroe RG, Gamble WJ, Hauck AJ, Nadas AS: The clinical usefulness of hydrogen gas as an indicator of left-to-right shunts. Circulation 28:542–551, 1963.
12. Kern MJ, Deligonul U, Gudipati C (eds): Hemodynamic and ECG data. In "The Cardiac Catheterization Handbook." St. Louis: Mosby Year Book, Inc., 1991, pp 119–177.
13. Yang SS, Bentivoglio LG, Maranhâo V, Goldberg H: Assessment of cardiovascular shunts. In "From Cardiac Catheterization Data to Hemodynamic Parameters," 3rd ed. Philadelphia: FA Davis Co, 1988, pp 166–188.
14. Shumacker HB Jr, Glover J: Congenital aneurysms of the ventricular septum. Am Heart J 66:405–408, 1963.
15. Hillis LD, Winniford MD, Jackson JA, Firth BG: Measurement of left-to-right intracardiac shunting in adults: Oximetric versus indicator dilution techniques. Cathet Cardiovasc Diagn 11:467–472, 1985.
16. Castillo CA, Kyle JC, Gilson WE, Rowe GG: Simulated shunt curves. Am J Cardiol 17:691, 1966.
17. Swan HJC, Burchell HB, Wood EH: The presence of venoarterial shunts in patients with interatrial communications. Circulation 10:705–713, 1954.

Index